Injury & Trauma Sourcebook

Learning Disabilities Sourcebook, 3rd Edition

Leukemia Sourcebook

Liver Disorders Sourcebook

Medical Tests Sourcebook, 4th Edition

Men's Health Concerns Sourcebook, 3rd Edition

Mental Health Disorders Sourcebook, 4th Edition

Mental Retardation Sourcebook

Movement Disorders Sourcebook, 2nd Edition

Multiple Sclerosis Sourcebook

Muscular Dystrophy Sourcebook

Obesity Sourcebook

Osteoporosis Sourcebook

Pain Sourcebook, 3rd Edition

Pediatric Cancer Sourcebook

Physical & Mental Issues in Aging Sourcebook

Podiatry Sourcebook, 2nd Edition

Pregnancy & Birth Sourcebook, 3rd Edition

Prostate & Urological Disorders Sourcebook

Prostate Cancer Sourcebook

Rehabilitation Sourcebook

Respiratory Disorders Sourcebook, 2nd Edition

Sexually Transmitted Diseases Sourcebook, 4th Edition

Sleep Disorders Sourcebook, 3rd Edition

Smoking Concerns Sourcebook

Sports Injuries Sourcebook, 4th Edition

Stress-Related Disorders Sourcebook, 2nd Edition

Stroke Sourcebook, 2nd Edition

Surgery Sourcebook, 2nd Edition

Thyroid Disorders Sourcebook

Transplantation Sourcebook

Traveler's Health Sourcebook

Urinary Tract & Kidney Diseases & Disorders Sourcebook, 2nd Edition

Vegetarian Sourcebook

Women's Health Concerns Sourcebook, 3rd Edition

Workplace Health & Safety Sourcebook

Worldwide Health Sourcebook

## Teen Health Series

Abuse & Violence Information for Teens

Accident & Safety Information for Teens

Alcohol Information for Teens, 2nd Edition

Allergy Information for Teens

Asthma Information for Teens, 2nd Edition

Body Information for Teens

Cancer Information for Teens, 2nd Edition

Complementary & Alternative Medicine Information for Teens

Diabetes Information for Teens, 2nd Edition

Diet Information for Teens, 3rd Edition

Drug Information for Teens, 3rd Edition

Eating Disorders Information for Teens, 2nd Edition

Fitness Information for Teens, 2nd Edition

Learning Disabilities Information for Teens

Mental Health Information for Teens, 3rd Edition

Pregnancy Information for Teens, 2nd Edition

Sexual Health Information for Teens, 3rd Edition

Skin Health Information for Teens, 2nd Edition

Sleep Information for Teens

Sports Injuries Information for Teens, 2nd Edition

Stress Information for Teens

Suicide Information for Teens, 2nd Edition

Tobacco Information for Teens, 2nd Edition

# Autism
## and Pervasive Developmental Disorders
# SOURCEBOOK

*Second Edition*

## Health Reference Series

*Second Edition*

# Autism
# and Pervasive
# Developmental
# Disorders
# SOURCEBOOK

*Basic Consumer Health Information about Autism Spectrum Disorders (ASD) Including Autistic Disorder, Asperger Syndrome, Rett Syndrome, Childhood Disintegrative Disorder, and Pervasive Developmental Disorder Not Otherwise Specified (PDDNOS)*

*Along with Facts about Causes, Symptoms, Assessment, Interventions, Treatments, and Education, Tips for Family Members and Teachers on the Transition to Adulthood, a Glossary of Related Terms, and a Directory of Resources for More Information*

**Edited by**
**Joyce Brennfleck Shannon**

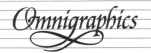

*Omnigraphics*

P.O. Box 31-1640, Detroit, MI 48231

Bibliographic Note
Because this page cannot legibly accommodate all the copyright notices, the Bibliographic Note portion of the Preface constitutes an extension of the copyright notice.

Edited by Joyce Brennfleck Shannon

*Health Reference Series*

Karen Bellenir, *Managing Editor*
David A. Cooke, MD, FACP, *Medical Consultant*
Elizabeth Collins, *Research and Permissions Coordinator*
Cherry Edwards, *Permissions Assistant*
EdIndex, Services for Publishers, *Indexers*

\* \* \*

Omnigraphics, Inc.

Matthew P. Barbour, *Senior Vice President*
Kevin M. Hayes, *Operations Manager*

\* \* \*

Peter E. Ruffner, *Publisher*

Copyright © 2011 Omnigraphics, Inc.

ISBN 978-0-7808-1146-1

Library of Congress Cataloging-in-Publication Data

Autism and pervasive developmental disorders sourcebook : basic consumer health information about autism spectrum disorders (ASD) including autistic disorder, Asperger syndrome, Rett syndrome, childhood disintegrative disorder, and pervasive developmental disorder not otherwise specified (PDDNOS); along with facts about causes, symptoms, assessment, interventions, treatments, and education, tips for family members and teachers on the transition to adulthood ... / edited by Joyce Brennfleck Shannon. -- 2nd ed.
    p. cm.
Includes bibliographical references and index.
Summary: "Provides basic consumer health information about the causes, risk factors, symptoms, and diagnosis of autism spectrum disorders and related conditions, along with facts about interventions and treatments, educational guidelines, and coping tips for families. Includes index, glossary, and other resources"-- Provided by publisher.
ISBN 978-0-7808-1146-1 (hardcover : alk. paper) 1. Autism in children--Popular works. 2. Developmental disabilities--Popular works. I. Shannon, Joyce Brennfleck.
RJ506.A9A8929 2011
618.92'85882--dc22

2011003831

∞

Printed in the United States

# *Table of Contents*

Visit www.healthreferenceseries.com to view *A Contents Guide to the Health Reference Series*, a listing of more than 15,000 topics and the volumes in which they are covered.

## Part II: Causes and Risk Factors Associated with Autism Spectrum Disorder

## Part III: Identifying and Diagnosing Autism Spectrum Disorders

## Part IV: Conditions That May Accompany Autism Spectrum Disorders

## Part V: Interventions and Treatments for Autism Spectrum Disorder

ix

## Part VI: Education and Autism Spectrum Disorder

## Part VII: Living with Autism Spectrum Disorder and Transitioning to Adulthood

## Part VIII: Additional Help and Information

# *Preface*

## *About This Book*

The Centers for Disease Control and Prevention (CDC) reports that roughly one in 90 children aged 3–17 received a diagnosis of autism spectrum disorder (ASD) in 2007. ASD includes autistic disorder, Asperger syndrome, Rett syndrome, childhood disintegrative disorder, and pervasive developmental disorder not otherwise specified. Studies indicate that the prevalence of these neurodevelopmental disabilities, which cause significant problems with social interaction and communication, is increasing. Researchers believe genes, brain dysfunction, and environmental factors play a role in causing ASD. Although there is no cure, early diagnosis and evidence-based interventions currently provide the best long-term outcomes.

*Autism and Pervasive Developmental Disorders Sourcebook, Second Edition* provides updated information about the specific types of autism spectrum disorders. It explains symptoms, assessment, and diagnosis of ASD and describes the importance of early interventions. Evidence-based behavior, communication, and biomedical interventions are presented, along with educational guidelines for teachers and parents of children with ASD. Support, safety, transition, mental health, and employment information for families and individuals affected by ASD is also provided. The book concludes with a glossary of related terms and a directory of resources offer additional help and information.

## How to Use This Book

This book is divided into parts and chapters. Parts focus on broad areas of interest. Chapters are devoted to single topics within a part.

*Part I: Overview of Autism Spectrum Disorder (ASD)* describes autistic disorder, Asperger syndrome, Rett syndrome, childhood disintegrative disorder, and pervasive developmental disorder not otherwise specified. A separate chapter reviews the increasing prevalence of autism spectrum disorders in the United States.

*Part II: Causes and Risk Factors Associated with Autism Spectrum Disorder* reviews findings on brain development and dysfunction and presents current research about the many genes linked to ASD. Risk factors for ASD—including diseases, vaccines, and premature birth—are discussed.

*Part III: Identifying and Diagnosing Autism Spectrum Disorders* describes the range of symptoms and developmental milestones and delays that indicate a need for further assessment. Developmental screening, medical and genetic tests, and other assessments are explained. A separate chapter reviews options for moving forward after receiving an ASD diagnosis.

*Part IV: Conditions That May Accompany Autism Spectrum Disorders* provides information about communication difficulties, non-verbal learning disability, seizures, and osteoporosis. Genetic disorders that co-occur with ASD—such as fragile X syndrome, Landau-Kleffner syndrome, and Prader-Willi syndrome—are also described.

*Part V: Interventions and Treatments for Autism Spectrum Disorder* gives detailed information about practices that are often effective for individuals with ASD. Topics include early intervention for children with developmental delays and interventions for individuals with Asperger syndrome. Communication and behavior therapies—such as applied behavior analysis, verbal therapy, and pivotal response treatment—are described. Medical treatments and research study participation are also discussed.

*Part VI: Education and Autism Spectrum Disorder* describes the special education process and offers tips for teaching students with ASD, managing challenging ASD behavior, and promoting social interaction. Separate chapters address secondary school experiences, preparing ASD students for postsecondary education, and teaching lifetime goals.

*Part VII: Living with Autism Spectrum Disorder and Transitioning to Adulthood* provides practical information about safety and support for ASD adults focusing on specific concerns such as depression and toilet training. It also offers facts about transition plans, finding housing, career planning, and job accommodations for adults in the autism spectrum.

*Part VIII: Additional Help and Information* provides a glossary of terms related to autism spectrum disorders. A directory of organizations with additional information about autism spectrum disorders is also included.

## *Bibliographic Note*

This volume contains documents and excerpts from publications issued by the following U.S. government agencies: Centers for Disease Control and Prevention (CDC); National Institute of Child Health and Human Development (NICHD); Genetics Home Reference; National Dissemination Center for Children with Disabilities (NICHCY); National Institute of Environmental Health Sciences (NIEHS); National Institutes of Health (NIH); National Institute of Mental Health (NIMH); National Institute of Neurological Disorders and Stroke (NINDS); National Institute on Deafness and Other Communication Disorders (NICDC); U.S. Department of Education; and the U.S. Environmental Protection Agency (EPA).

In addition, this volume contains copyrighted documents from the following organizations and individuals: ADAM, Inc.; American Speech-Language-Hearing Association; Angelman Syndrome Foundation; Asperger's Association of New England; Autism Research Institute; Autism Society; Autism Speaks; Autistic Self Advocacy Network; Beach Center on Disability at University of Kansas; Center for Autism and Related Disabilities at University of Central Florida; Barbara T. Doyle; Elsevier Health Sciences Publications; Families of Advocates Partnership for Education; First Signs, Inc.; HealthDay/ScoutNews LLC; Emily Doyle Iland; Indiana Resource Center for Autism; International Society for Augmentative and Alternative Communication; Kennedy Krieger Institute; MAAP Services for Autism and Asperger Syndrome; Maine Department of Health and Human Services; May Institute; National Autism Center; National Autistic Society; National Collaborative on Workforce and Disability for Youth; Nemours Foundation; Nova Science Publishers, Inc.; Ohio State University; Organization for Autism Research; Research Autism; Sage Publications; Simons Foundation Autism Research Initiative; Stuttering Foundation of America; Joycelyn

Taylor; Tuberous Sclerosis Alliance; University of Missouri; Vanderbilt University Medical Center; and Yale Child Study Center.

## Acknowledgements

In addition to the listed organizations, agencies, and individuals who have contributed to this *Sourcebook*, special thanks go to managing editor Karen Bellenir, research and permissions coordinator Liz Collins, and prepress services provider WhimsyInk for their help and support.

## About the Health Reference Series

The *Health Reference Series* is designed to provide basic medical information for patients, families, caregivers, and the general public. Each volume takes a particular topic and provides comprehensive coverage. This is especially important for people who may be dealing with a newly diagnosed disease or a chronic disorder in themselves or in a family member. People looking for preventive guidance, information about disease warning signs, medical statistics, and risk factors for health problems will also find answers to their questions in the *Health Reference Series*. The *Series*, however, is not intended to serve as a tool for diagnosing illness, in prescribing treatments, or as a substitute for the physician/patient relationship. All people concerned about medical symptoms or the possibility of disease are encouraged to seek professional care from an appropriate health care provider.

## A Note about Spelling and Style

*Health Reference Series* editors use *Stedman's Medical Dictionary* as an authority for questions related to the spelling of medical terms and the *Chicago Manual of Style* for questions related to grammatical structures, punctuation, and other editorial concerns. Consistent adherence is not always possible, however, because the individual volumes within the *Series* include many documents from a wide variety of different producers and copyright holders, and the editor's primary goal is to present material from each source as accurately as is possible following the terms specified by each document's producer. This sometimes means that information in different chapters or sections may follow other guidelines and alternate spelling authorities. For example, occasionally a copyright holder may require that eponymous terms be shown in possessive forms (Crohn's disease *vs.* Crohn disease) or that British spelling norms be retained (leukaemia *vs.* leukemia).

## Locating Information within the Health Reference Series

The *Health Reference Series* contains a wealth of information about a wide variety of medical topics. Ensuring easy access to all the fact sheets, research reports, in-depth discussions, and other material contained within the individual books of the *Series* remains one of our highest priorities. As the *Series* continues to grow in size and scope, however, locating the precise information needed by a reader may become more challenging.

*A Contents Guide to the Health Reference Series* was developed to direct readers to the specific volumes that address their concerns. It presents an extensive list of diseases, treatments, and other topics of general interest compiled from the Tables of Contents and major index headings. To access *A Contents Guide to the Health Reference Series*, visit www.healthreferenceseries.com.

## Medical Consultant

Medical consultation services are provided to the *Health Reference Series* editors by David A. Cooke, MD, FACP. Dr. Cooke is a graduate of Brandeis University, and he received his MD degree from the University of Michigan. He completed residency training at the University of Wisconsin Hospital and Clinics. He is board-certified in Internal Medicine. Dr. Cooke currently works as part of the University of Michigan Health System and practices in Ann Arbor, MI. In his free time, he enjoys writing, science fiction, and spending time with his family.

## Our Advisory Board

We would like to thank the following board members for providing guidance to the development of this *Series*:

- Dr. Lynda Baker, Associate Professor of Library and Information Science, Wayne State University, Detroit, MI
- Nancy Bulgarelli, William Beaumont Hospital Library, Royal Oak, MI
- Karen Imarisio, Bloomfield Township Public Library, Bloomfield Township, MI
- Karen Morgan, Mardigian Library, University of Michigan-Dearborn, Dearborn, MI
- Rosemary Orlando, St. Clair Shores Public Library, St. Clair Shores, MI

## Health Reference Series Update Policy

The inaugural book in the *Health Reference Series* was the first edition of *Cancer Sourcebook* published in 1989. Since then, the *Series* has been enthusiastically received by librarians and in the medical community. In order to maintain the standard of providing high-quality health information for the layperson the editorial staff at Omnigraphics felt it was necessary to implement a policy of updating volumes when warranted.

Medical researchers have been making tremendous strides, and it is the purpose of the *Health Reference Series* to stay current with the most recent advances. Each decision to update a volume is made on an individual basis. Some of the considerations include how much new information is available and the feedback we receive from people who use the books. If there is a topic you would like to see added to the update list, or an area of medical concern you feel has not been adequately addressed, please write to:

Editor
*Health Reference Series*
Omnigraphics, Inc.
P.O. Box 31-1640
Detroit, MI 48231-1640
E-mail: editorial@omnigraphics.com

# Part One

# Overview of Autism Spectrum Disorder (ASD)

# Chapter 1

# *What Are ASD and Autistic Disorder?*

Autism spectrum disorder (ASD) is a range of complex neurodevelopment disorders characterized by social impairments; communication difficulties; and restricted, repetitive, and stereotyped patterns of behavior. Autistic disorder, sometimes called autism or classical ASD, is the most severe form of ASD, while other conditions along the spectrum include a milder form known as Asperger syndrome, the rare condition called Rett syndrome, childhood disintegrative disorder, and pervasive developmental disorder not otherwise specified (usually referred to as PDDNOS). Although ASD varies significantly in character and severity, it occurs in all ethnic and socioeconomic groups and affects every age group. Experts estimate that three to six children out of every 1,000 will have ASD. Males are four times more likely to have ASD than females.

### *What are some common signs of autism?*

The hallmark feature of ASD is impaired social interaction. A child's primary caregivers are usually the first to notice signs of ASD. As early as infancy, a baby with ASD may be unresponsive to people or focus intently on one item to the exclusion of others for long periods of time. A child with ASD may appear to develop normally and then withdraw and become indifferent to social engagement.

---

This chapter includes text excerpted from "Autism Fact Sheet," National Institute of Neurological Disorders and Stroke (NINDS), NIH Publication No. 09–1877, updated May 14, 2010; and "Myths of Autism," © 2009 Autistic Self Advocacy Network (www.autisticadvocacy.org). Reprinted with permission.

Children with ASD may fail to respond to their names and often avoid eye contact with other people. They have difficulty interpreting what others are thinking or feeling because they cannot understand social cues, such as tone of voice or facial expressions, and don't watch other people's faces for clues about appropriate behavior. They lack empathy.

Many children with ASD engage in repetitive movements such as rocking and twirling, or in self-abusive behavior such as biting or head-banging. They also tend to start speaking later than other children and may refer to themselves by name instead of "I" or "me." Children with ASD do not know how to play interactively with other children. Some speak in a sing-song voice about a narrow range of favorite topics, with little regard for the interests of the person to whom they are speaking.

Children with ASD appear to have a higher than normal risk for certain co-occurring conditions, including fragile X syndrome (which causes mental retardation), tuberous sclerosis (in which tumors grow on the brain), epileptic seizures, Tourette syndrome, learning disabilities, and attention deficit disorder. About 20%–30% of children with ASD develop epilepsy by the time they reach adulthood. While people with schizophrenia may show some autistic-like behavior, their symptoms usually do not appear until the late teens or early adulthood. Most people with schizophrenia also have hallucinations and delusions, which are not found in autism.

### How is autism diagnosed?

ASD varies widely in severity and symptoms and may go unrecognized, especially in mildly affected children, or when it is masked by more debilitating handicaps. Very early indicators that require evaluation by an expert include:

- no babbling or pointing by age one,
- no single words by 16 months or two-word phrases by age two,
- no response to name,
- loss of language or social skills,
- poor eye contact,
- excessive lining up of toys or objects,
- no smiling or social responsiveness.

Later indicators include:

- impaired ability to make friends with peers,

- impaired ability to initiate or sustain a conversation with others,
- absence or impairment of imaginative and social play,
- stereotyped, repetitive, or unusual use of language,
- restricted patterns of interest that are abnormal in intensity or focus,
- preoccupation with certain objects or subjects,
- inflexible adherence to specific routines or rituals.

Health care providers will often use a questionnaire or other screening instrument to gather information about a child's development and behavior. Some screening instruments rely solely on parent observations, while others rely on a combination of parent and doctor observations. If screening instruments indicate the possibility of ASD, a more comprehensive evaluation is usually indicated.

A comprehensive evaluation requires a multidisciplinary team, including a psychologist, neurologist, psychiatrist, speech therapist, and other professionals who diagnose children with ASD. The team members will conduct a thorough neurological assessment and in-depth cognitive and language testing. Because hearing problems can cause behaviors that could be mistaken for ASD, children with delayed speech development should also have their hearing tested.

Children with some symptoms of ASD but not enough to be diagnosed with classical autism are often diagnosed with PDDNOS. Children with autistic behaviors but well-developed language skills are often diagnosed with Asperger syndrome. Much rarer are children who may be diagnosed with childhood disintegrative disorder in which they develop normally and then suddenly deteriorate between the ages of 3–10 years and show marked autistic behaviors. Girls with autistic symptoms may have Rett syndrome, a sex-linked genetic disorder characterized by social withdrawal, regressed language skills, and hand wringing.

### *Do symptoms of autism change over time?*

For many children, symptoms improve with treatment and with age. Children whose language skills regress early in life—before the age of three years—appear to have a higher than normal risk of developing epilepsy or seizure-like brain activity. People with ASD usually continue to need services and supports as they get older, but many are able to work successfully and live independently or within a supportive environment.

## *How is autism treated?*

There is no cure for ASD. Therapies and behavioral interventions are designed to remedy specific symptoms and can bring about substantial improvement. The ideal treatment plan coordinates therapies and interventions that meet the specific needs of individual children. Most health care professionals agree that the earlier the intervention, the better.

## Myths of Autism

**Myth: All autistics are savants.** Only about 10% of all autistics are savants. Most autistics (the other 90%) are not savants.

**Myth: Autistics do not attend college or other postsecondary education.** Autistics can and do attend college/university and other schooling pursuits after high school (for example: vocational training, trade schools). Several books and many articles have been written about autism and college. Many colleges are implementing greater support for their autistic students due to increasing attendance from students who identify as being on the autism spectrum.

**Myth: Only children are autistic. Autism disappears after childhood.** Autism is lifelong. Autistic children become autistic adolescents and autistic adults. The neurological diversity of autism does not disappear over time or age.

**Myth: All autistics are visual thinkers and have advanced visual-spatial skills.** Some autistics face challenges in tasks that rely heavily on visual-spatial thinking, such as navigation, modeling, and geometry.

**Myth: All autistics are geniuses.** Some autistics are geniuses, but many are not.

**Myth: Autism is not genetic and does not run in families.** Autism is in fact highly heritable. Past studies have suggested that the concordance of autism in maternal (identical) twins is likely to be between 60% and 90%. The concordance of autism among paternal (nonidentical) twins and siblings is likely to be between 5% and 25%.

**Myth: Autistics do not fly on airplanes or travel on buses and trains, and they cannot drive cars.** Autistics travel on all forms of public transportation, including airplanes, buses, and trains. Although some autistics do not drive, there are also some who do.

**Myth: You will not see and meet autistics in your local community. They do not work, shop, buy groceries, bank, or walk around town.** Autistics do work and do participate in their local community. Most people have seen and met countless autistics over the years and not known it.

# Chapter 2

# *Asperger Syndrome (High-Functioning Autism)*

Parents usually sense there is something unusual about a child with Asperger syndrome (AS) by the time of his or her third birthday, and some children may exhibit symptoms as early as infancy. Unlike children with autism, children with AS retain their early language skills. Motor development delays—crawling or walking late, clumsiness—are sometimes the first indicator of the disorder. The incidence of AS is not well established, but experts in population studies conservatively estimate that two out of every 10,000 children have the disorder. Boys are three to four times more likely than girls to have AS. Studies of children with AS suggest that their problems with socialization and communication continue into adulthood. Some of these children develop additional psychiatric symptoms and disorders in adolescence and adulthood.

Although diagnosed mainly in children, AS is being increasingly diagnosed in adults who seek medical help for mental health conditions such as depression, obsessive-compulsive disorder (OCD), and attention deficit hyperactivity disorder (ADHD). No studies have yet been conducted to determine the incidence of AS in adult populations.

This chapter includes excerpts from "Asperger Syndrome Fact Sheet," National Institute of Neurological Disorders and Stroke (NINDS), NIH Publication No. 05–5624, updated May 14, 2010; and, an excerpt from "Asperger Syndrome Fact Sheet," Centers for Disease Control and Prevention (CDC), 2010.

## Why is it called Asperger syndrome?

In 1944, an Austrian pediatrician named Hans Asperger observed four children in his practice who had difficulty integrating socially. Although their intelligence appeared normal, the children lacked non-verbal communication skills, failed to demonstrate empathy with their peers, and were physically clumsy. Their way of speaking was either disjointed or overly formal, and their all-absorbing interest in a single topic dominated their conversations. Dr. Asperger called the condition autistic psychopathy and described it as a personality disorder primarily marked by social isolation.

Asperger's observations, published in German, were not widely known until 1981, when an English doctor named Lorna Wing published a series of case studies of children showing similar symptoms, which she called Asperger syndrome. Wing's writings were widely published and popularized. AS became a distinct disease and diagnosis in 1992, when it was included in the tenth published edition of the World Health Organization's diagnostic manual, *International Classification of Diseases (ICD-10)*, and in 1994 it was added to the *Diagnostic and Statistical Manual of Mental Disorders (DSM-IV)*, the American Psychiatric Association's diagnostic reference book.

## Some Common Signs and Symptoms

The most distinguishing symptom of AS is a child's obsessive interest in a single object or topic to the exclusion of any other. Some children with AS have become experts on vacuum cleaners, makes and models of cars, even objects as odd as deep fat fryers. Children with AS want to know everything about their topic of interest and their conversations with others will be about little else. Their expertise, high level of vocabulary, and formal speech patterns make them seem like little professors. Children with AS will gather enormous amounts of factual information about their favorite subject and will talk incessantly about it, but the conversation may seem like a random collection of facts or statistics, with no point or conclusion. Their speech may be marked by a lack of rhythm, an odd inflection, or a monotone pitch. Children with AS often lack the ability to modulate the volume of their voice to match their surroundings.

Unlike the severe withdrawal from the rest of the world that is characteristic of autism, children with AS are isolated because of their poor social skills and narrow interests. In fact, they may approach other people, but make normal conversation impossible by inappropriate or eccentric behavior, or by wanting only to talk about their singular interest.

Children with AS usually have a history of developmental delays in motor skills such as pedaling a bike, catching a ball, or climbing outdoor play equipment. They are often awkward and poorly coordinated with a walk that can appear either stilted or bouncy.

Many children with AS are highly active in early childhood, and then develop anxiety or depression in young adulthood. Other conditions that often co-exist with AS are: attention deficit hyperactivity disorder (ADHD), tic disorders (such as Tourette syndrome), depression, anxiety disorders, and OCD.

### AS Causes

Current research points to brain abnormalities as the cause of AS. Using advanced brain imaging techniques, scientists have revealed structural and functional differences in specific regions of the brains of normal versus AS children. These defects are most likely caused by the abnormal migration of embryonic cells during fetal development that affects brain structure and "wiring" and then goes on to affect the neural circuits that control thought and behavior.

Scientists have always known that there had to be a genetic component to AS and the other autism spectrum disorders (ASDs) because of their tendency to run in families. A specific gene for AS, however, has never been identified. Instead, the most recent research indicates that there are most likely a common group of genes whose variations or deletions make an individual vulnerable to developing AS. This combination of genetic variations or deletions will determine the severity and symptoms for each individual with AS.

### Diagnosis

The diagnosis of AS is complicated by the lack of a standardized diagnostic screen or schedule. In fact, because there are several screening instruments in current use (each with different criteria), the same child could receive different diagnoses, depending on the screening tool the doctor uses. The diagnosis of AS is a two-stage process. The first stage begins with developmental screening during a well-child check-up with a family doctor or pediatrician. The second stage is a comprehensive team evaluation to either rule in or rule out AS.

### Treatment

The ideal treatment for AS coordinates therapies that address the three core symptoms of the disorder: poor communication skills, obsessive or repetitive routines, and physical clumsiness. There is no single best treatment package for all children with AS, but most professionals agree that the earlier the intervention, the better.

### Do children with AS get better? What happens when they become adults?

With effective treatment, children with AS can learn to cope with their disabilities, but they may still find social situations and personal relationships challenging. Many adults with AS are able to work successfully in mainstream jobs, although they may continue to need encouragement and moral support to maintain an independent life. With appropriate services and support, people with Asperger syndrome can make progress in managing or overcoming these challenges and can learn to emphasize their strengths.

## Asperger Syndrome Information from the Centers for Disease Control and Prevention (CDC)

### How is Asperger syndrome different from other autism spectrum disorders?

Children with Asperger syndrome do not have a language delay and, by definition, must have an average or above average intelligence quotient (IQ). Children with other autism spectrum disorders may have a language delay and can have an IQ at any level.

### What can I do if I think my child has Asperger syndrome?

Talk with your child's doctor or nurse. If you or your doctor thinks there could be a problem, ask for a referral to see a specialist such as a developmental pediatrician or psychologist. Talk with your child's teacher or school counselor, too.

Your child might benefit from intensive social skills training at school or in the community. Your child also might need speech therapy to learn how to talk with other people, or medicine to help with anxiety and attention problems. Other therapies including physical and occupational therapy also might be helpful depending on your child's needs.

It is very important to begin this intervention as early as possible in order to help your child reach his or her full potential. Acting early can make a real difference.

# Chapter 3

# *Rett Syndrome*

Rett syndrome is a neurodevelopmental disorder that affects girls almost exclusively. It is characterized by normal early growth and development followed by a slowing of development, loss of purposeful use of the hands, distinctive hand movements, slowed brain and head growth, problems with walking, seizures, and intellectual disability. The disorder was identified by Dr. Andreas Rett, an Austrian physician who first described it in a journal article in 1966. It was not until after a second article about the disorder, published in 1983 by Swedish researcher Dr. Bengt Hagberg, that the disorder was generally recognized.

The course of Rett syndrome, including the age of onset and the severity of symptoms, varies from child to child. Before the symptoms begin, however, the child generally appears to grow and develop normally, although there are often subtle abnormalities even in early infancy, such as loss of muscle tone (hypotonia), difficulty feeding, and jerkiness in limb movements. Then, gradually, mental and physical symptoms appear. As the syndrome progresses, the child loses purposeful use of her hands and the ability to speak. Other early symptoms may include problems crawling or walking and diminished eye contact. The loss of functional use of the hands is followed by compulsive hand movements such as wringing and washing. The onset of this period of regression is sometimes sudden.

---

This chapter is excerpted from "Rett Syndrome Fact Sheet," National Institute of Neurological Disorders and Stroke (NINDS), NIH Publication No. 09–4863, updated October 26, 2010.

13

Apraxia, the inability to perform motor functions, is perhaps the most severely disabling feature of Rett syndrome, interfering with every body movement, including eye gaze and speech. Children with Rett syndrome often exhibit autistic-like behaviors in the early stages. Other symptoms may include walking on the toes, sleep problems, a wide-based gait, teeth grinding and difficulty chewing, slowed growth, seizures, cognitive disabilities, and breathing difficulties while awake such as hyperventilation, apnea (breath holding), and air swallowing.

## Stages of the Disorder

Scientists generally describe four stages of Rett syndrome. Stage I, called early onset, typically begins between 6–18 months of age. This stage is often overlooked because symptoms of the disorder may be somewhat vague, and parents and doctors may not notice the subtle slowing of development at first. The infant may begin to show less eye contact and have reduced interest in toys. There may be delays in gross motor skills such as sitting or crawling. Hand-wringing and decreasing head growth may occur, but not enough to draw attention. This stage usually lasts for a few months but can continue for more than a year.

Stage II, or the rapid destructive stage, usually begins between ages one and four, and may last for weeks or months. Its onset may be rapid or gradual as the child loses purposeful hand skills and spoken language. Characteristic hand movements such as wringing, washing, clapping, or tapping, as well as repeatedly moving the hands to the mouth often begin during this stage. The child may hold the hands clasped behind the back or held at the sides, with random touching, grasping, and releasing. The movements continue while the child is awake but disappear during sleep. Breathing irregularities such as episodes of apnea and hyperventilation may occur, although breathing usually improves during sleep. Some girls also display autistic-like symptoms such as loss of social interaction and communication. Walking may be unsteady and initiating motor movements can be difficult. Slowed head growth is usually noticed during this stage.

Stage III, or the plateau or pseudo-stationary stage, usually begins between ages two and ten, and can last for years. Apraxia, motor problems, and seizures are prominent during this stage. However, there may be improvement in behavior, with less irritability, crying, and autistic-like features. A girl in stage III may show more interest in her surroundings and her alertness, attention span, and communication skills may improve. Many girls remain in this stage for most of their lives.

Stage IV, or the late motor deterioration stage, can last for years or decades. Prominent features include reduced mobility, curvature of the spine (scoliosis) and muscle weakness, rigidity, spasticity, and increased muscle tone with abnormal posturing of an arm, leg, or top part of the body. Girls who were previously able to walk may stop walking. Cognition, communication, or hand skills generally do not decline in stage IV. Repetitive hand movements may decrease and eye gaze usually improves.

## Causes

Nearly all cases of Rett syndrome are caused by a mutation in the methyl CpG binding protein 2, or MECP2 (pronounced meck-pea-two) gene. Scientists identified the gene—which is believed to control the functions of many other genes—in 1999. Not everyone who has an MECP2 mutation has Rett syndrome. Scientists have identified mutations in the CDKL5 and FOXG1 genes in individuals who have atypical or congenital Rett syndrome, but they are still learning how those mutations work. Although Rett syndrome is a genetic disorder, less than one percent of recorded cases are inherited or passed from one generation to the next. Most cases are spontaneous, which means the mutation occurs randomly.

## Incidence

Rett syndrome is estimated to affect one in every 10,000 to 15,000 live female births and in all racial and ethnic groups worldwide. Prenatal testing is available for families with an affected daughter who has an identified MECP2 mutation. However, since the disorder occurs spontaneously in most affected individuals, the risk of a family having a second child with the disorder is less than one percent. Genetic testing is also available for sisters of girls with Rett syndrome who have an identified MECP2 mutation to determine if they are asymptomatic carriers of the disorder, which is an extremely rare possibility.

## Diagnosis

Doctors clinically diagnose Rett syndrome by observing signs and symptoms during the child's early growth and development, and conducting ongoing evaluations of the child's physical and neurological status. Scientists have developed a genetic test to complement the clinical diagnosis, which involves searching for the MECP2 mutation on the child's X chromosome.

Examples of essential diagnostic criteria or symptoms include having apparently normal development until between the ages of 6–18 months and a normal head circumference at birth followed by a slowing of the rate of head growth with age (between three months and four years). Other essential diagnostic criteria include severely impaired expressive language, repetitive and stereotypic hand movements, and gait abnormalities, including toe-walking, or an unsteady, wide-based, stiff-legged walk.

Supportive criteria are not required for a diagnosis of Rett syndrome but may occur in some individuals. In addition, these symptoms—which vary in severity from child to child—may not be observed in very young girls but may develop with age. A child with supportive criteria but none of the essential criteria does not have Rett syndrome. In addition to the essential diagnostic criteria, a number of specific conditions enable physicians to rule out a diagnosis of Rett syndrome. These are referred to as exclusion criteria.

## Treatment

There is no cure for Rett syndrome. Treatment for the disorder is symptomatic—focusing on the management of symptoms—and supportive, requiring a multidisciplinary approach.

## Prognosis

Despite the difficulties with symptoms, most individuals with Rett syndrome continue to live well into middle age and beyond. Because the disorder is rare, very little is known about long-term prognosis and life expectancy.

# Chapter 4

# *Childhood Disintegrative Disorder*

## *Yale Child Study Center: Childhood Disintegrative Disorder (CDD)*

This rather rare condition was described many years before autism (Heller, 1908) but has only recently been officially recognized. With childhood disintegrative disorder (CDD), children develop a condition which resembles autism but only after a relatively prolonged period (usually two to four years) of clearly normal development (Volkmar, 1994). This condition apparently differs from autism in the pattern of onset, course, and outcome (Volkmar, 1994). Although apparently rare the condition probably has frequently been incorrectly diagnosed.

### *Criteria and Clinical Features*

Both *The Diagnostic and Statistical Manual of Mental Disorders (4ᵗʰ ed., rev.) (DSM-IV)* and *International Codes of Diagnosis, 2010 (ICD-10)* provide criteria for this condition. The criteria are rather similar in both, although some differences between the two systems are apparent. The condition develops in children who have previously seemed perfectly normal. Typically language, interest in the social environment, and often toileting and self-care abilities

---

This chapter begins with "Childhood Disintegrative Disorder," © 2010 Yale Child Study Center (http://childstudycenter.yale.edu). Reprinted with permission. It concludes with "Childhood Disintegrative Disorder," © 2010 A.D.A.M., Inc. Reprinted with permission.

are lost, and there may be a general loss of interest in the environment. The child usually comes to look very autistic, for example, the clinical presentation (but not the history) is then typical of a child with autism.

### History

A special educator in Vienna, Theodore Heller, proposed the term dementia infantilis to account for the condition. Few papers on the topic appeared and these were mostly case reports. The presumption until recently was that this condition was always associated with some specific neuropathological process. However, current data do not support this, and in most cases after even very extensive testing, no specific medical cause for the condition is found. As with autism, children who suffer from this condition are at increased risk for seizures.

### Etiology/Cause

The etiology is unknown but several lines of evidence suggest that it arises as a result of some form of central nervous system pathology.

### Epidemiology

More boys than girls appear to be affected. Childhood disintegrative disorder is perhaps ten times less common than more strictly defined autism (Volkmar, 1994).

### Case Illustration

John's early history was within normal limits. By age two he was speaking in sentences, and his development appeared to be proceeding appropriately. At age 30 months he was noted to abruptly exhibit a period of marked behavioral regression shortly after the birth of a sibling. He lost previously acquired skills in communication and was no longer toilet trained. He became uninterested in social interaction, and various unusual self-stimulatory behaviors became evident. Comprehensive medical examination failed to reveal any conditions that might account for this development regression. Behaviorally he exhibited features of autism. At follow-up at age 12 he still was not speaking, apart from an occasional single word, and had been placed in a school for the severely disabled.

# National Library of Medicine CDD Information from A.D.A.M., Inc.

Childhood disintegrative disorder is a condition in which children develop normally through age three or four. Then, over a few months, children lose language, motor, social, and other skills that they already learned.

## Causes

The cause of childhood disintegrative disorder is unknown, but it has been linked to brain and nervous system problems. A child who is affected loses:

- communication skills,
- nonverbal behaviors,
- skills they had already learned.

The condition is similar to autistic disorder (autism).

## Symptoms

- Delay or lack of spoken language
- Impairment in nonverbal behaviors
- Inability to start or maintain a conversation
- Lack of play
- Loss of bowel and bladder control
- Loss of language or communication skills
- Loss of motor skills
- Loss of social skills
- Problems forming relationships with other children and family members

## Exams and Tests

The health care provider will determine whether the child has this disorder, or a similar condition such as childhood schizophrenia or pervasive developmental disorder (autism).

The most important sign of childhood disintegrative disorder is the loss of developmental milestones. Generally, the diagnosis is made if the child has lost function in at least two areas of development.

## Treatment

Treatment is the same as for autistic disorder (autism) because the two disorders are similar. One experimental treatment uses steroid medications to slow the progression of the condition.

## Outlook (Prognosis)

The outlook for this disorder is poor. Most children with the condition have an impairment similar to that of children with severe autism by age ten.

## When to Contact a Medical Professional

Call your provider if your child has any delays in development or starts to lose developmental abilities.

## Alternative Names

Disintegrative psychosis; Heller syndrome

## Reference

Shah PE, Dalton R, Boris NW. Pervasive developmental disorders and childhood psychosis. In: Kliegman RM, Behrman RE, Jenson HB, Stanton BF, eds. *Nelson Textbook of Pediatrics. 18th ed.* Philadelphia, Pa: Saunders Elsevier; 2007: chap 29.

# Chapter 5

# *Pervasive Developmental Disorder Not Otherwise Specified (PDDNOS)*

Pervasive developmental disorder not otherwise specified—it's a mouthful, a long and laborious phrase. What it means, in truth, is "kind of like autism, but not meeting enough criteria to qualify for the autism diagnosis." Unlike the other pervasive developmental disorders, such as autistic disorder and Asperger syndrome, there is no lengthy list of criteria for PDDNOS. Its description is covered in a single paragraph which mainly asserts what it is not:

"This category should be used when there is severe and pervasive impairment in the development of reciprocal social interaction associated with impairment in either verbal or nonverbal communication skills or with the presence of stereotyped behavior, interests, and activities, but the criteria are not met for a specific pervasive developmental disorder, schizophrenia, schizotypal personality disorder, or avoidant personality disorder. For example, this category includes atypical autism—presentations that do not meet the criteria for autistic disorder because of late age at onset, atypical symptomatology, or sub-threshold symptomatology, or all of these."[1]

### *Who ends up with this awkward designation? And what are the consequences of receiving it?*

If a person has autistic-like behaviors and ways of taking in the world that impact functioning, but does not fully meet the criteria for

"PPD-NOS." Reprinted with permission from the Interactive Autism Network (IAN) Community (www.iancommunity.org), © 2007 Kennedy Krieger Institute.

21

autistic disorder or Asperger syndrome, he may receive the PDDNOS diagnosis. PDDNOS may be thought of as sub-threshold autism, or a diagnosis one can give a person who has atypical symptomatology.[2] In other words, when someone has an autistic "flavor" but some of their symptoms are mild, or they have severe symptoms in one area (like social deficits), but none in another key area (like restricted, repetitive behaviors), they may be given the PDDNOS label.

On the positive side, the existence of the PDDNOS category provides a way to name and include people who are on the autism spectrum but do not quite fit elsewhere. Some parents may even prefer the label, feeling it to be less stigmatizing than autism.

On the negative side, PDDNOS is rather non-specific. If you stick too many variations of something in the same pot, you risk making the category less and less meaningful. For instance, researchers have found that clinicians can much more reliably diagnose autistic disorder and Asperger syndrome as compared to PDDNOS.[3] "Reliable" here means that different clinicians, making an independent assessment of the same case, are likely to come up with the same diagnosis. The fact that they could not reliably diagnose PDDNOS means that a parent who has received a diagnosis of PDDNOS for their child, and seeks a second opinion, is not terribly likely to receive the same diagnosis again. In short, the category itself is not easy to pin down resulting in maximum confusion around diagnostic issues.

This fuzziness may impact other areas as well. Parents who were glad to receive a "less stigmatizing" PDDNOS label for their child may find there is a downside: less understanding of the label by institutions, and a harder fight for services.

What might a person who has received a diagnosis of PDDNOS look like? That will vary, of course, but in one study, researchers found that those with PDDNOS could be placed in one of three very different subgroups:[4]

- A high-functioning group (24%) who resembled people with Asperger syndrome but had transient language delay or mild cognitive impairment (such that they could not receive the Asperger diagnosis which requires no speech or cognitive delay).

- A group (24%) who resembled people with autism but who had a late age of onset, or otherwise did not meet the criteria for autism.

- A group (52%) who were autistic-like, but displayed fewer stereotyped and repetitive behaviors.

Research is needed to further investigate whether specific autism spectrum conditions, as yet unnamed, can be teased out of the catch-all category currently called PDDNOS. There is no question that there are such conditions, that PDDNOS (or whatever conditions we are bunching in that category for the moment) exists.

On the hypothetical autism spectrum, writes one researcher: "PDD-NOS is a paradoxical clinical entity. Despite its amorphous clinical boundaries and the subtlety of the clinical presentation, PDDNOS is one of the most important pervasive developmental disorders. Its importance stems from its relationship to autism, its prevalence, and most of all, the impairment that it imparts to those who have it."[5]

## *References*

1.  American Psychiatric Association. (2000). *Diagnostic and statistical manual of mental disorders (4th ed., rev.)*. Washington DC: Author. (Pg. 84).

2   Mesibov, G.B. (1997). Ask the Editor: What is PDD-NOS and how is it diagnosed? *Journal of Autism and Developmental Disorders, 27(4)*, 497–498.

3.  Mahoney, W.J., Szatmari, P., MacLean, J.E., Bryson, S.E., Bartolucci, G., Walter, S.D., Jones, M.B., and Zwaigenbaum, L. (1998). Reliability and accuracy of differentiating pervasive developmental disorder subtypes. *Journal of the American Academy of Child and Adolescent Psychiatry, 37(3)*, 278–285.

4.  Walker, D.R., Thompson, A., Zwaigenbaum, L, Goldberg, J., Bryson, S.E., Mahoney, W.J., Strawbridge, C.P., and Szatmari, P. (2004). Specifying PDD-NOS: A comparison of PDD-NOS, Asperger syndrome, and autism. *Journal of the American Academy of Child and Adolescent Psychiatry, 43(2)*, 172–80.

5.  Towbin, K.E. (2005). Pervasive developmental disorder not otherwise specified. In F. Volkmar et al. (Eds.), *Handbook of Autism and Pervasive Developmental Disorders* (pp.165–200). Hoboken, NJ: John Wiley and Sons. (pg.166).

# Chapter 6

# *Statistics on ASD in the United States*

## *Chapter Contents*

25

## Section 6.1

# *ASD Prevalence Is Increasing*

Excerpted from "NIMH's Response to New HRSA Autism Prevalence
Estimate," by Thomas Insel, National Institute of Mental Health
(NIMH), October 15, 2009.

On October 5, 2009, researchers with the Health Resources and Services Administration (HRSA), Centers for Disease Control and Prevention
(CDC), and Massachusetts General Hospital published a new estimate of
the prevalence of autism spectrum disorders (ASD) among children in the
United States (U.S.). The new estimate that roughly one in ninety U.S.
children ages 3–17 were given an ASD diagnosis in 2007 is significantly
higher than previous reports. But, this finding is consistent with previous reports that the prevalence—the number of people diagnosed with a
particular condition at a given time—of ASD is increasing. Epidemiological studies and surveys from the early 1990s estimated that one in 1500
children had autism. In 2002, this figure increased to one in 150.

The prevalence rate of one in 90 is based on telephone interviews
of parents who were asked about a diagnosis of ASD. Children were
not assessed independently to verify the parents' reports. There were
no earlier figures using this survey approach for comparison, although
a separate survey conducted by the CDC also reports roughly one in
100 children with the diagnosis in 2006, up from earlier reports in
2002. There are many possible explanations for this trend, including
a change in study methods to include a wider range of ASD diagnoses,
improved screening and diagnostic tools which may allow healthcare
providers to identify more cases of ASD and at earlier ages, as well
as increased public awareness which may encourage more parents
to bring their children in for diagnosis when they suspect their child
has ASD. This new estimate does not necessarily indicate a rising
incidence—the number of new cases over a given time span—for ASD.
Specifically, it is unclear from the October 2009 report in *Pediatrics*
whether the one in 90 estimate is measuring a true increase in ASD
cases or improvements in our ability to detect it.

The question is not whether diagnosis and awareness has changed,
but how much of the reported increase can be explained by changes

in diagnosis and awareness, and how much of the reported increase is due to a rising incidence. One recent study using disability services data for California estimated that 24% of the increase in prevalence can be attributed to the changing diagnostic criteria for ASD, including its use with other developmental disabilities.* While other factors appear to explain additional fractions of the increase in prevalence, there is still no complete explanation for the increase from one in 1500 to potentially one in 100 based on any of these factors. Thus, we cannot exclude the possibility that reports of increased prevalence reflect real increases in the numbers of children affected. Additional research will need to investigate this possibility using careful, consistent clinical assessments, carried out over a period of time in a well-defined population.

Regardless of whether the rate is one in 150 or one in 100, ASD presents a major challenge to public health. As more children are labeled or diagnosed with these disorders, there is a need to ensure they have access to and receive appropriate and personalized medical, educational, occupational, and social services throughout their lives.

*King M, Bearman P. Diagnostic change and the increased prevalence of autism. *Int J Epidemiol*. 2009 Oct;38(5):1224–34. Epub 2009 Sep 7. PubMed PMID: 19737791.

## Section 6.2

# *Risk Factors and Economic Costs of ASD*

This section includes excerpts from "Data and Statistics: Autism Spectrum Disorders," Centers for Disease Control and Prevention (CDC), May 13, 2010.

## *Risk Factors and Characteristics*

- Studies have shown that among identical twins, if one child has an autism spectrum disorder (ASD), then the other will be affected about 60–96% of the time. In non-identical twins, if one child has an ASD, then the other is affected about 0–24% of the time.[1]

- Parents who have a child with an ASD have a 2%–8% chance of having a second child who is also affected.[1]

- It is estimated that about 10% of children with an ASD have an identifiable genetic, neurologic or metabolic disorder, such as fragile X or Down syndrome. As we learn more about genetics, the number of children with an ASD and an identifiable genetic condition will likely increase.

- A report published by the Centers for Disease Control and Prevention (CDC) in 2009, shows that 30–51% (41% on average) of the children who had an ASD also had an intellectual disability or impairment defined as intelligence quotient less than or equal to 70. Data on cognitive functioning are reported for sites having intelligence quotient (IQ) test scores available on at least 75% of children who met the ASD case definition. The proportion of children with ASDs who had test scores indicating cognitive impairment (IQ less than 70) ranged from 29.3% in Colorado to 51.2% in South Carolina (average: 41%). In four of the six sites (Alabama, Arizona, North Carolina, and South Carolina), a higher proportion of females with ASDs had cognitive impairment compared with males, although Arizona was the only site for which the proportions differed significantly.

- Studies show that 5% of people with an ASD are affected by fragile X and 10% to 15% of those with fragile X show autistic traits.

- One to four percent of people with ASD also have tuberous sclerosis.

- About 40% of children with an ASD do not talk at all. Another 25%–30% of children with autism have some words at 12 to 18 months of age and then lose them. Others may speak, but not until later in childhood.[2]

## Economic Costs

- Recent studies have estimated that the lifetime cost to care for an individual with an ASD is $3.2 million.

- Individuals with an ASD had average medical expenditures that exceeded those without an ASD by $4,110–$6,200 per year. On average, medical expenditures for individuals with an ASD were 4.1–6.2 times greater than for those without an ASD. Differences in median expenditures ranged from $2,240 to $3,360 per year with median expenditures 8.4–9.5 times greater.

## References

1.  Boyle C, Van Naarden Braun K, Yeargin-Allsopp M. The Prevalence and the Genetic Epidemiology of Developmental Disabilities. In: *Genetics of Developmental Disabilities*. Merlin Butler and John Meany eds. 2005.

2.  Johnson, C.P. Early Clinical Characteristics of Children with Autism. In: Gupta, V.B. ed: *Autistic Spectrum Disorders in Children*. New York: Marcel Dekker, Inc., 2004:85–123.

## Section 6.3

# *Diagnoses of ASD Made at Earlier Ages*

This section includes an excerpt from "Data and Statistics: Autism Spectrum Disorders," Centers for Disease Control and Prevention (CDC), May 13, 2010; and Table 6 from "Prevalence of Autism Spectrum Disorders—Autism and Developmental Disabilities Monitoring Network, United States, 2006," *Morbidity and Mortality Weekly Report (MMWR) Surveillance Summaries, 58*(SS10), Centers for Disease Control and Prevention (CDC), December 18, 2009.

## *Diagnosis*

- The median age of earliest autism spectrum disorder (ASD) diagnosis is between 4.5 and 5.5 years, but for 51–91% of children with an ASD, developmental concerns had been recorded before three years of age.

- Studies have shown that about one third of parents of children with an ASD noticed a problem before their child's first birthday, and 80% saw problems by 24 months.

- Research has shown that a diagnosis of autism at age two can be reliable, valid, and stable. But despite evidence that ASDs can often be identified at around 18 months, many children do not receive final diagnoses until they are much older. (Source: Boyle C, Van Naarden Braun K, Yeargin-Allsopp M. The Prevalence and the Genetic Epidemiology of Developmental Disabilities. In: *Genetics of Developmental Disabilities*. Merlin Butler and John Meany eds. 2005.)

**Table 6.1.** Number of children aged eight years with autism spectrum disorder (ASD), by median age in months at earliest known diagnosis—Autism and Developmental Disabilities Monitoring Network, 11 Sites, United States, 2002 and 2006.

| Site | 2002 Age (in months) of earliest ASD diagnosis on record | | | 2006 Age (in months) of earliest ASD diagnosis on record | | | Change in age of earliest ASD diagnosis on record, 2002 to 2006 |
|---|---|---|---|---|---|---|---|
| | Total no. with ASDs | Median | Range | Total no. with ASDs | Median | Range | |
| Alabama | 116 | 66 | (10–101) | 212 | 51 | (22–99) | -15 |
| Arizona | 280 | 63 | (20–101) | 504 | 59 | (5–104) | -4 |
| Colorado | 65 | 62 | (12–100) | 54 | 60 | (23–97) | -2 |
| Georgia | 337 | 58 | (23–103) | 474 | 53 | (2–101) | -5 |
| Maryland | 199 | 60 | (21–105) | 243 | 58 | (18–105) | -2 |
| Missouri | 205 | 56 | (20–106) | 321 | 53 | (10–102) | -3 |
| North Carolina | 135 | 53 | (21–99) | 230 | 50 | (15–106) | -3 |
| Pennsylvania | 111 | 58 | (24–94) | 150 | 52 | (19–105) | -6 |
| South Carolina | 140 | 60* | (14–103) | 196 | 54 | (13–103) | -6 |
| Wisconsin | 181 | 54 | (11–104) | 257 | 53 | (18–106) | -1 |

*Data published previously for 2002 (Centers for Disease Control and Prevention [CDC]. Prevalence of autism spectrum disorders—autism and developmental disabilities monitoring network, 14 sites, United States, 2002. In Surveillance Summaries, February 9, 2007. *MMWR 2007;56*[No. SS-1]:12–28) reported South Carolina's earliest age of diagnosis at age 64 months. These data have been updated to include the earliest known ASD diagnosis reported in the records.

# Part Two

# Causes and Risk Factors Associated with Autism Spectrum Disorder

Chapter 7

# Brain Dysfunction in ASD

## Chapter Contents

# Section 7.1

# *Mirror Neuron System and Autism*

Excerpted from "Mirror Neuron System and Autism," by Nouchine Hadjik-hani, *Progress in Autism Research* (Paul C. Carlisle, ed), pp 151–156. © 2007 Nova Science Publishers Inc. Reprinted with permission. To view the complete text of this chapter including references, visit http://www.nmr.mgh .harvard.edu/nouchinelab/pdfs/Hadjikhani_MNS&autism_chapter.pdf.

## *The Mirror Neuron System*

Resonance behavior, defined as a neural activity spontaneously generated during movement, gestures, or action, and that is also elicited when the individual observes another individual making similar movements, gestures, or actions, has its underlying neural substrate in mirror neuron system (MNS). The MNS was discovered serendipitously in the monkey, by a group of Italian researchers, G. Rizzolatti, L. Fogassi, and V. Gallese. These scientists were performing electrophysiological recording in area F5 of the monkey, a region specialized for the control of hand action. The recorded neurons were firing when the monkey was grasping objects (food)—but to their surprise, they noticed that the same neurons would also fire when the experimenter was performing the same grasping action. These neurons 'mirror' the behavior of other animal/human, as though the observer were performing the action; they are not involved in imitation, but rather in action understanding: by allowing a direct matching between the visual description of an action and its execution, the results of the visual analysis of an observed action can be translated into an account that the individual is able to understand. In the monkey, mirror neurons have been found in the ventral premotor cortex (F5), in the inferior parietal lobule, and in the superior temporal sulcus (STS).

The MNS is also present in humans as evidenced by many imaging studies, including transcranial magnetic stimulation (TMS), electroencephalographic (EEG), and magnetoencephalographic (MEG).

Studies using functional magnetic resonance imaging (fMRI) have further studied the function and location of the MNS: The MNS is composed of a network of areas comprising the pars opercularis of the inferior frontal gyrus (BA 44) and its adjacent ventral area 6 (inferior frontal cortex, [IFC]), the inferior parietal lobule (IPL), and the superior temporal sulcus (STS). These areas show activation during mental representation of one's own action, and mental representation and observation of another person's action. The MNS is also activated during imitation of action and reciprocal imitation, including face imitation. The MNS is most probably the substrate of action understanding by having the same neural substrate being activated by both action observation and action execution, the MNS provides an automatic simulated re-enactment of the same action.

In addition to action understanding, there are evidences that the MNS is involved in understanding others' intentions, and in the prediction of other people's action goals. In a recent study, Falk-Ytter and colleagues tested the hypothesis that if the MNS is involved in social cognition, then it should be functional at the time before children achieve communication by means of gesture or language, around 8–12 months of life. Using an elegant paradigm, they searched for the presence of proactive goal-directed eye movements at six months and at twelve months. They showed that when observing actions, twelve-month-old infants focus on a goal in a way similar to that of adults, whereas five-month old infants do not, and concluded that the MNS underlies the ability to predict the outcome of others' actions and is mediating processes related to social cognition.

This model of action understanding through shared representation may also be applied in the domain of emotion, and the MNS has been hypothesized by several groups as being the possible basis of "mind reading," imitation learning, and empathy, and a neural substrate for human social cognition. According to this model, emotions are understood when implicitly mapped onto our motor representation through mirror mechanisms. This model was illustrated by the work of Leslie et al. in 2004, who found a common substrate subserving both facial expression and hand gesture observation and imitation in healthy controls, with a right hemispheric dominance for facial expression passive observation.

## Facial Expression Mimicry

Facial expressions of emotion have a biological basis and are generated by biologically given affect programs that are independent of conscious cognitive processes. Humans have a natural predisposition to react emotionally to facial stimuli and to have facial reactions to facial expressions.

Dimberg et al. have shown that subjects exposed to facial expressions of anger or happiness tend to activate muscles that are normally involved in the production of these facial expressions, implying mimicry of the facial stimulus occurring as early as 300 milliseconds (ms) after stimulus onset. The same facial electromyographic reactions can even be elicited when people are unconsciously exposed to facial emotional expression, using short duration stimulus exposure (30ms) and a backward-masking, showing that emotional reactions can be unconsciously evoked. Moreover, a significant interaction has been reported between facial muscle reaction, self-reported feelings, and emotional empathy.

Imitation and observation of emotional facial expressions activate a similar network of areas, including the IFC, the STS, the insula, and the amygdala, suggesting that we understand other's feeling by a mechanism of action representation, and facial mimicry can be understood as a feedback system in which the facial muscle activity provides proprioceptive information and influences the internal emotional experience.

There is a large degree of overlap between neural substrates of emotion perception and emotional experience, and deficits in the production of an emotion and deficits in the face-based recognition of that emotion reliably co-occur: patients with insula damage, an area implicated in the experience of disgust, are also impaired at facial recognition of disgust; similarly, patients with bilateral amygdala damage, a region involved with experience and recognition of fear, have trouble recognizing facial expression of fear. Lesion of the somatosensory cortex in the face area impairs face emotion. Conversely, voluntary facial action generates emotion-specific autonomic nervous system activity.

All these above observations are in line with Damasio's somatic marker hypothesis describing the mechanism by which we acquire, represent and retrieve the values of our actions. According to this model, the feeling of emotions relies on the activation of internal activation of sensory maps that create a representation of the changes experienced by the body in response to an emotion. A similar mechanism for empathy can be postulated, by which the same sensory maps are activated when observing emotions in others via a mirror system mechanism.

In conclusion, the MNS may be neuronal substrate of imitative behavior and empathy, and a system allowing us to understand others' goals and actions. Imitation, empathy, and the understanding of other's goal all seem to be abilities that are challenged in autism. What evidences do we have that these might be the consequences from a deficient MNS?

## Autism and MNS

### *Imitative Deficits in Autism*

Several studies have found imitative deficits in autism. Autistic children have deficits in imitating simple body movements and actions with symbolic meaning. In infants, Charman et al. have found that compared with developmentally delayed and normally developing children, 20-month-old infants with autism were specifically impaired on some aspects of empathy, joint attention, and imitation, pointing to a basic-level imitation impairment in autism. Individuals with autism tend to have limitations in imitating the style of another person's action, and they tend to lack the natural preference for imitation in a mirror-image fashion. Moreover, children with autism have an impairment in imitation of facial expression of emotion.

**Anatomical and functional studies of MNS in autism:** The hypothesis of a deficient MNS in autism was first formulated in 1999 by Riitta Haris' group and two years later Williams et al., published the first review on imitation, mirror neurons, and autism. In this paper, Williams and colleagues underline the role of a deficit in early imitation as part of the autistic development, and point to the important resemblances that exist between imitation and the attribution of mental states, as both involve the translation from one perspective to the other. They offer a series of testable predictions that flow from their hypothesis of a deficient MNS in autism—and anatomical and functional studies have been done for the past four years that support their proposition.

**Anatomical studies:** The anatomical substrate of autism is still unknown. Our group conducted a magnetic resonance imaging (MRI) study in a group of autistic adults carefully matched for gender, age, intelligence quotient, and handedness. The technique we used allows a precise measure of the thickness of the cortical mantle, validated by histological measures. We found that adults with high functioning autism (HFA) display significantly reduced cortical thickness in areas of the MNS, including the pars opercularis of the inferior frontal gyrus, the IPL, and the STS. In addition, the degree of cortical thickness decrease was correlated with the severity of communicative and social symptoms of the subjects.

Our data represent a snapshot in time, and prospective studies are needed to understand the direction of the causality between MNS function and symptomatology. However, from these data we can postulate that an early dysfunction of the MNS may be the *primum movens* of the deficits in imitation, empathy, and experiential sharing present in autism.

**Magnetoencephalographic studies:** Magnetoencephalography (MEG) is a method which allows us to measure the minute magnetic field changes associated with brain electrical activity non-invasively with a millisecond resolution. The spatial resolution is enhanced compared to electroencephalography (EEG) due to the skull not smearing MEG signals. MEG directly relates to neural activity and yields dynamic images that inform us about the speed of the neural processes as well as their sequence in the different brain areas involved. This allows separate examination of the integrity of the different components of a network and their individual role in brain activation.

The first study testing the hypothesis of a deficient MNS in autism was performed using MEG by Hari's group in Finland. The results of this first study, however, were negative, and no differences could be found between autism subjects and the controls. However, in 2003 the same group pursued this hypothesis and showed in a behavioral experiment that Asperger subjects, unlike normal controls, did not profit from mirror-image movement of others during an imitation task. A year later they published another MEG study showing delayed and weaker activation of the inferior frontal lobe and of the primary motor cortex in Asperger subjects during imitation of still pictures of lip forms, providing evidence of MNS dysfunction.

**Transcranial magnetic stimulation studies:** Transcranial magnetic stimulation (TMS) uses rapidly changing magnetic fields to induce electric fields in the brain. With TMS, cortical excitability in chosen areas of the brain can be temporally modulated to test hypotheses relative to their involvement in task performance. Theoret et al. applied TMS over the primary motor cortex (MI) during observation of intransitive meaningless finger movements. They revealed an impairment in the system matching action observation and execution in autism, with a failure of the observation of movement to modulate the excitability of the motor cortex, and concluded that a dysfunction of the MNS could underlie the social deficits characteristics of autism.

**Electroencephalographic studies:** Two electroencephalographic (EEG) studies have been conducted so far examining the MNS in autism, and they both concluded to the existence of MNS dysfunction in autism. The study by Oberman et al. examined the responsiveness of EEG oscillations at the mu frequency (8–13 hertz [Hz]) to actual and observed movement. In normal controls, it is known that mu power is reduced both when the individuals perform as well as when they observe an action, reflecting an observation/execution system. In adults and teenagers with autism, they observed that while mu power was reduced during action performance, it was unchanged during action observation, supporting the hypothesis of a dysfunctional MNS in autism. The same data were observed by Lepage et al. in children with autism.

**Functional MRI studies:** Two fMRI studies have recently been published examining the function of the MNS in autism. In the study by Dapretto et al., children with autism were examined during observation and imitation of facial emotional expressions and compared with typically developing children. Both groups were able to perform the imitation task; however, only the typically developing children showed enhanced activation in the pars opercularis of inferior frontal gyrus, while the autism children had no mirror neuron activity in that area. The same pattern was observed during passive observation of facial expressions. In addition, and similarly to the findings of the anatomical study described, an inverse correlation was found between the level of brain activity in the pars opercularis of inferior frontal gyrus and the severity of symptoms in the social domain, further suggesting a relationship between MNS dysfunction and social deficits in autism.

Our study (Hadjikhani et al., 2006) was the follow up of our first examination of face perception in autism (Hadjikhani et al., 2004). In our first study, we had challenged the findings of other groups reporting no "face area activation" (FFA) in autism subjects when viewing faces. By introducing a fixation cross in the eye-region of the face and asking the subject to fixate it, we ensured that the subjects were actually looking at the faces—it is indeed well known that autistic subjects tend to avoid looking at faces, especially at the eye region. By using this strategy, we were able to show robust activation in the FFA of autistic subjects that did not differ from that of normal controls. However, it is known that autistic subjects have behavioral deficits with faces, and that they have difficulty recognizing facial expressions. To identify the substrate of this deficit, we examined another group of adults with autism, using the same stimuli as in our first study. However, this time we acquired data covering the entire brain as opposed to only examining the visual regions as we had done previously.

We replicated our initial results of robust FFA activation during face perception in autism. But we found that areas of the MNS were hypoactivated in the HFA compared to controls. We also found hypoactivation in right motor and somatosensory cortex corresponding to the face representation. Furthermore, and similarly to the findings of

Dapretto et al., we found an inverse correlation between the activation in the IFC and the severity of the social symptoms.

In addition to these findings, we found that the hypoactivated areas in the HFA group that were overlapping with areas of cortical thinning observed in another group of HFA patients in the anatomical study described. We concluded that areas belonging to the MNS are involved in the face-processing disturbances in autism.

**Electromyographic studies:** Individuals with autism are delayed in comprehending the meaning of facial expression and communicative gestures, and the ability of autistic children to imitate facial expression of emotion is limited. A recent electromyographic (EMG) study casts light on both fMRI results described. McIntosh et al. examined automatic and voluntary mimicry of facial expressions of emotions in adolescents and adults with autism, using the same protocols as those used by Dimberg et al. They found that while both autistic subjects and controls were able to produce voluntary mimicry, autistic subjects did not show any automatic mimicry of facial expression.

The production of voluntary and automatic emotional facial movements depends on two dissociated neural circuits, that can selectively be affected. Selective loss of voluntary facial expression, Foix-Chavany-Marie syndrome, is a classical clinical finding in stroke; but, the selective loss of emotional facial movement while voluntary facial movement are preserved has also been described. Emotional facial mimicry is an automatic process that relies on the MNS, and the emotion deficits present in autism could be explained by a basic deficit in the MNS system.

In summary, a number of anatomical and functional studies all seem to point to dysfunctions of the MNS in autism.

### *Implication for Treatment*

As mentioned in the introduction, most of the studies presented here, showing evidence of MNS dysfunction, were conducted in a subgroup of autism spectrum disorders (ASD), namely HFA or Asperger syndrome, and they may not pertain to mentally retarded autistic subjects. However, a dysfunction of the MNS in HFA may open interesting therapeutic approaches.

The brain is a plastic organ, and training can modify its structure and its function. This has been shown in the animal model: motor skill learning increases cortical thickness in rats, implying that the repetitive environmental demand leads to structural changes in the brain. Similar results have recently been shown in humans: increases in gray matter have been shown in volunteers learning to juggle, in musicians, and in bilingual individuals. In all these cases, brain gray matter increase corresponds to skill-training, and was probably due to an increase in the number of connections in the neuronal population.

An approach consisting in a training of imitative skill may be a valid way to develop not only imitation per se, but also socio-cognitive aspects in autism. Recent data from Wallen and Bulkeley showing that three sessions of adult imitation increased some appropriate social behaviors of young children with autism supports this hypothesis.

## Section 7.2

# *Environment and the Developing Brain*

This section begins with an excerpt from "Environment and the Developing Brain," National Institute of Environmental Health Sciences (NIEHS), April 2010; and concludes with questions excerpted from "Autism and Neurodevelopmental Disorders," Environmental Protection Agency (EPA), August 5, 2010.

Neurodevelopment refers to how the brain and nervous system develops. Scientists have made tremendous progress in understanding how the brain works, and are gaining new insight into the role that early environmental exposures may play in the development of a broad spectrum of childhood and adult disorders, including autism, attention deficit disorder, and learning and movement disorders. Research supported by the National Institute of Environmental Health Sciences (NIEHS) has clearly shown that it is not just genetics that impacts the risk of neurodevelopmental disorders, but also the interplay of genes and the environment. Researchers are making progress in tackling hard questions about the vulnerability of the developing brain as they look at timing and level of exposures, including low-dose exposures in utero and during childhood, to unravel some of the mysteries of impaired neurodevelopment.

### *What environmental exposures may play a role in the development of autism?*

Research from the University of California (UC) at Davis Children's Center has connected thimerosal (ethyl mercury) with immune system dysfunction in mice. This study provides the first evidence that dendritic cells (DCs) in the immune system show sensitivity to thimerosal, resulting in fundamental changes in the immune system's ability to respond to external factors. Also, UC Davis researchers have developed a new method to culture DCs in normoxic atmosphere and in the absence of 2-mercaptoethanol typically present in DC growth media, as this would confound interpretation of results with mercury.

Developmental exposure to non-coplanar polychlorinated biphenyls (PCBs) enhances excitability of the hippocampus and significantly alters seizure threshold. This is significant as children with autism are known to have a very high rate (about 30%) of seizure disorder. Also, the finding that PCBs induce apoptosis in cultured hippocampal neurons via ryanodine receptor (RyR) activation and increased reactive oxygen species (ROS) provides a biologically plausible link between the molecular actions of PCBs and their neurotoxic effects in humans exposed during early development.

Lead exposure to cortical precursors in cell culture enhanced neurite outgrowth at two days of age and increased cell survival at four days. This has implications for autism because autistic children generally show increased postnatal head growth.

Exposure to methylmercury (MeHg) shows population-specific toxicity in newborn rat pups, reducing deoxyribonucleic acid (DNA) synthesis by 50% in the hippocampus. This raises concerns about chemical-induced teratogenesis.

## *What susceptibility factors may contribute to the development of autism?*

- The UC Davis Children's Center has shown an association between delayed adaptive development and difficulty with sleep onset and maintenance.

- Elevated leptin levels have been identified in early onset autism.

- Children with autism and/or their parents show a higher incidence of at least two newly identified gene deletions or polymorphisms that may make them more susceptible to environmental chemicals.

- A study at the University of Medicine and Dentistry of New Jersey (UMDNJ) Children's Center tested the hypothesis that children with autism have increased oxidative stress. 8-iso-PGF2alpha levels, a biomarker of oxidative stress, were significantly higher in children with autism. The majority of autistic subjects showed a moderate increase in isoprostane levels while a smaller group of autistic children showed dramatic increases in their isoprostane levels. These results suggest that the lipid peroxidation biomarker is increased in this cohort of autistic children, especially in the subgroup of autistic children.

## Section 7.3

# *People with Autism Have Trouble with the Distinction between Self and Others*

"People with autism stumble on self-other distinctions," by Virginia Hughes, © 2010 Simons Foundation Autism Research Initiative (SFARI). Reprinted with permission.

**Self-unconscious:** During self-reflective thought, people with autism show lower activation in brain regions involved in decision-making compared with healthy controls.

In 1943, psychiatrist Leo Kanner described 11 children who preferred to be alone and ignored people around them. Some of the children didn't respond to direct questions, others used the pronouns "you" or "he," instead of "I." Kanner called the children autistic, from the Greek word *autos*, or self.

A team of cognitive scientists at University of Cambridge has uncovered a brain signature of this abnormal self-representation in people with autism. Using functional magnetic resonance imaging, the team found that when thinking about themselves, adults with autism have lower activity in two specific brain regions important for decision-making and social interactions than do healthy controls. What's more, individuals with autism have weaker connections between one of these areas, the ventromedial prefrontal cortex (vMPFC), and regions harboring mirror neurons, cells that fire either when a person performs or observes a given action. The report—only the second imaging study to address the concept of self in people with autism—was published in the February 2010 issue of *Brain*.[1]

"On the face of it, it looks as if [people with autism] are not attending to the key difference between themselves and others," notes lead investigator Simon Baron-Cohen, professor of developmental psycho-pathology at University of Cambridge. "The results of this study may provide one more piece of the puzzle in helping to explain the core impairments in social understanding and communication that characterize autism."

For decades, psychologists have brooded over the autistic self. As Kanner first pointed out, people with the disorder can seem highly self-absorbed, lost in their own world. Their conversations with others tend to be one-sided, focused entirely on topics that interest them. Yet some experiments suggest that people with autism have an abnormally low self-interest. For example, studies of the younger siblings of children with autism have shown that those who go on to develop the disorder don't respond to their own name at 12 months old—even if they have normal language abilities.[2] Similarly, unlike typical children, those with autism don't preferentially remember words associated with themselves.[3,4]

"How do we resolve the fact that they can be impaired at thinking about themselves, yet highly egocentric and thinking about themselves all the time?" asks Michael Lombardo, a graduate student in Baron-Cohen's lab who did the research. "That's the paradox, and I think a lot of autism researchers scratch their heads about that." Hoping to find a neural explanation, the researchers scanned the brains of 29 men with high-functioning autism and 33 healthy controls while they answered a series of questions about their own preferences and those of Queen Elizabeth. For instance, the researchers asked, "How likely is the Queen to think that keeping a diary is important?" In the healthy controls, two regions lit up more when participants thought about their own thoughts than when they thought of the Queen's: the vMPFC—part of the frontal lobe known to be involved in decision-making—and the middle cingulate cortex (MCC), which sits deeper in the brain and is active during social interactions. In contrast, in men with autism, the vMPFC responded equally when participants thought about themselves and about the Queen; and the MCC was more active when thinking about the Queen.

## Self Versus Other

Dampened vMPFC activity during self-thought in autism is somewhat predictable, notes Antonia Hamilton, a lecturer in psychology at University of Nottingham who was not involved in the work. That's because many studies have shown that the region is important for "Theory of Mind," the ability to infer what someone else is thinking, which is drastically impaired in people with autism. However, lower activity of the MCC in autistic participants is more surprising, she says. "No one's paid very much attention to this region in social cognition," she notes, although it seems to be cropping up as significant in the latest research.

Scientists fingered the MCC in the first imaging study of the self in autism, published in *Neuron* in 2008.[5] In that work, researchers from Baylor College of Medicine in Houston, Texas, scanned people with autism while they played a complex trust game with another person. Compared with healthy controls, participants with autism show a marked decrease in MCC activity when deliberating their own decisions, the researchers found.

Hamilton has other preliminary data suggesting that the MCC is involved in thinking about others. She has found MCC activation in healthy adults when they watch people picking up an object, but not when they watch the same object moving on its own. Adults with autism, in contrast, have no MCC activity during the task, she says.

Bolstering the idea that a misrepresentation of self can cause social problems, the new study also links the magnitude of abnormal brain activation with the severity of the participants' social impairments. Participants with autism who show the greatest difference in vMPFC activity between "self" questions and "Queen" questions—that is, those whose brain activity looks most like the control group's—were less socially impaired as children than those whose brains show little distinction between self and other.

## Brain Biomarkers

"The most intriguing finding is that there's this correlation with the clinical condition," says Marco Iacoboni, who was not involved in the new study. If the association is verified in a larger sample, clinicians could use it as a biomarker of autism, suggests Iacoboni, professor of psychiatry and biobehavioral sciences at University of California, Los Angeles. "It's useful because if you have a very reliable parameter that tells you a lot about the condition of this particular individual, then in principle, you could use it for evaluating interventions, evaluating treatments, and so on," he says.

The new study also analyzed how the vMPFC talks to other brain regions when thinking about the self. The researchers found that participants with autism have weaker connections between the vMPFC and two cortical regions in the parietal lobe: the ventral premotor cortex and the somatosensory cortex. These regions are activated when an individual takes action, and are thought to contain mirror neurons.

Iacoboni and colleagues in 2006 first suggested that the mirror neuron system is disrupted in autism,[6] preventing children with the disorder from imitating other people and developing normal social relationships. The new study supports this idea, Iacoboni says. "It's another example of these two systems, one on the external side of the brain and one on the internal side, that are talking to each other. They are probably both very important to understanding the conditions in which social cognition becomes problematic, like autism."

Other experts agree, noting that these frail connections could underlie the lack of eye contact or gestures in people with autism. "A very common symptom in autism, for example, would be a lack of facial expression. If you smile, they don't automatically smile back," notes Justin Williams, a senior lecturer in child and adolescent psychiatry at University of Aberdeen in Scotland. "Thinking about people's thoughts is based in the parts of brain that enact those thoughts. But in autism, that connection is not there." It would be interesting to investigate whether this abnormal brain signature changes in the presence of certain brain chemicals, such as serotonin, Williams says. "If we can find out how we can manipulate such a difference, then we might have an important direction for treatment."

## References

1. Lombardo M.V. et al. *Brain* Epub ahead of print (2009) PubMed.

2. Nadig A.S. et al. *Arch. Pediatr. Adolesc. Med. 161*, 378–383 (2007) PubMed.

3. Toichi M. et al. *Am. J. Psychiatry 159*, 1422–1424 (2002) PubMed.

4. Henderson H.A. et al. *J. Child Psychol. Psychiatry 50*, 853–861 (2009) PubMed.

5. Chiu P.H. et al. *Neuron 57*, 463–473 (2008) PubMed.

6. Dapretto M. et al. *Nat. Neurosci. 9*, 28–30 (2006) PubMed.

## Section 7.4

# *Autism Is Not a Fundamental Problem of Attention*

"Autism not a fundamental problem of attention, study says," by Amanda Leigh Mascarelli, © 2010 Simons Foundation Autism Research Initiative (SFARI). Reprinted with permission.

**Driven to distraction:** When looking straight at a face, children with autism switch their gaze to other objects, such as a star, more quickly than healthy children do.

Toddlers with autism pay less attention to faces than do healthy controls, but both groups give equal attention to objects, according to a study published February 1, 2010 in the *Archives of General Psychiatry*.[1] Individuals with autism have impaired social interactions and tend to avoid eye contact. These symptoms led to the controversial sticky attention hypothesis, which says that people with autism get their attention stuck on objects, and that the disorder is associated with a fundamental impairment in the brain systems responsible for attention.[2]

The new findings challenge this idea, suggesting instead that individuals with autism struggle with how to attend to social stimuli, such as information from faces, researchers say. "[The study] suggests that there's something about social information, per se, that's not capturing the children's attention," says Geraldine Dawson, research professor of psychiatry at the University of North Carolina, Chapel Hill, and chief science officer at Autism Speaks, an advocacy organization that funds autism research. Dawson was not involved with the study. The participants in the study ranged from 15 months to nearly five years old, a broad range intended to control for the effect of age.

"It is quite likely that the phenomenon that we are tapping into is very basic and well preserved in development, and likely it is present already in the first year of life," says lead investigator Katarzyna Chawarska, assistant professor of psychology at the Yale Child Study Center. Identifying the earliest point in development at which this abnormality occurs could help children at risk receive behavioral interventions before they develop more overt symptoms, she says.

Researchers have suspected for several decades that individuals with autism have difficulties processing social information from faces. In 2003, Chawarska's team suggested that this abnormality is connected to impaired attention.[3] In that study, researchers placed two-year-old children in car seats in front of computer monitors displaying either a face or an object. After about 1.5 seconds, the face or object disappears, and an image of a toy appears on one side of the screen. The researchers measured how long it takes for a child to look at the toy. When children with autism look at faces, they divert their attention to the toy in the periphery faster than their healthy peers do, the researchers found. But the study did not address whether this abnormality is specific to autism, or is shared by children with other developmental disorders. Because the faces vanished from the screen just before the non-social stimulus appeared, the study also didn't adequately simulate real life.

In the new work, Chawarska's team studied 42 toddlers with autism spectrum disorder, 31 with other development or language delays and 46 healthy controls. This time, the faces remained on the screen throughout the trial, better simulating actual social interactions. Once again, researchers found that toddlers with autism shift their eyes away from faces to peripheral objects more quickly than do either the typically developing toddlers or those with an array of developmental disorders. And again, there was no measurable difference in the time it takes each group to divert attention from non-social stimuli to a peripheral object.

## In the Eyes

Based on these findings, the researchers speculate that when healthy or developmentally delayed children see a face, they begin making complex brain computations such as: Is this face new or familiar? Is this person nice or mean? Is he or she happy or sad? "These children are trying to extract as much information about this face as possible, thereby creating a more elaborate representation of the face in their memory," Chawarska says. "Next time the child sees this face, it's easier for the child to recognize it."

In contrast, children with autism might focus on physical aspects of a face, such as: Is this a man or a woman? or, Does this person have red hair or gray hair?, rather than processing facial gestures and expressions. Because children with the disorder encode fewer facial features, they might process information more superficially and spend less time looking at faces than do control groups. Children with autism may also have trouble remembering faces, which could result from less attention and more superficial processing of social information.

Last year, Chawarska and her colleague Frederick Shic found that toddlers with autism have difficulty recognizing faces, and that these deficits in recognition are associated with a tendency to look more at external facial features—such as cheeks and forehead—than at the eyes, nose, or mouth.[4] In 2008, co-investigator Ami Klin and his group also reported that when looking at a face, toddlers with autism prefer to look at the mouth than the eyes.[5] Children with autism might be able to shift their attention away from faces more quickly because they engage less with eyes, says Klin, head of autism research at the center.

The new study suggests that children with autism don't reap the same social rewards from looking at faces as healthy children do, notes Dawson. Her research has found that behavioral interventions can teach very young children with autism to find social interactions more rewarding and engaging.[6]

Learning more about these differences could also help address the problem much earlier in infancy, notes John Constantino, professor of psychiatry and pediatrics at Washington University in St. Louis. "What these researchers are after is finding the earliest fundamental thing that distinguishes these children, with the hope that someday we could actually target that and reverse it, so that it doesn't result in this cascade of deteriorated social function," Constantino says.

Chawarska says that it is still too early to predict how her findings will influence therapeutic approaches to autism. She is studying siblings of children with autism with the hope of identifying face-processing skills that are either preserved or impaired in babies who later develop autism. "Once we understand the mechanisms, then we hope to intervene and not only diminish the symptoms, but also hopefully prevent new symptoms or secondary symptoms from developing," Chawarska says.

## References

1. Chawarska K. et al. *Arch. Gen. Psychiatry 67*, 178–185 (2010) Abstract.

2. Landry R. and S.E. Bryson *J. Child Psychol. Psychiatry 45*, 1115–1122 (2004) PubMed.

3. Chawarska K. et al. *Child Dev. 74*, 1108–1122 (2003) PubMed.

4. Chawarska K. and F. Shic *J. Autism Dev. Disord. 39*, 1663–1672 (2009) PubMed.

5. Jones, W. et al Arch. *Gen. Psych. 65*, 946–954 (2008) PubMed.

6. Dawson G. et al. *Pediatrics 125*, e17–e23 (2010) PubMed.

## Section 7.5

# *Brain Proteins with Links to Nicotine Addiction and Autism*

"Researchers Find Link between Nicotine Addiction and Autism,"
November 17, 2008, Ohio State University Research Communications.
© 2008 Ohio State University. Reprinted with permission.

Scientists have identified a relationship between two proteins in the brain that has links to both nicotine addiction and autism. The finding has led to speculation that existing drugs used to curb nicotine addiction might serve as the basis for potential therapies to alleviate the symptoms of autism.

The discovery identified a defining role for a protein made by the neurexin-1 gene, which is located in brain cells and assists in connecting neurons as part of the brain's chemical communication system. The neurexin-1 beta protein's job is to lure another protein, a specific type of nicotinic acetylcholine receptor, to the synapses, where the receptor then has a role in helping neurons communicate signals among themselves and to the rest of the body.

This function is important in autism because previous research has shown that people with autism have a shortage of these nicotinic receptors in their brains. Meanwhile, scientists also know that people who are addicted to nicotine have too many of these receptors in their brains.

"If we were to use drugs that mimic the actions of nicotine at an early time in human brain development, would we begin to help those and other circuits develop properly and thus significantly mitigate the deficits in autism? This is a novel way of thinking about how we might be able to use drugs to approach autism treatment," said Rene Anand, associate professor of pharmacology in Ohio State University's College of Medicine and principal investigator of the research. "It would not be a complete cure, but right now we know very little and have no drugs that tackle the primary causes of autism."

The drugs in question are known as cholinergic agents, which interact with the brain to counter nicotine addiction. Anand said the medications could be retailored for use in children in an effort to increase the level of neurexin-1 beta protein in the brains of people with autism. More neurexin would in turn not only enhance the presence of nicotinic acetylcholine receptors, but also a host of other proteins that are important for the proper formation and maturation of synapses. Proper synapse function is critical to the nervous system's ability to connect to and control other systems of the body.

"Now that these associations have been made, we believe that nicotine in smokers' brains possibly increases the level of neurexin-1 and, as a consequence, helps bring more receptors to the synapses and makes those circuits highly efficient, reinforcing the addiction. In autism, we have the opposite problem. We have a lack of these receptors, and we speculate that neurexin levels are lower," he said. "Our research reveals how changes in the functions of neurexin could affect the guidance of nicotinic acetylcholine receptors to their functional destinations in nerve cells, perhaps increasing receptors in tobacco addicts while decreasing them in autistic individuals, thus increasing susceptibility to these devastating neurological disorders."

Autism symptoms include impaired social interaction, problems with verbal and nonverbal communication, and repetitive or severely limited activities and interests. An estimated three to six of every 1,000 children are diagnosed with autism, and boys are four times more likely than girls to have the disorder, according to the National Institute of Neurological Disorders and Stroke.

Anand and colleagues were studying drug abuse and addiction when they discovered the neurexin-1 beta protein's relationship to a certain type of nicotinic receptor. The timing of the discovery was key, as it built upon two other research groups' previous observations: The brains of people with autism and other neurological disorders that were examined after their death showed a 60%–70% decrease in specific nicotinic receptors, and some patients with autism have mutations in the neurexin-1 gene that suggest the gene's improper functions could play a role in the disorder.

"These have all been 'association studies.' None has been able to prove what causes autism," Anand said. "And then we accidentally discovered that neurexin-1 and nicotinic receptors tangle. So we knew that there was a genetic link to the process leading to synapse formation, and we had nicotinic receptors that had disappeared in the brains of autistic patients. Our finding filled a gap by saying there is a physical and functional association between these two things occurring in the brain."

Neurexin has implications for tobacco addicts, as well, Anand said. Yet another group of researchers recently found that people with a mutation in the neurexin-1 gene were more likely to be smokers, meaning changes in the gene's functions that lead to excess levels of the nicotinic receptors might make people more susceptible to nicotine addiction.

"Our research reveals how changes in the functions of neurexin could affect the guidance of nicotinic acetylcholine receptors to their functional destinations in nerve cells, perhaps increasing receptors in tobacco addicts while decreasing them in autistic individuals, thus increasing susceptibility to these devastating neurological disorders," Anand said. The finding also has implications for nicotine addiction because drugs known to alter neurexin's guidance of nicotinic receptors within nerve cells could be used to suppress tobacco addiction.

# Chapter 8

# *Genetics Impact ASD*

## *Chapter Contents*

## Section 8.1

# *Genes Involved with Autism*

This section begins with text excerpted from "Autism and Genes," National Institute of Child Health and Human Development (NICHD), NIH Pub. No. 05–5590, May 2005, updated in October 2010 by David A. Cooke, MD, FACP; and, concludes with excerpts from "Autism Risk Higher in People with Gene Variant," *NIH News*, National Institutes of Health (NIH), January 10, 2008.

Scientists don't know exactly what causes autism. Much evidence supports the idea that genetic factors—that is, genes, their function, and their interactions—are one of the main underlying causes of autism spectrum disorders (ASD). But, researchers aren't looking for just one gene. Current evidence suggests that as many as 12 or more genes on different chromosomes may be involved in autism to different degrees.

Unlike some diseases like sickle cell anemia or cystic fibrosis, most cases of autism do not appear to be caused by a single gene. Rather, a person must have several different genes for autism to occur. Some genes may place a person at greater risk for autism, called susceptibility. Other genes may cause specific symptoms or determine how severe those symptoms are. Or, genes with mutations might add to the symptoms of autism because the genes or gene products aren't working properly. In addition, interactions between a person's genes and other factors are probably important in determining whether autism develops. Research has also shown that environmental factors, such as viruses, may also play a role in autism. Researchers are looking at possible neurological, infectious, metabolic, and immunologic factors that may be involved in autism.

**Studies of twins with autism:** Analyses of twin study suggest that about 90% of autism is genetically determined, with other factors accounting for the remaining 10%.

**Family studies of autism:** Studies of family histories show that the chances a brother or sister of someone who has autism will also have autism is between 2% and 8%, which is much higher than in the general population.

**Diagnosable disorders and autism:** In about 5% of autism cases, another single-gene disorder, chromosome disorder, or developmental disorder is also present. This type of co-occurrence helps researchers who are trying to pinpoint the genes involved in autism.

## *What have researchers found by studying genes and autism?*

Although some analyses suggest that as many as 12 genes might be involved in ASD, the strongest evidence points to areas on:

**Chromosome 2:** Scientists know that areas of chromosome 2 are the neighborhoods for homeobox or HOX genes, the group of genes that control growth and development very early in life. Expression of these HOX genes is critical to building the brain stem and the cerebellum, two areas of the brain where functions are disrupted in ASDs.

**Chromosome 7:** Researchers have found a very strong link between this chromosome and autism. Their investigations now focus on a region called AUTS1, which is very likely associated with autism. Most of the genome studies completed to date have found that AUTS1 plays some role in autism.

**Chromosome 13:** In one study, 35% of families tested showed linkage for chromosome 13. Researchers are now trying to replicate these findings with other populations of families affected by autism.

**Chromosome 15:** Genome-wide screens and cytogenetic studies show that a part of this chromosome may play a role in autism. Genetic errors on this chromosome cause Angelman syndrome and Prader-Willi syndrome, both of which share behavioral symptoms with autism. Cytogenetic errors on chromosome 15 occur in up to 4% of patients with autism.

**Chromosome 16:** Genes found on this chromosome control a wide variety of functions that, if disrupted, cause problems that are similar or related to symptoms of autism.

**Chromosome17:** A study found the strongest evidence of linkage on this chromosome among a set of more than 500 families whose male members were diagnosed with autism. Missing or disrupted genes on this chromosome can cause problems such as galactosemia, a metabolic disorder that if left untreated can result in mental retardation. Chromosome 17 also contains the gene for serotonin transporter, which allows nerve cells to collect serotonin.

**The X chromosome:** Two disorders that share symptoms with autism—fragile X syndrome and Rett syndrome—are typically caused by genes on the X chromosome, which suggests that genes on the X chromosome may also play a role in ASD.

## Autism Risk Higher in People with Gene Variant: Difference in Gene Appears to Pose More Risk When Inherited from Mothers

Scientists have found a variation in a gene that may raise the risk of developing autism, especially when the variant is inherited from mothers rather than fathers. Inheriting the gene variant does not mean that a child will inevitably develop autism. It means that a child may be more vulnerable to developing the disease than are children without the variation.

The gene, CNTNAP2, makes a protein that enables brain cells to communicate with each other through chemical signals and appears to play a role in brain cell development. Previous studies have implicated the gene in autism, and in this study researchers were able to link a specific variation in its structure to the disease.

Results of the study were reported online January 10, 2008 in the *American Journal of Human Genetics*, by Aravinda Chakravarti, PhD, Dan E. Arking, PhD, and colleagues from the Johns Hopkins University School of Medicine, with Edwin Cook, MD, and colleagues from the University of Illinois at Chicago.

The assertion that the CNTNAP2 gene appears to be involved is strengthened by the fact that each of the different analytical approaches the researchers used in this study led to the same conclusion. Results were replicated in a second, larger group of participants, further implicating the gene. Together, the two groups of participants comprised one of the largest autism studies reported to date. "CNTNAP2 is an excellent candidate gene for autism," Chakravarti said. "It encodes a protein that's known to mediate interactions between brain cells and that appears to enable a crucial aspect of brain-cell development. A gene variant that altered either of these activities could have significant impact."

## Section 8.2

# *Spontaneous Gene Mutations May Boost ASD Risk*

Text in this section is excerpted from "Tiny, Spontaneous Gene Mutations May Boost Autism Risk," National Institute of Mental Health (NIMH), March 15, 2007.

Tiny gene mutations, each individually rare, pose more risk for autism than had been previously thought. These spontaneous deletions and duplications of genetic material were found to be ten times more prevalent in sporadic cases of autism spectrum disorders than in healthy control subjects—but only twice as prevalent in autism cases from families with more than one affected member. The results implicate the anomalies as primary, rather than just contributory, causes of the disorder in most cases when they are present, according to the researchers. Although they might share similar symptoms, different cases of autism could thus be traceable to any of 100 or more genes, alone or in combination. Drs. Jonathan Sebat, Michael Wigler, Cold Spring Harbor Laboratory (CSHL), and 30 colleagues from several institutions, reported on their discovery online, March 16, 2007 in *Science Express*.

"These structural variations are emerging as a different kind of genetic risk for autism than the more common sequence changes in letters of the genetic code that we've been looking for," explained National Institute of Mental Health director Thomas Insel, MD.

"Our results show conclusively that these tiny glitches are frequent in autism, occurring in at least ten percent of cases, and primarily in the sporadic form of the disease, which accounts for 90% of affected individuals," added Sebat. "Understanding such sporadic autism will require different genetic approaches and stepped-up recruitment of families in which only one individual has the disease."

## Section 8.3

# *Risk of Autism Tied to Genes That Influence Brain Cell Connections*

This section is excerpted from "Risk of Autism Tied to Genes That Influence Brain Cell Connections," National Institute of Neurological Disorders and Stroke (NINDS), April 28, 2009.

In three studies, including the most comprehensive study of autism genetics to date, investigators have identified common and rare genetic factors that affect the risk of autism spectrum disorders. The results point to the importance of genes that are involved in forming and maintaining the connections between brain cells.

"These findings establish that genetic factors play a strong role in autism spectrum disorder," says Acting National Institutes of Health Director Raynard Kington, MD, PhD.

"Previous studies have suggested that autism is a developmental disorder resulting from abnormal connections in the brain. These three studies suggest some of the genetic factors which might lead to abnormal connectivity," says Thomas Insel, MD, director of the National Institute of Mental Health (NIMH).

All three studies were genome-wide association studies, which are undertaken to find clues about the causes of complex disorders. The largest study, reported in *Nature*, involved more than 10,000 subjects, including individuals with autism spectrum disorder (ASD), their family members, and other volunteers from across the United States (U.S.). The study was led by Hakon Hakonarson, MD, PhD, a professor at the University of Pennsylvania School of Medicine and director of the Center for study.

In their large study, Dr. Hakonarson and his colleagues found several genetic variants that were commonly associated with ASD, all of them pointing to a spot between two genes on chromosome 5, called CDH9 and CDH10. Both genes encode cadherins—cell surface proteins that enable cells to adhere to each other. The researchers also found that a group of about 30 genes that encode cell adhesion proteins (including cadherins and neurexins) were more strongly associated with ASD than all other genes in their data set. In the developing brain,

60

cell adhesion proteins enable neurons to migrate to the correct places and to connect with other neurons.

In a second study, Margaret Pericak-Vance, PhD, a professor at the University of Miami Miller School of Medicine and director of the Miami Institute for Human Geonomics, completed an independent search for small genetic variants associated with ASD, in collaboration with Jonathan Haines, PhD, of Vanderbilt University Medical Center in Nashville. Published in the *Annals of Human Genetics* in April 2009, the study provides a striking confirmation that ASD is associated with variation near CDH9 and CDH10.

Finally, in a third study, reported in *Nature*, April 2009, Dr. Hakonarson and Gerard D. Schellenberg, PhD, professor at the University of Pennsylvania School of Medicine, led a search for genes that were duplicated or deleted in individuals with ASD. Previous, smaller genetic studies reported a connection between male-only autism and CNTNAP2, a type of neurexin. Together, the three new studies suggest that genetic differences in cell-to-cell adhesion could influence susceptibility to ASD on a large scale.

## Section 8.4

# *Silenced Gene for Social Behavior Found in Autism*

Text in this section is excerpted from "Silenced Gene for
Social Behavior Found in Autism," National Institute of Mental
Health (NIMH), December 3, 2009.

For the first time, inherited disruption of gene expression in a brain
system for social behavior has been implicated in autism. Margaret
Pericak-Vance, PhD, at the University of Miami and Simon Gregory, PhD,
at Duke University, and a multinational team of researchers found evidence for such epigenetic effects on the gene for the oxytocin receptor—
part of a brain system that mediates social behaviors disturbed in autism.
The findings suggest a potential genetic biomarker for the disorder.

### Findings of This Study

The researchers found a deletion in the oxytocin receptor gene in a
person with autism and his mother, who had obsessive compulsive disorder (OCD). OCD shares with autism symptoms of repetitive behaviors.
Oxytocin receptor genes were similarly silenced—but by methylation—
in a sibling with autism who lacked the deletion. That is, two separate mechanisms of gene expression regulation resulted in the same
outcome—loss of oxytocin receptor expression—in the same family.

Following up in blood cells and temporal cortex brain tissue of people
with autism, the researchers pinpointed higher levels of methylation—
about 70% versus the normal 40%—at an epigenomic site known to
regulate the oxytocin receptor. They also found decreased expression
of the receptor in the temporal cortex tissue, an area previously linked
to autism.

### Significance

Excess methylation of the oxytocin receptor could render people
with autism less sensitive to the social hormone's effects. Gene expression most likely became altered in very early gestation (between

fertilization and implantation), suggest the researchers. This could increase vulnerability of the oxytocin receptor gene to environmental insults during the first few weeks of pregnancy, they say. The results suggest that such epigenetic misregulation of the oxytocin receptor gene may be an important factor in the development of autism.

## Section 8.5

# *Gene Linked to Autism and Gastrointestinal (GI) Disorders*

"Gene linked to autism, GI disorders," March 6, 2009, Vanderbilt University Medical Center *Reporter*, © 2009. Reprinted with permission.

A single gene variant may be responsible for both autism and gastrointestinal (GI) disorders in some children, according to a new Vanderbilt Medical Center study. The study, published in the journal *Pediatrics*, suggests that disrupted signaling of the MET protein may contribute to the co-occurring medical conditions in some families. It is well known that GI conditions are common among individuals with autism, but not known if co-occurring GI conditions represent a unique autism subgroup.

Some speculate that GI dysfunction impacts brain development, or that altered nervous system development affects GI function. The MET protein participates in both brain development and GI repair, suggesting that disruption of its signaling may contribute to both medical conditions. "For too long, people have been debating the validity of GI problems in children with autism," said co-author and Pat Levitt, PhD, Vanderbilt Kennedy Center's director and professor of Pharmacology. "GI disorders don't cause autism. Autism is a disorder of brain development. However, our study brings together genetic risk for autism and co-occurring GI disorders in a way that provides a biologically plausible explanation for why they are seen so often together," Levitt said.

Lead author Daniel Campbell, PhD, said the research is mounting evidence that the broad term autism will soon be divided into separate, more specific categories. "Among individuals with autism, 30% to 70%

also have GI problems, including chronic constipation and chronic diarrhea," Campbell said. "And, because many of these patients have difficulties with communication, they may act out rather than be able to communicate that their tummy hurts."

A total of 918 individuals from 214 Autism Genetics Resource Exchange families were studied, each with a complete medical history including GI condition report. The MET rs1858830 C allele was associated with both autism and GI conditions in 118 families containing at least one child with co-occurring autism and GI conditions. In contrast, there was no association of the MET polymorphism with autism in the 96 families lacking a child with co-occurring autism and GI conditions.

Researchers concluded that a functional genetic variant in the MET gene is more strongly associated with autism, specifically in those families where an individual had co-occurring autism and a GI condition.

## Section 8.6

# *Facial Recognition Is a Distinct Genetic Skill*

Text in this section is from "Face recognition is distinct genetic skill, studies find," by Victoria Stern, © 2010 Simons Foundation Autism Research Initiative (SFARI). Reprinted with permission.

**About face:** Identical twins score more similarly on standard tests of facial recognition—such as determining whether a face is misaligned— than do fraternal twins. ꞏ

The ability to recognize faces and interpret facial expressions is programmed partly by genes and inherited separately from other traits, according to three independent studies published this year. The findings suggest that the ability to recognize faces is separate from general intelligence[1] and, along with the ability to interpret emotional expressions, may be hardwired into genes.[2] They might also help explain why an individual with autism retains some cognitive skills—such as reading maps or solving puzzles—and loses others, and why individuals with autism can have remarkably different behaviors.

"If cognitive skills like face recognition are inherited separately, our study results may very indirectly explain why there is such a wide spectrum of symptoms and severity in autism," says Nancy Kanwisher, professor of cognitive neuroscience at Massachusetts Institute of Technology and lead investigator of one of the new studies. The results may also spur a broader investigation of whether other cognitive abilities—such as spatial navigation and language—are independently heritable, researchers say.

In the most recent study, published online February 21, 2010 in *Proceedings of the National Academy of Sciences*,[3] researchers assessed how well identical and fraternal same-sex adult twins score on the Cambridge Face Memory Test. This test measures an individual's ability to learn faces and then recognize them at different angles and in different lightings. Identical twins—who share 100% of their genes—are more than twice as similar to each other in their ability to recognize faces than are fraternal twins, who share about half their genes, the researchers found. This suggests that there is a strong genetic component to face recognition.

To confirm that the results are specific to face recognition and not a more general aspect of memory, the researchers compared the ability to recognize faces with that of remembering word-pairings and images of abstract art. Twin and non-twin participants memorized 25 word pairs and 50 abstract art images and were then tested on their ability to recall them. For all participants, the researchers found that an individual's scores on face recognition and word or art recognition do not correlate, suggesting that face recognition is genetically independent from these other cognitive abilities.

Kanwisher's team reported similar results in children in the January 26, 2010 issue of *Current Biology*. She and her collaborators in China gave three classic tests of face recognition to 51 pairs of identical twins and 35 pairs of fraternal twins, all healthy and aged 7–19. In the first task, participants saw black-and-white images on a computer screen for one second each, and were asked whether each picture was a face or a house. In the other two tests, participants determined whether a face was upright or upside-down, and whether it was one complete face or a mash-up of the top of one face and the bottom of another. In all three tests, the researchers found that identical twins have more similar accuracy scores than do fraternal twins.[4]

## *Waves of Recognition*

By comparing the performance of the identical and fraternal twins, the researchers calculated precisely how much influence genes have in determining an individual's accuracy score. They found that genes account for 25% to 39% of the variation in face recognition ability between identical and fraternal twins; the remainder is a result of either environmental influences or errors in measurement. For instance, extroverts may be better at recognizing faces than introverts because extroverts see more faces in their daily life, says investigator Jia Liu, a professor of cognitive neuroscience at Beijing Normal University in China.

There were no differences between the range of scores in identical twins and fraternal twins in other cognitive abilities, such as sharpness of vision, object recognition and memory. "Our data show at least one cognitive ability—face recognition ability—is independently heritable," says Liu. "We don't know whether the 25% to 39% is low or high, but from our statistical estimates, it seems reasonably high."

Genes might also predict specific patterns of brain activity during face processing, according to an independent study published online February 3, 2010 in *Behavioral Genetics*. Andrey Anokhin and colleagues at Washington University School of Medicine examined how 47 pairs of identical twins and 51 pairs of fraternal twins, all 12 years of age, responded to images of happy, fearful, or neutral facial expressions. About once every second, the researchers replaced each photo with a new one of the same person sporting a different facial expression. Participants wore electrodes on their scalp that measured their changing brain waves during the task.

Anokhin's team found that identical twins have more similar brainwave patterns than do fraternal twins. They estimate that 36% to 64% of the individual differences in processing emotional expressions are a result of the difference in genes. "To my knowledge, this is one of the first studies to show that processing of emotional expressions [is] largely determined by genetic factors," says Anokhin.

The new studies are consistent with previous research implicating a genetic component in facial recognition, notes Michael Tarr, co-director of the Center for the Neural Basis of Cognition at Carnegie Mellon University, who was not involved in the new studies. For instance, individuals with an inherited condition known as congenital prosopagnosia, or face blindness, cannot recognize faces, even though they retain the ability to identify many other classes of objects.[5]

Although the genetic influence is substantial, the studies highlight the fact that environmental factors and epigenetic changes—those that turn genes on or off without changing the underlying deoxyribonucleic acid (DNA) code—also contribute to facial recognition. "This is consistent with what we know from studies on autism as well," says Mustafa Sahin, professor of neuroscience at Harvard University, who was not involved in either study. Genes play a greater role in the risk of autism than in any other common neurodevelopmental disorder, with a reported heritability of about 90%.[6] Still, this means that environmental and epigenetic factors probably play a role in at least 10% of cases, he says.

To find out whether specific genetic factors cause the face-processing deficits seen in autism, researchers would need to repeat the studies in infants with and without the disorder, Sahin says. "Studies in young children could allow early detection of abnormalities in visual processing."

## References

1. Kanwisher N. *Nat. Neurosci. 3*, 759–763 (2000) PubMed.

2. Anokhin A. et al. *Behav. Genet.* Epub ahead of print (2010) PubMed.

3. Wilmer J. et al. *PNAS* Epub ahead of print (2010).

4. Zhu Q. et al. *Curr Biol. 20*, 137–142 (2010) PubMed.

5. Thomas C. et al. *Nat. Neurosci. 12*, 29–31 (2009) PubMed.

6. Geschwind D. *Annu. Rev. Med. 60*, 367–380 (2009) PubMed.

## Section 8.7

# *Possible Genetic Overlap between Attention Deficit Hyperactivity Disorder (ADHD) and Autism*

This section includes text from " Researchers probe genetic overlap between ADHD, autism," by Andrea Anderson, © 2010 Simons Foundation Autism Research Initiative (SFARI). Reprinted with permission.

**Puzzling link:** More than half of children with attention deficit hyperactivity disorder meet the diagnostic criteria for autism spectrum disorders.

Attention deficit hyperactivity disorder (ADHD) and autism may have more in common than childhood onset and a few similar symptoms. New research suggests the conditions share genetic roots. Children with ADHD often have problems staying still, and easily get bored or distracted while working on tasks. In contrast, individuals with autism tend to have social and communicative impairments, and frequently show repetitive behaviors.

Although these core diagnostic symptoms do not overlap, behavioral differences between the two disorders can be subtle, and doctors often mistake one for the other. For instance, social withdrawal in a child with autism is sometimes mistaken for inattention associated with ADHD. Likewise, children with autism may be hyperactive as youngsters but become calmer and more withdrawn with age.

Autism and ADHD also tend to crop up in the same families, and both disorders may include aggression, disruptive behavior, or problems in school. Overall, an estimated 30% to 80% of children with autism have ADHD,[1,2] and more than half of children with ADHD meet the diagnostic criteria for autism spectrum disorders. Despite increasing awareness of this overlap, no one has found genetic variants in individuals who have both conditions. Researchers investigating each disorder separately, however, are turning up clues suggesting that the two share some genetic risk variants, brain patterns, and neuropsychological features, such as cognitive, motor, and language impairments. The puzzling link is described in a review published in the February

2010 issue of *European Child and Adolescent Psychiatry*.[3] "There is a lot more to discover about the genetics of both [conditions]," notes Philip Asherson, professor of molecular psychiatry at King's College London, who studies ADHD.

Researchers don't yet know whether the same genes are at play when the disorders are present separately and together. The overlap has been poorly studied, in part because doctors have historically been reluctant to diagnose both conditions in the same individual. The American Psychiatric Association's *Diagnostic and Statistical Manual of Mental Disorders,* the *DSM-IV*, does not allow ADHD and autism to be diagnosed together, reflecting the view that ADHD symptoms in autism could be temporary or simply a consequence of autism's complex and variable presentation.

In addition, because of the hierarchical nature of the DSM guidelines, diagnosis with a so-called pervasive developmental disorder such as autism trumps an ADHD diagnosis. That may change as some push for ADHD and autism to be co-diagnosed. Members of the DSM-V Autism Work Group are debating recommending the co-diagnoses in the next version of the guidelines, set to debut in May 2013. "Most clinicians—most people working with those with ADHD and autism—know that you see features of one in the other," Asherson says.

## Twin Insights

Analyzing parental questionnaires, Asherson and colleagues in February 2010 reported overlap between ADHD and autism behaviors in 312 sets of two-year-old identical and fraternal twins. They found the correlation between ADHD and autism behaviors to be fairly modest: behaviors resembling ADHD or autism overlap nearly as often in fraternal twin pairs, who share about half their genes, as they do in identical twins, who share all their genes.[4]

Earlier studies found that the overlap between the two disorders is more pronounced in older children. When researchers assessed eight-year-old twins from 6,771 families, for example, they found that identical twins are nearly twice as likely to show an overlap as are fraternal twins. Based on their observations, the researchers estimated that more than half of the genes involved in one condition also influence the other.[5] These results may reflect the fact that ADHD and autism symptoms can become more pronounced with age, notes Angelica Ronald, a lecturer in psychological sciences at the University of London and first author of both twin studies. The genes affected in both disorders— perhaps related to brain development and behavior—may be activated with age, she says. Other studies have found an abundance of autism symptoms in children diagnosed with ADHD.

Using parent and teacher questionnaires and interviews, researchers from the International Multi-Centre ADHD Genetics consortium evaluated autism symptoms in 821 five- to seventeen-year-old children with ADHD, 1,050 siblings and 149 healthy controls. Individuals with ADHD score higher on tests for autism-like symptoms, such as the Social Communication Questionnaire, than do their siblings or controls, the researchers reported last year.[6] Male siblings of children with ADHD score higher on the tests than do children in the general population. Although the researchers don't know why brothers are affected more than sisters, the results highlight the overlap of these conditions within families and support the notion that the conditions share some genetic underpinnings.

## *Variants Common and Rare*

Because both ADHD and autism appear to involve abnormal signaling between nerve cells in the brain, the promising candidates for the overlap act in pathways related to the neurotransmitters dopamine and serotonin. For instance, the dopamine transporter gene DAT1 and the dopamine receptor genes DRD4 and DRD5 are among the genes most strongly associated with ADHD.[7] Several teams are exploring the role of dopamine genes in autism, which has so far been linked to one gene in the pathway, the dopamine receptor gene DRD3.[8]

Meanwhile, genome-wide association studies of individuals diagnosed with ADHD have turned up more than a dozen single-letter variations, or single-nucleotide polymorphisms (SNP), that have been separately implicated in autism.[9] Conversely, dozens of SNPs associated with autism have been independently implicated in ADHD.[3]

There is debate over whether these common variants are the causal factors in either ADHD or autism, or whether rare variants are to blame. For example, in a study of 335 children with ADHD and their parents, Peter White and colleagues at the University of Pennsylvania identified hundreds of rare copy number variations (CNVs)—deoxyribonucleic acid (DNA) deletions or duplications—in ADHD families that are absent in 2,026 unaffected controls.[10]

Among the 222 CNVs detected in ADHD families, four include genes previously implicated in autism: A2BP1, AUTS2, CNTNAP2 and IMMP2L. CNVs fingered in the study also affect 15 genes linked to schizophrenia and two genes associated with Tourette syndrome, a neurological condition characterized by involuntary and repetitive movements and vocalizations. What's more, the overlapping genes tend to contribute to brain function and development. For example, a mouse study published in January 2010 suggests that the AUTS2 gene codes for a protein found in several developing brain regions, including the frontal cortex, hippocampus, and cerebellum.[11] Even the most frequent ADHD-related CNVs show up in only about one percent of individuals tested, however.

Getting to the bottom of the genetics behind ADHD and autism co-morbidity will require studying families in which both conditions are present, says Nanda Rommelse, assistant professor of psychiatry at Radboud University in the Netherlands and first author of the new review. "As yet, there are no established findings at all in the genetic overlap between ADHD and autism spectrum disorders," Rommelse says. "It's still an area of research that has been largely ignored." Her team intends to genetically screen as many as 300 families over the next few years, and has already recruited 80, for an effort called the Biology of Autism project. The project aims to explore the role of both common polymorphisms and CNVs in co-morbid ADHD and autism cases. The researchers also plan to do neuropsychological tests aimed at finding endophenotypes, cognitive traits that can predict an individual's risk of developing one or both conditions.

## *References*

1. Simonoff E. et al. *J. Am. Acad. Child Adolesc. Psychiatry 47*, 921–929 (2008) PubMed.

2. Lee D.O. and O.Y. Ousley J. *Child Adolesc. Psychopharmacol. 16*, 737–746 (2006) PubMed.

3. Rommelse N.N. et al. *Eur. Child. Adolesc. Psychiatry* Epub ahead of print (2010) PubMed.

4. Ronald A. et al. *J. Abnorm. Child Psychol. 38*, 185–196 (2010) PubMed.

5. Ronald A. et al. *J. Child Psychol. Psychiatry 49*, 535–542 (2008) PubMed.

6. Mulligan A. et al. *J. Autism Dev. Disord. 39*, 197–209 (2009) PubMed.

7. Gizer I.R. et al. *Hum. Genet. 126*, 51–90 (2009) PubMed.

8. de Krom M. et al. *Biol. Psychiatry 65*, 625–630 (2009) PubMed.

9. Franke B. et al. *Hum. Genet. 126*, 13–50 (2009) PubMed.

10. Elia J. et al. *Mol. Psychiatry* Epub ahead of print (2009) PubMed.

11. Bedogni F. et al. *Gene Expr. Patterns 10*, 9–15 (2010) PubMed.

# Chapter 9

# *Diseases, Vaccines, and ASD*

## Chapter Contents

## Section 9.1

# *Can Diseases and Vaccines Cause ASD*

"An introduction to possible biomedical causes and treatments for autism spectrum disorders," by Marcie Wheeler. © 2008 Indiana Resource Center for Autism. Reprinted with permission.

An increasing number of parents are seeking biomedical interventions for their children on the autism spectrum. Various theories on biomedical treatments exist. Making the decision to explore biomedical interventions more difficult are the unique differences among individuals, the cost involved for evaluations, testing and treatments, the lack of knowledgeable professionals to consult, and the relatively small amount of easily accessible and understandable research and information available to review.

Current opinion is that there are many potential causes of autism spectrum disorders. Most agree that there are multiple factors involved. Research on the possible genetic basis of autism spectrum disorders is expanding along with research on biomedical triggers. In the majority of cases, there is likely a complex relationship between a genetic predisposition and an environmental trigger that results in the behavioral symptoms of an autism spectrum disorder diagnosis.

This section will briefly highlight the biomedical theories of causation and the associated biomedical interventions that are more commonly pursued by families. This brief article cannot begin to address all the important issues and information related to biomedical treatments. It is merely an attempt to provide basic information. The information contained in this section is not to be considered a recommendation or endorsement for a particular theory or approach for treatment. It is important to understand the status of research and carefully examine treatment options and interventions whether they are educational, therapeutic, or biomedical in nature.

## *Some Biomedical Based Causal Theories of Autism Spectrum Disorders*

There is no universally accepted theory of causation. It appears there is a complex interplay of factors that can result in symptoms leading to a diagnosis of an autism spectrum disorder. There is now believed to be a number of genetic and environmental causes. The purpose of this article is not to focus on genetic theories of causation. Here, the only focus will be on the most commonly cited biomedical concerns thought to be implicated. Later, the more commonly cited interventions which address these biomedical concerns will be shared.

Currently, there are four broad areas of focus which conceptualize the possible biomedical causes of autism spectrum disorders. Most researchers and practitioners feel that all four areas are intertwined and that each affects the other. Gastrointestinal abnormalities, immune dysfunctions, detoxification abnormalities, and/or nutritional deficiencies or imbalances have all been suggested as potential biomedical triggers for autism spectrum disorders. It is hard to determine which scenario came first. It is felt that one problem is connected to the next that follows. But deciding which came first seems to be another part of the puzzle to address for each individual.

Gastrointestinal abnormalities, immune dysfunctions, detoxification irregularities, and nutritional deficiencies or imbalances may cause some of the same symptoms. Often a problem in one of the four biomedical areas impacts one or more of the other areas. However, for purposes of simplification and clarity, each of these will be discussed separately.

For children on the autism spectrum, symptoms of gastrointestinal problems may include: diarrhea, constipation, reflux, food cravings, bloating, fatigue, aggression, sleep difficulties, spaciness, agitation, inappropriate laughing and stim behaviors including hand movements, toe walking, and spinning objects or self. Gastrointestinal abnormalities may be due to the following ailments:

- Bacteria, yeast, or fungus overgrowth (Shaw, 1998)

- Leaky gut defined as increased permeability of the intestinal lining, often caused by chronic inflammation that is often due to yeast and/or the inability to break down proteins from casein (dairy products) and gluten (wheat, barley, rye, oats, and other grains) which then leak into the bloodstream and travel to and impact various tissues, including the brain, possibly causing an opiate affect in the brain (McCandless, 2002)

- Alteration of intestinal flora as a result of antibiotic use for common childhood infections such as earaches (Shaw, 1998)

- Enterocolitis, a unique inflammation due to the presence of the measles virus in the intestinal tract: ileal hyperplasia (McCandless, 2002)

Signs of impaired immunity in children on the autism spectrum may include: cyclic fevers, compulsive behaviors, skin rashes or eczema, impulsivity, aggression, and bowel problems such as diarrhea, constipation, impaction, and/or blood and mucus in stools. There are also anecdotal stories of children with autism who spike a high fever that result in a dramatic increase in awareness as well as communication and social abilities (Blakeslee, 2005). This effect is lost again when the fever subsides. This is thought to relate to differences in the immune system. Immune system dysfunctions are believed to impact brain development or functioning in susceptible individuals.

Immune dysfunction is thought to be a result of the following genetically linked or environmentally acquired ailments:

- Viruses that are present that may or may not be detected according to the symptoms presented (McCandless, 2002)
- Leaky gut (McCandless, 2002)
- Infections treated with antibiotics that over time alter the immune system (Shaw, 1998)
- Genetic predisposition to autoimmune diseases in the family (McCandless, 2002)
- Allergies or sensitivities to foods (Marohn, 2002)

Children on the autism spectrum may show signs of impaired detoxification such as: sensory issues, sleep difficulties, stimming, impulsivity, aggression, compulsive behaviors, night sweats, anxiety, dilated pupils, and lack of speech or pica (ingestion of inedible items). Detoxification abnormalities may be related to a genetically linked susceptibility or an environmentally acquired condition such as the following:

- Methionine cycle abnormalities; part of the body's required sulfation process (James, 2005)
- Methylation may be impaired for some individuals; this is a process by which organic chemicals are made available for various important body functions (Marohn, 2002)
- Glutathione synthesis abnormalities; glutathione naturally rids the body of heavy metals (James, 2005)
- Metallothionein (MT) dysfunction has been seen in some individuals; zinc-copper balance and detoxification of heavy metals are key roles of MT, a protein in the body (McCandless, 2002)
- Oxidative stress is damage caused by build-up of metabolic byproducts often due to glutathione depletion (James, 2005)

Detoxification abnormalities are thought to contribute to the build-up of heavy metals in the tissues including the brains of individuals on the autism spectrum. Symptoms of heavy metal exposure are similar to many of the symptoms of autism spectrum disorders.

Nutritional deficiencies or imbalances are a fourth major biomedical area of concern that families and professionals address. Common symptoms of nutritional abnormalities in children on the autism spectrum may include: underweight or overweight, anxiety, mood swings, sensory issues, lack of speech, stimming, aggression, impulsivity, eye poking, dry hair or skin, and pica (ingestion of inedible items).

Whether nutritional deficiencies and imbalances are a cause of or a result of an autism spectrum disorder is not clear. Nutritional problems can result from malabsorption of nutrients and/or problems with digestion that may be associated with the gastrointestinal, immune, and detoxification problems.

## Some Potential Biomedical Treatments

There continue to be disagreements about biomedical treatment options. This is due the limited published research. And, for various reasons, there is also controversy as to the significance of the research that has been published. This disagreement and controversy then carries over to discussion of biomedical-related interventions. There are a limited number of professionals in Indiana as well as elsewhere who are informed about biomedical theories and treatments. Some may be willing and interested to learn more. Even among those professionals that are using biomedical treatments with patients, there seem to be many differences in knowledge and approaches used.

There is disagreement for example as to which area to begin addressing first; the gastrointestinal issues, the immune dysfunction, the detoxification needs, or the nutritional imbalances. There are different testing protocol used among professionals and also disagreement about how to interpret the testing results. There is a network of doctors that families often access called DAN! practitioners. DAN! is an acronym for Defeat Autism Now! DAN! practitioners may include other medical personal such as nurses, nurse practitioners, and homeopaths, as well as physicians. The Autism Research Institute (ARI) offers a registry of DAN! practitioners who provide biomedical treatments for children and adults with autism spectrum disorders. ARI does not endorse, certify, or guarantee the knowledge or skills of any individual listed. These practitioners are not screened or held to any standard of knowledge or experience. As of January 2008, there are two lists, one for licensed healthcare providers and one for others such as naturopaths and homeopaths that are not required by the laws of their state to have a license. For an individual to be listed they must attend a DAN! Clinician Seminar at least once every two years and sign a statement that he or she conducts their practice following the DAN! philosophy. Further information about the Defeat Autism Now! philosophy and practitioners is available at: http://www.autism.com/dan/index.htm. Many families and practitioners who are successfully pursuing biomedical treatments do belong to a network (such as DAN!), an internet Listserv, or other informal group interested in biomedical approaches for the treatment of individuals with autism spectrum disorders.

Currently, the prevailing thought among doctors is to start biomedical interventions by healing the gut (digestive system). This may include the following:

- Gluten-free/casein-free (gf/cf) diet or possibly the specific carbohydrate diet. The gf/cf diet eliminates most common grains (gluten) and dairy products. This does take some time and effort as these ingredients are often hidden in pre-packaged foods. Attention has to be given to preparing meals that are nutritionally balanced and appealing. This can be hard and time consuming at first.

- Allergy testing is often done to check for allergies to common foods and additives in the diet such as corn, soy, and eggs. Any additional food allergies are also addressed.

- Medication may be considered for acid reflux.

- Bacteria, yeast, or fungal overgrowth, or parasites in the gut is often treated with probiotics, anti-fungal medication, and/or specific antibiotics that may be used for many months or longer.

- Viral inflammation will be treated with an anti-viral medication. Treatment for viruses may take months, a year, or more.

- Digestive enzymes are often considered. There are special formulations of enzymes that a few suppliers offer especially for children with autism spectrum disorders (McCandless, 2002).

- Nutritional, mineral, and vitamin supplements will usually be considered; as with enzymes, there are a number of mail order supplement suppliers that specialize in products for individuals with an autism spectrum disorder (Marohn, 2002).

As the diet, enzymes, and medication heal the gut and the supplements work to treat nutritional deficiencies, the immune system may be helped. There are other, more invasive, or alternative biomedical treatments that are used by some to boost the immune system:

- Transfer factor therapy: molecules produced by white blood cells used to transfer immunity to the recipient (McCandless, 2002)

- IVIG therapy (intravenous immune globulin) is a blood plasma product containing antibodies used to treat immune deficiency (McCandless, 2002)

- Treatment of allergies may consist of traditional treatments or NAET (Nambudripad's allergy elimination techniques) named after the doctor who developed this treatment of healing techniques combining homeopathy, acupuncture, chiropractic, kinesiology, and nutrition (Nambudripad, 1999)

After the gut and immune system are ready, there may be metabolic system treatments considered and introduced. Certain detoxification protocols are most often, but not always, the last phase of biomedical intervention to be implemented. There is continued debate about which detoxification protocol to follow. More caution is followed because not enough is known about the path of heavy metals out of the body and brain when using certain protocols for detoxification of heavy metals.

- Methylcobalamin, which is one type of vitamin B-12, is often used to help activate biochemical pathways related to sulfur detoxification as well as methylation. The common way to administer Methyl B-12 is by subcutaneous injection (Neubrander, 2005).

- Chelation is a treatment to rid the body of heavy metals. In healthy individuals, the kidneys and other organs do this appropriately. There are various substances and programs used to chelate. Information on this is very diverse and somewhat controversial (Green, 2006).

- Intravenous glutathione might be used to treat a glutathione deficiency (McCandless, 2002).

- Metabolic imbalances including oxidative stress may be treated with various supplements, vitamins, minerals, and amino acids (James et. al, 2004).

- Metallothionein defects, in some cases, may be successfully treated with supplements (Marohn, 2002).

More and more families are pursuing alternative treatments for their children. Some who are using biomedical interventions are seeing a lot of positive results despite the limited published double-blind, placebo-controlled research studies on many of these biomedical interventions. There is more anecdotal evidence which continues to grow along with clinical trials that support some of the biomedical treatments for autism spectrum disorders. Though most current clinical trials do not follow the rigorous double-blind, placebo controlled standard, the results are still considered important by many and used as a basis for treatment decisions.

At this time, there are many biomedical treatments in various stages of acceptance and use by families and professionals. However, not everyone sees results with biomedical treatments and there is little available to help predict who might benefit from a particular biomedical intervention. There is disagreement, too, about the significance of side effects and how to proceed if side effects are seen. There is still so much that needs to be learned. This article is merely an introduction to the current biomedical theories of causation and treatment. No endorsement of any theory or treatment should be implied. Not all biomedical theories and treatments related to autism spectrum disorders are represented here. Those interested in learning more are encouraged to do so. The references and resources cited can be used to help gather further information.

## References

Blakslee, S. (2005). Focus narrows in search for autism's cause. *New York Times*, February 8, 2005.

Green, J. (2006). Overview: Detoxification through chelation therapy. *Autism Research Review International, 20,* (1), 3.

James, S.J. (2005). *Pathogenic implications of low glutathione levels and oxidative stress in children with autism: Metabolic biomarkers and genetic predisposition,* Presented 04/05.

James, S.J. et. al. (2004). Metabolic biomarkers of increased oxidative stress and impaired methylation capacity in children with autism. *American Journal of Clinical Nutrition, 80,* p. 1611–7.

Marohn, S. (2002). *The natural medicine guide to autism*. Charlottesville, VA: Hampton Roads Publishing Company.

McCandless, J. (2002). *Children with starving brains: A medical treatment guide for autism spectrum disorders*. North Bergen, NJ: Bramble Books.

Nambudripad, D.S. (1999). *Say good-bye to allergy-related autism*. Buena Park, CA: Delta Publishing Company.

Neubrander, J.A. (2005). *Methyl-B-12: Making it work for you!* Presented 5/29/2005.

Shaw, W. (1998). *Biomedical treatments for autism and POD*. Kansas City, KS: Great Plains Laboratory.

Wheeler, M. (2008). *An introduction to possible biomedical causes and treatments for autism spectrum disorders*. Bloomington, IN: Indiana Resource Center for Autism.

## Section 9.2

# *Vaccines Are Not Associated with ASD*

Excerpted from "Autism Spectrum Disorders: Related Topics,"
Centers for Disease Control and Prevention (CDC), May 13, 2010.

### *Do vaccines cause autism spectrum disorders (ASDs)?*

Many studies have looked at whether there is a relationship between vaccines and autism spectrum disorders (ASDs). To date, the
studies continue to show that vaccines are not associated with ASDs.
However, the Centers for Disease Control and Prevention (CDC) knows
that some parents and others still have concerns. To address these
concerns, CDC is part of the Inter-Agency Autism Coordinating Committee (IACC), which is working with the National Vaccine Advisory
Committee (NVAC) on this issue. The job of the NVAC is to advise
and make recommendations regarding the National Vaccine Program.
Communication between the IACC and NVAC will allow each group to
share skills and knowledge, improve coordination, and promote better
use of research resources on vaccine topics.

### *Is there a link between mitochondrial diseases and ASDs?*

In mitochondrial diseases, the mitochondria cannot efficiently turn
sugar and oxygen into energy, so the cells do not work the way they
should. There are many types of mitochondrial disease, and they can affect different parts of the body: the brain, kidneys, muscles, heart, eyes,
ears, and others. Not everyone with a mitochondrial disease will show
symptoms. However, among the mitochondrial diseases that tend to affect
children, symptoms usually appear in the toddler and preschool years.

A child with an ASD may or may not have a mitochondrial disease.
When children have both an ASD and a mitochondrial disease, they
sometimes have other problems too, including epilepsy, problems with
muscle tone, or movement disorders. More research is needed to find
out how common it is for people to have an ASD and a mitochondrial
disease. Right now, it seems rare. In general, more research about
mitochondrial disease and ASDs is needed.

## Section 9.3

# *Autism, Asthma, Inflammation, and the Hygiene Hypothesis*

Excerpted from "Autism, asthma, inflammation, and the hygiene hypothesis," by Kevin G. Becker. Reprinted from *Medical Hypotheses*, Volume 69, Issue 4, pp 731–40, 2007. Copyright 2007 Elsevier, Ltd. All rights reserved. Reprinted with permission. The complete text of this document including references is available at http://www.grc.nia.nih.gov/branches/rrb/dna/pubs/aaihh.pdf.

## *Introduction*

Autism is an enigmatic childhood disorder of unknown origin. It is characterized by developmental, language, and social deficits, ranging in severity from patients with profound deficits to individuals that are high functioning. Although the underlying etiological basis of autism has eluded researchers, the genetic heritability of autism is quite strong. Specifically what genes are involved and how they contribute to the disease phenotype is unclear.

Many theories regarding the biological basis of autism have been suggested, including neurodevelopmental, exposure to environmental toxins, particularly to mercury, and immune hypotheses. More recently, theories of hyper-systemizing and assortative mating and hyperdopamine have been proposed. At this time there is little definitive evidence to support any single theory of the fundamental biological nature of autism.

Numerous reports have described imbalances in immune and inflammatory processes in autistic patients, including aberrations in antibody levels, cytokines, and cellular subsets. Additionally, recent reports have described an increased frequency of HLA-A2 and HLA-DR4 antigens in autism. Interestingly, epidemiological studies have provided evidence for the association of asthma and allergies or autoimmune disorders in families with autistic children. The exact significance of immune abnormalities and the relationship of infections, immunizations, allergies, inflammation, or other aspects of immune response to disease etiology are unclear and controversial. Alterations of immune and inflammatory processes in autism have recently been reviewed.

One of the challenges in the early study of the molecular basis of classical autoimmune disorders was the attempt to establish the relevance of highly variable and fluctuating immune serum proteins and cell populations to disease etiology. That is, are fluctuations in any set of cytokines, immune mediators, or T cell populations, causative; or, are they epiphenomena due to peripheral effects of target tissue destruction, transient common infections, or more importantly, are they echoes of long ago infections? There is an ever present "which came first, the chicken or the egg" nature in the study of highly variable immune mediators. Are oligoclonal antibody bands found in the cerebrospinal fluid (CSF) of multiple sclerosis patients related to the etiology of the disease; or, are they end stage phenomena? Do alterations in cytokines from a patient with systemic lupus erythematosus have a role in disease etiology; or, are they late stage responses to tissue destruction brought on by other mechanisms? Similarly, are immune aberrations in autism disease causing; or, are they epiphenomena?

## Other Comparisons of Autism to Asthma and Autoimmune/Inflammatory Disorders

In addition to imbalances in immune molecular mediators, there are other seemingly unrelated parallels in the study of immune and inflammatory disorders as compared to autism that, when viewed collectively, may provide additional support for shared aspects of disease etiology between immune and inflammatory disorders and autism. These include: sex bias, birth order, age-of-onset, neonatal head circumference, increasing prevalence in the population, rural versus urban disease comparisons, and shared molecular and genetic markers.

**Disease onset and sex bias:** In asthma and in autism presentation is in early childhood. Both disease types have an age of onset in early childhood; 2–4 years for children with autistic disorder and 3–6 for wheeze and asthma. In addition, both autism and asthma display a skewed sex bias toward boys. This bias is approximately 4:1 boys to girls in autism and approximately 2:1 in asthma. It is well known that in most adult autoimmune and inflammatory disorders, including asthma, there is a predominance of adult women with the diagnosis. However, less well known is that prior to puberty this skewing is toward boys. This male bias prior to puberty may be true in other immune mediated disorders as well such as multiple sclerosis, Type 1 diabetes, and thyroiditis.

**Birth order:** Some studies have shown birth order to be relevant in atopic disorders as well as autism. In both cases, being first born may carry a greater risk for disease than later births. In a large study of 11,371 Italian young men, those with no siblings had the highest level of serum immunoglobulin E (IgE) sensitization. An inverse association was observed between number of siblings at time of testing and prevalence of high atopy P less than 0.0001. Similar findings have been shown for atopic disease in Crete; asthma, eczema-urticaria, and hay fever in Scotland; asthma with allergic rhinitis in Denmark; and, asthma, allergy, and eczema in the Netherlands. These observations are thought to be related to increased transmission of childhood infections due to a growing family size in the context of the hygiene hypothesis. Similarly, the risk of autism has been shown in some cases to be related to birth order in the same direction as asthma and atopic disorders, with risk decreasing with a greater number of older siblings in the United States, Western Australia, and England.

**Increased neonatal head circumference:** Increased neonatal head circumference has been found in both autism and asthma. Increases in neonatal head circumference have been associated with asthma and atopy. In particular, head circumference has been associated with elevated serum IgE levels and hay fever disorders. Increased neonatal head circumference or macrocephaly is a robust finding in autism with the largest effect between the ages of 2–5. This brain size difference is largely back to normal by adolescence. The biological basis for this increase is unknown although genetic, infectious, and inflammatory mechanisms have been proposed.

**Increase in prevalence in the population—parallel epidemics:** Both autism and asthma have had reports of apparent increases in the population over the last 30 years. Numerous studies show general increases in prevalence in both asthma and autism, at roughly similar rates over the last 30 years. In both disease types, this has been often referred to as an epidemic. In both disease types, this apparent increase is controversial. Changes in diagnostic classifications and access to health care resources have confounded the interpretation of prevalence estimates in the study of asthma and autism. Significant increases in disease prevalence over a short time in evolutionary terms suggest that purely genetic mechanisms may not be solely responsible. Given the strong heritability of autism, changing environmental modifiers in the context of the background genetics of autism may be important over the past 30 years. There have been similar increases in the prevalence in classical autoimmune diseases over the same time span as well, including Type 1 diabetes.

**Rural versus urban disease distribution:** Both autism and asthma appear to show uneven geographical distributions in disease prevalence. Differential susceptibility or resistance to asthma and allergies is found in urban environments versus rural or farm environments. Although the exact mechanistic basis of the difference is not known, this distribution pattern of disease is thought to have an inverse relationship to infection and is central to the hygiene hypothesis.

The geographical distribution of autism is less clear although there is evidence that there may be an urban versus rural distribution. This has been found in epidemiological studies from multiple countries including Denmark, the United States (US), England, and Japan. Interestingly, in studies of autism that analyzed numerous familial risk factors, a major risk factor for autism was increasing degree of urbanization. In a study from the US, the urban versus rural distribution was attributable to mercury exposure in the environment; however, this may reflect an industrialized versus rural pattern as well.

The Inuit of northern Canada may provide an interesting population case study. This isolated rural population exists in crowded living conditions, with high levels of mercury and other environmental toxins in the diet. However, autism is essentially non-existent in the Inuit. In a recent report, Fombonne et al. state that no case of autism has ever been reported in an Inuit child in the past 15 years. In parallel, asthma and atopic disorders are uncommon in Inuit children, even with very high rates of lower respiratory infections prior to age two and particularly high rates of childhood smoking (31.9%).

**Molecular and genetic markers shared with inflammatory/ autoimmune diseases:** Like many common human disorders, autism, asthma, and autoimmune disorders have been studied using genetic linkage and genetic association approaches. The chromosomal regions identified in linkage studies and the specific variants of genes identified in genetic association studies are quite often not unique to any one disorder. Many, if not most, genes in the human genome have broad-based effects influencing different cells and tissues at different times of development under the influence of different environmental modifiers. In the context of common human disease, important regulatory genes may affect disease susceptibility differently when found in combination with different disease associated alleles.

**ADRB2, beta(2)-adrenergic receptor:** The gene for the beta(2)-adrenergic receptor encodes a member of the G protein-coupled receptor superfamily and is expressed on epithelial and endothelial cells of the lung, mast cells, as well as airway smooth muscle cells. ADRB2 activation is thought to work through increased intracellular cAMP levels. Polymorphisms in ADRB2, including the Glu27 allele, have been studied in multiple disease states including hypertension, atopic dermatitis, Grave disease, rheumatoid arthritis, obesity, and in particular, asthma. ADRB2 is of major interest in asthma as it may be involved in lung function as well as response to beta(2)-adrenergic agonists. ADRB2 polymorphisms may not influence asthma incidence or prevalence but may influence persistence of asthmatic symptoms. Importantly, the Glu27 allele of ADRB2 has recently been associated with autism in twins as well as in the AGRE autism cohort.

**PTEN-phosphatase and tensin homolog:** PTEN, phosphatase and tensin homolog, is central to phosphoinositide metabolism as an important autism, asthma, inflammation, and the hygiene hypothesis 3 regulatory checkpoint in the PI3K/ATK signaling pathway, effecting multiple downstream processes including immune function, cell growth, cell survival, and differentiation. PTEN has been shown to play a role in lymphocyte proliferation, systemic autoimmunity, and autoimmune disease, as well as in benign tumors of the gastrointestinal tract. In relation to disease, PTEN has been implicated in bronchial asthma and allergic inflammation.

Interestingly, PTEN has been implicated in macrocephaly (OMIM #153480) and Cowden disease (OMIM #158350). PTEN has been implicated in autism as well, in particular, within a subset of autistic individuals with macrocephaly. A recent report described a patient with a PTEN mutation having autistic features, macrocephaly as well as nodular lymphoid hyperplasia of the small and large intestinal mucosa. Moreover, a mouse model with specific deletions of PTEN in selected neuronal cell types resulted in macrocephaly, changes in social interactions, and increased responses to sensory stimuli, suggesting a model for autistic spectrum disorder.

**MET (met proto-oncogene):** The proto-oncogene MET, also known as hepatocyte growth factor receptor, encodes a tyrosine kinase receptor which has been shown to have pleiotropic effects, in myocardial infarction, ischemia, angiogenesis, and importantly in cancer progression. Recently, polymorphic variants that result in reduced expression of MET have been genetically associated with autism. MET also has been shown to effect the immune system, in particular it suppresses immune dendritic cell function. In addition, c-MET and its ligand HGF have been shown to be involved in multiple neuronal processes including synaptic plasticity in the hippocampus, development of cortical pyramidal dendrites, and synaptic organization.

**Genome wide scans:** Genome wide scans are genetic linkage studies that use evenly spaced polymorphic markers that span the entire human genome in an attempt to link disease phenotypes to specific regions in the human genome. In a comparison of genome wide linkage studies between autoimmune and inflammatory disorders and similar studies in autism and Tourette syndrome, overlap of polymorphic markers were found to be statistically significant (P = 0.01) in chromosomal regions originally independently identified in autism and Tourette syndrome, or in autoimmune and inflammatory disorders (http://www.grc.nia.nih.gov/branches/rrb/dna/pubs/cgoatad. pdf). This comparison was performed using the approach originally taken for autoimmune disorders. A more comprehensive listing of marker overlap between autoimmune/inflammatory disorders and autism and Tourette syndrome can be found online at http://www.grc. nia.nih.gov/branches/rrb/dna/atsmap.htm. Moreover, a subset of these markers found to be statistically significant in both disease classes is not due to simple coincidental overlap of genetic regions, but includes 144 identical polymorphic markers originally found to be statistically significant in both autism and autoimmune or inflammatory disorders, including asthma. For example, in the chromosomal region 17q25.3, the polymorphic marker D17S784 has been independently linked to psoriasis, Crohn disease, Tourette syndrome, and autism. A listing of markers independently found in both disease classes can be found online at https://www.quickbase.com/db/8qsiujvy.

## Summary of Disease Comparisons

The epidemiological, morphometric, molecular, and genetic comparisons between autism and inflammatory disorders highlight multiple lines of evidence in addition to humoral and cellular immune abnormalities with the goal to strengthen an etiological relationship between autism and autoimmune and inflammatory disorders. It is not suggested that these comparisons support any direct link between these disorders. However, these shared observations between autism and inflammatory disorders are used in support of the development of a hypothesis for the apparent rise in the prevalence of autism using the framework of the immune hygiene hypotheses.

## The Hygiene Hypothesis

The hygiene hypothesis is a widely held theory of the etiology of asthma and atopic disorders which builds on observations of rural versus urban distribution of disease. It suggests that cleaner environmental conditions in westernized countries, as compared to developing countries, play a role in the increase of the prevalence of these disorders in western countries. Moreover, low levels of asthma and allergies are found with early exposure to cats, being raised in a farm environment, larger family size, day-care attendance, and birth order.

Risk for asthma and atopy may be due to a lack of early immune challenge of the post-natal immune system by microbial or parasitic infection possibly including environmental saprophytes and gut commensal organisms, relative to the developing innate immune system. Alteration in the immune repertoire early in thymic development may lead to the establishment of immune hypersensitivity ultimately leading to inflammatory pathology.

In certain ways, the hygiene hypothesis is counterintuitive, in that less clean polluted environments were once thought to cause asthma. Moreover, it is common practice in western society to protect children from bacteria and microorganisms through isolation indoors and through overuse of antibacterial soaps. This practice may be harmful in not allowing robust immune challenge in early neonatal development. The hygiene hypothesis is not without criticism. The changes in the prevalence of atopic disorders may have more complex etiologies with regard to overall microbial load or helminth infection in the general population rather than with simple notions of personal or community hygiene practices.

### Autism and the Hygiene Hypothesis

As compared, similarities between autism, asthma, and inflammatory disorders raise the possibilities of shared mechanisms between these disease types. These include altered immune function in both types of disorders, a similar sex bias at diagnosis, similar birth order relationships, unexplained increased neonatal head circumference, a similar increase in prevalence rates during the last quarter century, a possible rural-urban distribution of the diagnosis with disease being more prevalent in urban environments, and shared molecular and genetic factors between autism and asthma. This adds multiple lines of evidence that mechanisms important in the etiology of immune and inflammatory processes may contribute to the etiology of autism.

It is proposed here that the hygiene hypothesis, a viable theory in the etiology of asthma, should be considered in the etiology of autism. Underlying factors important in the hygiene hypothesis, whether they are truly related to hygiene practices or to overall microbial or parasitic load, thought to be relevant to the increase in asthma and atopy, may contribute to the rise in the incidence of autism as well. Altered patterns of infant immune stimulation may hypersensitize the early immune system not toward allergic sensitivity and bronchial hypersensitivity but to inflammatory or cytokine responses affecting brain structure and function leading to autism. It is well documented that immune cytokines play an important role in normal brain development as well as pathological injury in early brain development. It is hypothesized that immune pathways altered by hygiene practices in western society may effect brain structure or function contributing to the development of autism.

## Section 9.4

## *Autism and Fragile X Syndrome Feature Immune Signatures*

This section includes text from "Autism and fragile X feature immune signatures," by Kelly Rae Chi," © 2010 Simons Foundation Autism Research Initiative (SFARI). Reprinted with permission.

**Signs of immunity:** Cytokines, molecular soldiers in the body's war against infection, seem to be improperly regulated in people with autism and fragile X syndrome.

Scientists have identified distinct blood signatures of cytokines—proteins that control communication between cells of the immune system—in individuals with developmental disorders. The study is the first to report cytokine profiles in people with fragile X syndrome, the most common single-gene cause of autism. The type and the number of cytokines vary depending on whether an individual is healthy, has fragile X syndrome, or has both fragile X syndrome and autism, the study found.[1]

The results, published January 25, 2010 in *Brain, Behavior, and Immunity*, add to research showing that certain cytokines are elevated, and others depleted, in people with autism.[2] Although scientists don't know yet if cytokine patterns could reliably predict fragile X or autism—in part because they measure cytokine levels in the blood and not in the brain—the study adds heft to a long-standing hypothesis that the immune system goes awry in both disorders. "The findings suggest that the immunological background of patients with fragile X and autism versus controls may be very different," says Carlos Pardo-Villamizar, associate professor of neurobiology and pathology at Johns Hopkins University, who was not involved in the study. Because the body's immune responses are known to affect thought and behavior, the cytokines may contribute to features of autism.

Several lines of evidence suggest a link between the immune system and autism. For instance, some individuals with the disorder have fewer total antibodies than do healthy controls. The lower the levels of some antibodies such as immunoglobulin G, the more severe are particular symptoms, such as irritability, repetitive behaviors, and hyperactivity.[3]

So far, no clear-cut cytokine patterns have emerged in individuals with autism. That is partly because studies have examined different tissues, such as blood, brain, and cerebrospinal fluid—the nutrient-rich solution that bathes the brain and spinal nerves—in individuals of different ages and with varying symptom severity. For instance, compared with healthy individuals, the cytokine transforming growth factor-$\beta$ is lower in the blood,[4] but higher in cerebrospinal fluid and brain tissue of people with the disorder.[5]

The immune system has also been implicated in fragile X syndrome, a disorder caused by mutations in the fragile X mental retardation 1 (FMR1) gene. Children with fragile X syndrome tend to get infections more easily than do healthy peers, according to some reports.[6] Anecdotal reports also attest that children with fragile X have recurring gastrointestinal woes, such as loose stools, which could arise if immune molecules in the gut are reacting to certain types of foods.

Problems with brain development and function in autism spectrum disorders may result from improper activation of T-cells, which secrete cytokines, according to a paper on Rett syndrome published in the April 2010 issue of *Molecular Psychiatry*.[7] Therapies that boost the immune system might address some of these anomalies, the researchers suggest.

The new study on fragile X is one of the first to look for molecular irregularities of the immune system in people with the syndrome. Scientists from the University of California, Davis, measured blood-plasma cytokines in 40 boys and men with fragile X syndrome and autism, 64 with fragile X syndrome alone and 19 healthy controls. A half-dozen of these molecules differ between the groups, the scientists found. For example, cytokines interleukin-1 and interleukin-12 show up in larger quantities in people with both fragile X and autism compared with those who have fragile X alone, and these proteins are higher in both groups than in controls.

Researchers should measure these cytokines not only in blood, but in brain tissue and cerebrospinal fluid, Pardo-Villamizar says. Because only some cytokines cross the barrier between blood and brain, and because the molecules have vastly different roles in each tissue, blood measures do not necessarily reflect neurodevelopment. "As a study of biomarkers, the findings are very interesting, and they are relevant for the neurobiology of the disease," Pardo-Villamizar says. "But I don't think that we can extrapolate all these findings to [cytokines in] the brain of these patients."

## *Spotlight on Interleukin-6 (IL-6)*

Researchers don't yet understand the pathological or behavioral consequences of these differences in cytokine levels. "There is really a dysregulation of these cytokines [in fragile X syndrome]," says investigator Flora Tassone, a full research biochemist at the University of California, Davis. "Now that there is a hint that something is going on, maybe people will start to look in more detail."

Much of the previous work on cytokines in autism focused on tumor necrosis factor-$\alpha$ (TNF-$\alpha$) and interleukin-6 (IL-6), which are elevated in the brains of people with autism spectrum disorders compared with controls. Both cytokines can directly influence the ability of neurons to change the strength of their connections, a basic mechanism of learning, memory, and neural development.[8]

In 2001, researchers collecting peripheral blood mononuclear cells, a type of immune cell, from 71 children with autism found that these cells produce excessive cytokines—such as TNF-$\alpha$, IL-6, and interleukin-1$\beta$, which are associated with innate immunity—compared with controls.[9] A subsequent report of 13 children with autism and 13 healthy controls also found elevated IL-6 and TNF-$\alpha$ in the blood of children with autism compared with controls, but the difference was not statistically significant.[10]

The new study found that IL-6 levels do not differ significantly between people with fragile X syndrome—with or without autism—and controls. But that doesn't mean the molecule is not important in autism. Comparing the new findings with those of people with classic autism is inappropriate because mutations in functional magnetic resonance imaging (fMRI) affect the transcription of hundreds of other genes, notes Paul Patterson, professor of biology at California Institute of Technology in Pasadena, who has done much of the work on IL-6 and autism. "The mutation that causes fragile X—we don't know what it does to the immune system," he adds. "So you can't necessarily extrapolate from autism to fragile X with autism."

In 2007, Patterson's team found that activating the immune system of pregnant mice produces offspring with autism-like behaviors, such as an unwillingness to explore open areas, in adulthood.[11] These behaviors improve when the offspring receive an injection of an antibody that inhibits IL-6, suggesting that the cytokine is critical for proper brain development. Tassone's group plans to expand the study's sample size and include a group of children with classic autism. They have already collected about 20 blood samples from two- to five-year-old children with the disorder.

The researchers found differences in cytokine levels in the children with autism, she says, but decided not to report them because the group's age varies drastically from that of controls. The healthy participants in the study are 15 years old, on average, but range from toddlers to adults. This wide age span is typical in human studies, and may be problematic because cytokine levels change with age. "Observational studies that are done in patients who are already out of neurodevelopmental stages are difficult to interpret," Pardo-Villamizar says. "In the future, the studies need to concentrate more on the first two or three years of age, when the brain is still undergoing development."

## *References*

1.   Ashwood P. et al. Brain Behav. *Immun.* Epub ahead of print (2010) PubMed.

2.   Goines P. and J. Van de Water Curr. Opin. *Neurol. 23*, 111–117 (2010) PubMed.

3.   Heuer L. et al. *Autism Res. 1*, 275–283 (2008) PubMed.

4.   Ashwood P. et al. *J. Neuroimmunol. 204*, 149–153 (2008) PubMed.

5.   Vargas D.L. et al. *Ann. Neurol. 57*, 67–81 (2005) PubMed.

6.   Hagerman R.J. et al. *Am. J. Dis. Child. 141*, 184–187 (1987) PubMed.

7.   Derecki N.C. et al. *Mol. Psychiatry* Epub ahead of print (2010) PubMed.

8.   Tonelli L.H. and T.T. Postolache *Neurol. Res. 27*, 67–84 (2005) PubMed.

9.   Jyonouchi H. et al. *J. Neuroimmunol. 120*, 170–179 (2001) PubMed.

10. Croonenberghs J. et al. *Neuropsychobiology 45*, 1–6 (2002) PubMed.

11. Smith S.E. et al. *J. Neurosci. 27*, 10695–10702 (2007) PubMed.

# Chapter 10

# *Premature Birth and Autism*

**Distinct syndrome:** Babies born early show developmental problems, but may also have symptoms, such as a small head, that aren't indicative of autism.

The proposed connection between premature birth and autism may be more complicated than it seems, according to a report published online January 5, 2010 in the *Journal of Pediatrics*.[1] Early birth may not cause classically defined autism but, rather, may predispose children to autism-like symptoms that are part of a larger syndrome, the researchers say. "When you come to a diagnosis of autism spectrum disorder in this population, you have to think very hard, actually, 'Is it the same condition?'" says lead investigator Neil Marlow, professor of neonatal medicine at University College London.

In the new study, Marlow and colleagues relied on clinical information and parental questionnaires and interviews to show that children born before 26 weeks gestation are more likely to have autistic traits at age 11 than are their classmates born at, or near, term. These findings echo several other studies completed over the past few years. But Marlow points out that research looking at brain development and other traits in this subset of children suggests a distinct phenotype. For instance, although past research has tied autism with increased head size, Marlow's new study found that premature children with the

This chapter includes text from "Studies challenge link between premature birth and autism," by Andrea Anderson, © 2010 Simons Foundation Autism Research Initiative (SFARI). Reprinted with permission.

smallest head sizes at 2.5 years old tend to have the most pronounced autistic symptoms. Although preterm males are still more likely to show autistic symptoms than females, the gender ratio for prevalence tends to be more balanced, hovering around 2:1 as compared with 4:1 for typical autism.[2]

Premature children also seem to be at higher risk of brain injury because of their early birth, which could potentially contribute to some autistic symptoms. "It's a really, really tricky area," Marlow says. For at least a decade, scientists have explored the connections between preterm birth or very low birth weight and neurodevelopmental,[3] academic,[4] social,[5] and cognitive and behavioral problems. [6,7,8] For instance, low birth weight individuals are less likely to finish high school than are peers born at normal weight.[4] Parents of children born between the 22nd and 32nd weeks of pregnancy report more hyperactivity, inattention, and other behavioral problems than do parents of those born at or near term.[8]

Studies over the past couple of years have shown that preterm babies are up to three times more likely to develop autistic traits in early childhood than are babies born at term. Researchers don't know how many of these children will go on to be formally diagnosed with the disorder, but some say that preterm birth could be a significant risk factor. "Being born preterm at least appears to be a larger risk than any others identified at this point," with the exception of specific genetic causes and syndromes, which are thought to cause up to 20% of autism cases, notes Karl Kuban, chief of Boston Medical Center's pediatric neurology division.

It is difficult to unravel whether premature birth is in and of itself a risk factor for autism, or whether other factors predispose to both preterm birth and autism. Because most experts believe the disorder develops in the first half of pregnancy, autism risk probably isn't just a consequence of being born early, Kuban argues. More likely, he says, it involves a combination of environmental and unrecognized genetic risk factors affecting the brain.

## Tricky Diagnoses

Understanding developmental consequences of preterm birth will only get more pressing in the years to come. Premature births are on the rise in the United States, growing from 9.5% in 1981 to 12.7% in 2007. Because of improved medical technology and infant care, babies can now survive birth as early as the 22nd week of pregnancy. "Today we have the sickest, smallest survivors," notes Catherine Limperopoulos, assistant professor of neurology and neurosurgery at McGill University and research associate in neurology at Harvard University.

In the first study looking specifically at early signs of autism in toddlers born very early in 2008, Limperopoulos and her colleagues studied two-year-old children born between 23 and 30 weeks gestation and weighing less than three pounds, three ounces.[9] The researchers screened 91 children for early indicators of autism using a parental questionnaire called the *Modified Checklist for Autism in Toddlers*, or M-CHAT, designed to identify children at elevated risk of developing autism spectrum disorders. The team found that 25% of the preterm children screened positive, compared with known rates of 5%–6% of children in the general population. That study showed that premature children tend to have so-called internalizing behavior, such as being socially withdrawn or suffering from anxiety or depression.

Kuban reported similar findings last April, in a study of 988 children born before the 28th week of pregnancy.[10] He and colleagues in the *Extremely Low Gestational Age Newborns (ELGAN) Study* group found that more than 21% of these premature babies tested positive on the M-CHAT at two years old.

The M-CHAT is quite sensitive, identifying most children at risk of autism. But, it also gives many false positives: only about one-tenth of the children who screen positive go on to be diagnosed with an autism spectrum disorder. Consequently, researchers say it's unlikely that most preterm children who test positive for early autism symptoms will go on to have a formal diagnosis of autism. "I do feel that these reports are somewhat preliminary," Limperopoulos says. The M-CHAT was designed to screen children in the general population and relates to a child's developmental state. Consequently, conditions such as cerebral palsy, vision and hearing problems, or low intelligence quotients—all more common in preterm children than in children in the general population—could muddle M-CHAT scores.

## Brain Trajectories

Still, after accounting for motor, visual, and hearing deficits, the ELGAN study found that 16% of preterm children still tested positive on the M-CHAT screen—almost three times the rate observed in the general population. "What's critical in all of these studies are the diagnostic follow-up tests," Limperopoulos says. She and her colleagues are completing follow-up testing for autism in preterm children around five years old who screened positive on M-CHAT when they were younger.

Researchers from the ELGAN study are also following children in their own preterm cohort and plan to look for autism and other outcomes when the children are nine years old. Prospective studies of autistic traits in children born early are consistent with previous epidemiological studies identifying risk factors—such as birth weight and gestational age and health complications at birth[11,12,13]—among children diagnosed with autism spectrum disorders. Despite the many studies hinting at links between autism and early birth, the biology underlying this apparent connection is unclear. Researchers don't know, for instance, whether the cause of the autistic symptoms also happens to increase the likelihood of preterm birth, or whether complications that typically come with preterm birth—such as the incomplete development of the brain and other organs—cause babies to develop autism. To explore such questions, researchers are taking a closer look at the brains of infants born early.

Limperopoulos and her team found that one-third of preterm children who test positive on M-CHAT have abnormal brain scan results—such as tissue loss or bleeding in the brain—when they are around ten months old. The researchers are investigating how injury to the cerebellum, a brain region involved in coordination, motor control, and some learning-related functions, might relate to autism risk in premature babies.

Others have also detected injury or impaired growth in brain scans of preterm children, particularly affecting the brain's white matter, the insulated nerve fibers that transmit messages between brain cells.[14,15,16,17] The ELGAN group proposes brain-imaging studies to look for potential white matter volume and white matter connectivity differences in their cohort of preterm children.

## References

1. Johnson S. et al. *J. Pediatr.* Epub ahead of print (2010) PubMed.

2. Schendel D. and T.K. *Bhasin Pediatrics 121*, 1155–1164 (2008) PubMed.

3. Johnson S. et al. *Pediatrics 124*, 249–257 (2009) PubMed.

4. Hack M. et al. *N. Engl. J. Med. 346*, 149–157 (2002) PubMed.

5. Dahl L.B. et al. *Pediatrics 118*, 449–459 (2006) PubMed.

6. Bhutta A.T. et al. *JAMA 288*, 728–737 (2002) PubMed.

7. Delobel-Ayoub M. et al. *Pediatrics 117*, 1996–2005 (2006) PubMed.

8. Delobel-Ayoub M. et al. *Pediatrics 123*, 1485–1492 (2009) PubMed.

9. Limperopoulos C. et al. *Pediatrics 121*, 758–765 (2008) PubMed.

10. Kuban K.C. et al. *J. Pediatr. 154*, 535–540 (2009) PubMed.

11. Larsson H.J. et al. *Am. J. Epidemiol. 161*, 916–925 (2005) PubMed.

12. Schendel D. and T.K. Bhasin *Pediatrics 121*, 1155–1164 (2008) PubMed.

13. Buchmayer S. et al. *Pediatrics 124*, 817–825 (2009) PubMed.

14. Kuban K., et al. *J. Pediatr. 134*, 539–546 (1999) PubMed.

15. O'Shea T.M. et al. *Early Hum. Dev. 85*, 719–725 (2009) PubMed.

16. Limperopoulos C. *Clin. Perinatol. 36*, 791–805 (2009) PubMed.

17. Dammann O. et al. *Neonatology 97*, 71–82 (2010) PubMed.

# Chapter 11

# *Early Development Risk Factors for ASD*

The Study to Explore Early Development (SEED) is a multi-year study funded by Centers for Disease Control and Prevention (CDC). It is currently the largest study in the United States to help identify factors that may put children at risk for autism spectrum disorders (ASDs) and other developmental disabilities. SEED is looking at three main areas:

- **Physical and behavioral characteristics of children with ASDs, children with other developmental disabilities, and children without a developmental delay or disability**: We want to learn more about why people with ASD are the way they are—how they behave, grow, think, and interact with the world around them.

- **Health conditions among children with and without ASDs:** SEED provides an opportunity to compare health conditions and health-related issues such as sleeping and eating patterns in children with ASD, in children with other developmental disabilities, and in children without a developmental delay or disability.

- **Factors associated with a child's risk for developing ASDs:** We hope that SEED will give us a better idea which of the many possible risk factors that we will be evaluating seem

Text in this chapter is excerpted from "Study to Explore Early Development (SEED)," and "SEED Frequently Asked Questions," Centers for Disease Control and Prevention (CDC), May 13, 2010.

to be associated with or related to ASDs. The risk factors may be related to genes, health conditions, experiences of the mother during pregnancy, and the health and development of the child during infancy and the first few years of life.

### Why are we looking at other developmental disabilities?

By comparing children with autism and children with other developmental disabilities, we will have a better sense of whether the physical traits, health conditions, and risk factors we find among children with autism are unique to autism or if they also are found among children with other developmental problems.

### How many children will be enrolled in SEED?

We plan to enroll 2,700 children. At each of the six Centers for Autism and Developmental Disabilities Research and Epidemiology (CADDRE) SEED sites, we plan to enroll 150 children in each of three groups: children with autism, children with other developmental problems, and children from the community whom are assumed to be developing normally. Children 2–5 years of age will be asked to take part in SEED.

### Why are we looking only at children 2–5 years of age?

The study is limited to this age group because we want to study the early development of children with and without autism. Also, children in this age group will be more likely to be near the beginning of treatment if they are already participating in developmental intervention programs. Finally, we are focusing on children who were born in and still reside in certain areas.

### When the study is done, will we know the causes of autism?

It is too soon to know that. The goal of the study is to give us a better idea of which risk factors seem to be important in causing autism. The causes might be related to genes, the environment, or both.

### Will this study find a way to prevent or cure autism?

At this time, we can't answer this question. But, we hope that the findings from SEED will lead to future studies specifically designed to test treatments among children with autism.

# Part Three

# Identifying and Diagnosing Autism Spectrum Disorders

# Chapter 12

# *Symptoms of ASD*

## *Chapter Contents*

## Section 12.1

# *Range of Symptoms*

Excerpted from "Signs and Symptoms, Autism Spectrum Disorders," Centers for Disease Control and Prevention (CDC), May 13, 2010.

Autism spectrum disorders (ASDs) affect each person in different ways and can range from very mild to severe. People with ASDs share some similar symptoms, such as problems with social interaction. But, there are differences in when the symptoms start, how severe they are, and the exact nature of the symptoms.

ASDs begin before the age of three and last throughout a person's life, although symptoms may improve over time. Some children with an ASD show hints of future problems within the first few months of life. In others, symptoms may not show up until 24 months or later. Some children with an ASD seem to develop normally until around 18 to 24 months of age and then they stop gaining new skills, or they lose the skills they once had. Studies have shown that one-third to half of parents of children with an ASD noticed a problem before their child's first birthday, and nearly 80%–90% saw problems by 24 months of age.

It is important to note that some people without an ASD might also have some of these symptoms. But, for people with an ASD, the impairments make life very challenging.

### Possible Red Flags

A person with an ASD might do the following:

- Not respond to their name by 12 months of age
- Not point at objects to show interest (point at an airplane flying over) by 14 months
- Not play pretend games (pretend to feed a doll) by 18 months
- Avoid eye contact and want to be alone
- Have trouble understanding other people's feelings or talking about their own feelings
- Have delayed speech and language skills

- Repeat words or phrases over and over (echolalia)
- Give unrelated answers to questions
- Get upset by minor changes
- Have obsessive interests
- Flap their hands, rock their body, or spin in circles
- Have unusual reactions to the way things sound, smell, taste, look, or feel

## Social Skills

Social issues are one of the most common symptoms in all of the types of ASD. People with an ASD do not have just social difficulties like shyness. The social issues they have cause serious problems in everyday life. Examples of social issues related to ASDs include these:

- Does not respond to name by 12 months of age
- Avoids eye-contact
- Prefers to play alone
- Does not share interests with others
- Only interacts to achieve a desired goal
- Has flat or inappropriate facial expressions
- Does not understand personal space boundaries
- Avoids or resists physical contact
- Is not comforted by others during distress
- Has trouble understanding other people's feelings or talking about own feelings

## Communication

Each person with an ASD has different communication skills. Some people can speak well. Others cannot speak at all or only very little. About 40% of children with an ASD do not talk at all. About 25%–30% of children with an ASD have some words at 12 to 18 months of age and then lose them. Others might speak, but not until later in childhood. Examples of communication issues related to ASDs include the following:

107

- Delayed speech and language skills
- Repeats words or phrases over and over (echolalia)
- Reverses pronouns (says me instead of I)
- Gives unrelated answers to questions
- Does not point or respond to pointing
- Uses few or no gestures (does not wave goodbye)
- Talks in a flat, robot-like, or sing-song voice
- Does not pretend in play (does not pretend to feed a doll)
- Does not understand jokes, sarcasm, or teasing

## Unusual Interests and Behaviors

Many people with an ASD have unusual interests or behaviors.

- Lines up toys or other objects
- Plays with toys the same way every time
- Likes parts of objects (wheels)
- Is very organized
- Gets upset by minor changes to normal daily patterns
- Has obsessive interests
- Has to follow certain routines
- Flaps hands, rocks body, or spins self in circles

Repetitive motions are actions repeated over and over again. They might repeatedly turn a light on and off or spin the wheels of a toy car. These types of activities are known as self-stimulation or stimming.

## Other Symptoms

Some people with an ASD have other symptoms. These might include the following:

- Hyperactivity (very active)
- Impulsivity (acting without thinking)
- Short attention span
- Aggression

- Causing self-injury
- Temper tantrums
- Unusual eating and sleeping habits
- Unusual mood or emotional reactions
- Lack of fear or more fear than expected
- Unusual reactions to the way things sound, smell, taste, look, or feel

## Development

Children with an ASD develop at different rates in different areas. They may have delays in language, social, and learning skills, while their ability to walk and move around are about the same as other children their age. They might be very good at putting puzzles together or solving computer problems, but they might have trouble with social activities like talking or making friends. Children with an ASD might also learn a hard skill before they learn an easy one. For example, a child might be able to read long words but not be able to tell you what sound a "b" makes.

## Section 12.2

# *Autism Symptoms Emerge in Infancy*

This section includes text from "Autism symptoms emerge in infancy, sibling study finds," by Sandeep Ravindran, © 2010 Simons Foundation Autism Research Initiative (SFARI). Reprinted with permission.

**Warning sign:** At 12 months of age, infants who are eventually diagnosed with autism look less often at faces than do typically developing controls.

At six months of age, babies who will later develop autism begin to lose some of their social skills and continue to regress until age three, according to a study published in March 2010 in the *Journal of the American Academy of Child & Adolescent Psychiatry*.[1] Unexpectedly, most parents do not notice this decline, suggesting that it happens gradually and without easily detectable dramatic changes. "The results really, really surprised us," says lead investigator Sally Ozonoff, professor of psychiatry at the University of California, Davis M.I.N.D. Institute.

The study highlights the need for better screening methods to identify children at risk for the disorder as early as possible, the researchers note. "We don't have any screeners right now that are useful for the 6- to 12-month period," says Sally Rogers, professor of psychiatry at the University of California, Davis M.I.N.D. Institute. Based on the findings of their study, the researchers are developing new screening tools.

The American Pediatric Association recommends that clinicians screen children for autism twice by age two. Given the new findings, these guidelines may need to be revised, Rogers adds. "It may really be that we're going to have to be recommending repeated screenings, maybe at every well-baby checkup, across the infant and preschool period if we really want to identify everybody."

Rogers' team followed younger siblings of children with autism from six months to three years of age. Many studies in the past few years have focused on these so-called baby sibs, who are ten to twenty times as likely to develop the disorder as are those without a family history, experts say.

None of these previous studies—which focused mostly on language, motor and sensory skills—found signs of autism in children younger than six months.[2,3] The same trend holds in the new study, the first to delve more thoroughly into baby sibs' social behaviors. Researchers compared 25 children who would later be diagnosed with autism with 25 healthy controls. Every three months, the scientists evaluated the children on a variety of measures, such as their ability to utter sounds, words or phrases, how often their gaze is directed either at faces or at objects, and how often they smile or laugh.

At six months, children who go on to develop autism score no differently than do controls. "This was the most important finding that we had, and the biggest surprise to us," Rogers says. "We were sure that we would be able to detect decreased social interaction, decreased social interest, and decreased eye contact in babies who were going to develop the behaviors of autism—and we could not find that."

## Direct Measures

The researchers did not detect differences between the two groups until the babies reached 12 months. At that age, baby sibs who go on to develop autism begin to spend less time looking at faces or vocalizing while doing so than do healthy baby sibs. By 18 months, baby sibs who develop autism show a similar decrease in the amount of time they spend smiling while looking at faces. As they get older, this group of children continues to lose skills and social behaviors.

This study is important because it is one of the first prospective studies to look for early onset of autism, notes Ami Klin, director of the Autism Program at Yale Child Study Center. Until recently, researchers relied either on retrospective reports or indirect measures, such as movies made by parents, when looking for early signs of autism. "This is a great advancement, in that people are now observing children directly," Klin says.

Still, he adds that the researchers' conclusions are a bit premature. "This study utilized basically brief observational measures of children obtained in a very constrained environment," he says. More sophisticated and quantifiable measures of behavior that appear early in development could help detect autism even earlier than six months, he says. For example, even two-day-old healthy infants show a preference for animated depictions of human motion compared with other animations. Klin's studies have shown that two-year old children with autism show no such preference.[4]

Other experts say they have qualms about the way the researchers measured and analyzed baby behaviors. Researchers at two sites videotaped the infants while they interacted with adults. For the final analyses, the researchers pooled observational data from both sites. Because some families missed visits and some video clips were unusable, however, the two sites evaluated a different number of infants in each age group.

The lack of a tightly controlled observational setting and the particular statistical analyses used make the data difficult to interpret, notes Mayada Elsabbagh, coordinator of the British Autism Study of Infant Siblings. "The findings may be robust as group data, but we need to be careful with how valid such measures are in individual children," she says.

## Regressive Debate

The findings about regression are somewhat more controversial. Researchers had previously hypothesized that there are two kinds of autism: one in which symptoms appear early and become more pronounced with age, and another in which children develop normally and then gradually lose skills.[5] But not all reports agree with the idea of a regressive autism phenotype. For example, a study that analyzed the brain waves of children with autism during sleep found epilepsy-like readings in 14% of children who had undergone regression, as opposed to 6% of children with early-onset autism.[6] A subsequent study, however, found no difference in brain activity between the two groups.[7]

The new study found that 86.4% of the infants who later develop autism show a clear decline in social communication. This differs from previous reports, based on which the researchers expected to see regression in only a small proportion of the children. "When the babies came in before 12 months, parents would say, 'I'm so happy to be sharing my normal baby with you'," Rogers says. "But then in the next year, that baby developed autism, which was just devastating." Parents noticed this regression in only four out of 19 cases, however. "It was very surprising. It's one of the most interesting things we've learned in these seven years of study," Rogers says.

Rogers previously reported that parents can detect early signs of autism by the time their children are 12 months old.[8] Taken with the new results, this suggests that children with autism lose social skills slowly over the first year. The decline is so subtle and gradual that parents don't notice it, the researchers suggest. Early-onset and regressive autism are probably part of the same continuum, says Rogers, adding that the timing of autism's onset may be random, with no bearing on the disorder's severity. She compares it to an infant catching a cold for the first time: "You're going to get a cold, and it probably doesn't mean anything whether it's at six months or at fifteen months."

Researchers will need more intensive follow-up studies using better measures of social development before drawing such strong conclusions about whether autism is regressive, Klin cautions. That's because social behaviors may serve different purposes at different times of development. For example, at six months, a smile could be an instinctive reaction to seeing other people, but at 12 or 18 months, it could indicate that the child is engaging socially with others. Without understanding the purpose of a specific behavior at a particular age, it's difficult to know whether a child loses social skills, or simply fails to develop them in the first place, Klin says.

To confirm the findings and address some of these limitations, the researchers plan to expand the study to include more children and evaluate them more frequently. They also plan to use different measures of early development, such as eye-tracking.

## *References*

1. Ozonoff, S. et al. *J. Am. Acad. Child Adolesc. Psychiatry* Epub ahead of print (2010) Abstract.

2. Landa, R. and E. Garrett-Mayer J. *Child. Psychol. Psychiatry* 47, 629–638 (2006) PubMed.

3. Bryson, S.E. et al. *J. Autism Dev. Disord. 37*, 12–24 (2007) PubMed.

4. Klin, A. et al. *Nature 459*, 257–261 (2009) PubMed.

5. Lord, C. et al. *J. Child Pychol. Psychiatry 45*, 936–955 (2004) PubMed.

6. Tuchman R.F. and I. Rapin *Pediatrics 99*, 560–566 (1997) PubMed.

7. Baird G. et al. *Dev. Med. Child Neurol. 48*, 604–608 (2006) PubMed.

8. Ozonoff, S. et al. *J. Dev. Behav. Pediatr. 30*, 367–375 (2009) PubMed.

## Section 12.3

## *Eye Response to Light a Possible Autism Biomarker*

Text in this section is from "Pupil response to light could be biomarker for autism," by Kelly Rae Chi. © 2009 Simons Foundation Autism Research Initiative (SFARI). Reprinted with permission.

The pupils of children with autism contract more slowly in response to flashes of light than those of their healthy peers, according to findings published in the November 2009 issue of the *Journal of Autism and Developmental Disorders*.1 If the result is confirmed in larger groups of children with autism, visual reactions could serve as a potential biomarker for the disorder, researchers say. "If this is part of the symptomatology, it means you should be able to use it as a measure for identifying kids who might be at risk for autism," says John Colombo, a professor of psychology at the University of Kansas in Lawrence who was not involved with the study.

Pupil size and responsiveness have long been used as a test of lower brain function, but only a handful of studies published in the past 40 years have examined pupils in children with autism. Researchers first observed in 1961 that the pupils of five children with autism constricted more slowly when first exposed to a lighted room, compared with those of four healthy controls.[2]

Autism research then moved away from pupil reflexes because researchers had other ideas about the underpinnings of autism, primarily involving higher centers of the brain such as the cortex. In recent years, however, researchers have renewed their interest in lower-brain function in autism, Colombo notes. In 2006, he and his colleagues observed that the pupils of children with autism constrict when they look at human faces, whereas those of both healthy and developmentally delayed controls widen.[3] His team also reported in March that pupils are generally larger in individuals with autism compared with controls.[4]

In the latest study, bioengineer Gang Yao and his colleagues at the University of Missouri in Columbia set out to test more refined measures of lower-brain function by asking whether the pupils of children with autism respond differently to flashes of light. The researchers tested 24 children with autism with an average age of 12 years, and 44 healthy controls with an average age of ten years. They examined the children's pupil responses while they spent time in each of two different environments: at least five minutes sitting in a well-lit room and 20 minutes in a dark room.

The scientists asked the children to first focus on a computer screen four feet away in order to capture the baseline pupil diameter, and compared it with the diameter after exposure to lights of two different levels of brightness. They measured pupil diameter and response time in each eye for ten seconds after 100-millisecond exposures, using a customized pupillograph device—similar to those used by eye doctors to check vision—that Yao's group created.

Compared with the pupils of healthy controls, pupils of children with autism are slower, by about 16 milliseconds, to respond to a low intensity light and 40 milliseconds slower to respond to a brighter flash. "We've got to figure out now what [this] means, and whether it's specific to autism," says collaborator Judith Miles, professor of pediatrics and pathology at the University of Missouri.

Based on their results, measurements in pupil reactivity may help researchers identify people with autism with roughly 92% accuracy, the researchers estimate. The team is planning to examine 100 additional children with autism. "In order for it to be a really useful biomarker, [the study] will have to be done in large number of kids," says Andrew Zimmerman, a pediatric neurologist at the Kennedy Krieger Institute in Baltimore.

## Fundamental Functions

Yao's group also plans to investigate whether there is a connection between pupillary reflexes and other symptoms associated with the disorder, such as problems with digestion or sleep. All of these physiological responses are controlled by the autonomic nervous system, which includes both the sympathetic and the parasympathetic nervous system. Sympathetic nerves trigger an animal's fight or flight response to threatening stimuli, whereas the parasympathetic nervous system regulates 'rest and digest' in a more peaceful environment.

Both systems, which are controlled by lower parts of the brain, regulate pupil size and are thought to be out of balance in some children with autism.[5] The findings bolster the idea that defects in lower parts of the brain, in addition to the higher cortical centers of the brain, contribute to autism, Colombo says. "That is very different from the kinds of the hypotheses that have been raised over the last decade," he says.

The new study uses only healthy children for comparison, but to hone in on the specificity of the light reflex, and to assess its true potential as a biomarker, it should be examined in different types of developmental disorders, such as fragile X syndrome and Rett syndrome, Zimmerman notes. "I would expect some overlap with other disorders," he adds. It will also be interesting to see whether differences in pupil reactivity are apparent in younger children, Zimmerman adds. That may require some behavioral training of toddlers, or an adaptation of the technology—such as incorporating the measuring device into a toy—to help them stay still during the test.

## References

1. Fan X. et al. *J. Autism Dev. Disord. 39*, 1499–1508 (2009) PubMed.

2. Rubin L.S. *J. Nerv. Ment. Dis. 133*, 130–142 (1961) Abstract.

3. Anderson C.J. et al. *J. Dev. Psychobiol. 51*, 207–211 (2009) PubMed.

4. Anderson C.J. et al. *J. Clin. Exp. Neuropsychol. 28*, 1238–1256 (2006) PubMed.

5. Ming X. et al. *Brain Dev. 27*, 509–516 (2005) PubMed.

# Section 12.4

# *Sensory Sensitivity and ASD*

## *Description*

Some people with autistic spectrum disorders—such as autism or Asperger syndrome—appear to sense the world in different ways to other people. Some seem to be hypersensitive and some appear to be hyposensitive. They misinterpret everyday sensory information, such as touch, sound, and movement. So some individuals may find certain sounds or colors disturbing, while other individuals may not even hear the sound or notice the color at all.

**Alternative terms:** Some people use the term sensory processing disorder or (SPD), or sensory integration dysfunction, to describe sensory sensitivity. The Sensory Processing Disorder Network, describes SPD as follows: "a complex disorder of the brain. People with SPD misinterpret everyday sensory information, such as touch, sound, and movement. This can lead to behavioral problems, difficulties with coordination, and many other issues."

### *Sub-Types*

**Hypersensitive:** People who are hypersensitive receive too much information via their senses, so their brains become overloaded. This means they may see, hear, feel, smell, or taste the world in a more extreme manner than other people. For example, they may find certain noises disturbing or frightening, not like to look at things if they are a certain color or shape, or not like to taste or smell certain things.

**Hyposensitive:** People who are hyposensitive receive too little information, so the brain struggles to make sense of what little information there is. This means they may see, hear, feel, smell, or taste the world in a more muted way than other people. For example, they may not be able to hear certain sounds, including other people, and may not feel pain the same way as other people.

## Related Problems

**Causes:** We have yet to identify any research which demonstrates what the causes of altered senses may be.

**Prevalence:** We have yet to identify how many people with autism suffer from sensory sensitivity. Kern et al. (2007) believe that because sensory processing dysfunction is common in autism it should be considered as part of the disorder. Conditions include Asperger syndrome, autism (autistic disorder), autism spectrum disorders, pervasive developmental disorder (not otherwise specified).

**Effects:** Sensory sensitivity can lead to behavioral problems, difficulties with coordination, and many other issues.

**Hypersensitive individuals may react in two main ways:** With inactivity because their brain can't make sense of what it is receiving; or, with hyperactivity because the brain doesn't like what it is receiving. In either case, they may become anxious and frustrated.

**Hyposensitive individuals may react in two main ways:** With inactivity because their brain can't make sense of what it is receiving; or, with hyperactivity because the brain wants more information. This may result in self-stimulation or inattention. In either case, they may become anxious and frustrated.

# Section 12.5

# *Regression in Autism*

This section includes "Study Provides New Insights into the Implications of Autism Onset Patterns," © 2010 Kennedy Krieger Institute (www.kennedy krieger.org). Reprinted with permission. And under a separate heading, "Contradictory results on 'regressive' autism divide researchers," by Virginia Hughes, © 2010 Simons Foundation Autism Research Initiative (SFARI). Reprinted with permission.

## *Study Provides New Insights into the Implications of Autism Onset Patterns*

Kennedy Krieger Institute announced new study results showing that when and how autism symptoms appear in the first three years of life has vital implications to a child's developmental, diagnostic, and educational outcomes. Published in the April 2010 *Journal of Autism and Developmental Disorders*, this study found children with early developmental warning signs may actually be at lower risk for poor outcomes than children with less delayed early development who experience a loss or plateau in skills.

Researchers collected data from 2,720 parents through the Interactive Autism Network (www.ianproject.org), the nation's largest online autism research project. Through custom questionnaires and standardized rating scales, researchers examined differences in early milestone achievement (for example: first words, walking, phrase speech, and so forth), autism symptom severity and diagnosis, and educational supports between children with three different patterns of autism symptom onset:

- **Regression (n=44%):** A loss of previously acquired social, communication, or cognitive skills prior to 36 months.

- **Plateau (n=17%):** Display of only mild developmental delays until the child experiences a gradual to abrupt developmental halt that restricts further advancement of skills.

- **No loss and no plateau (n=39%):** Display of early warning signs of autism spectrum disorders without loss or plateau.

119

Results from the study, currently the largest to have examined regression in autism spectrum disorders, provides strong evidence for poorer developmental outcomes in children who experienced regression, a controversial topic among autism researchers. More specifically, children with regression had a significant increase in severity of autism symptoms, the greatest risk for not attaining conversational speech, and were more likely than any other group to require increased educational supports. These findings were markedly worse for the children whose parents reported the regression as severe.

This study was also one of the first to examine the implications of developmental plateau, which tended to occur around the child's second birthday. When compared to children with "no loss and no plateau," these children were more likely to need educational supports and receive an autistic disorder diagnosis, which is typically more severe than other diagnoses on the autism spectrum (Asperger syndrome or pervasive developmental disorder not otherwise specified). Children with "no loss and no plateau" were at the least risk for poor outcomes.

"Children who plateau or regress have a later manifestation of autism, but when it manifests it devastates their development," said Dr. Paul Law, corresponding study author and Director of the Interactive Autism Network at Kennedy Krieger. "Children with developmental plateau are an especially under-researched group, and these findings have important implications for those designing and prioritizing clinical evaluations."

Previous studies have reached a variety of different conclusions concerning outcomes for children with regression. Some research has found these children fared worse in the long term, while other studies found no differences in outcome between these children and those without regression. In examining these discrepancies, the current study suggests researchers who require children to have near typical development prior to regression may be missing the most severely impaired children in their findings. In fact, 35% of parents in this study had concerns about their child's general development before they noticed the more obvious signs of skill loss.

"Parents have good instincts when it comes to their children," said Dr. Rebecca Landa, co-author and director of Kennedy Krieger's Center for Autism and Related Disorders. "If they're concerned, they shouldn't wait to see a professional for immediate in-depth screening and developmental surveillance. We know from other research that the sooner you can diagnose autism and start intervention, the better the child's outcomes."

# Contradictory Results on "Regressive" Autism Divide Researchers

## *Sharp Divide*

Scientists do not agree on whether children with regressive autism are more likely to have distinct features, such as electroencephalograms (EEGs) that indicate epilepsy. Children with autism may show signs of the disease when they are younger than a year old, say some scientists. But parents and pediatricians of some children with autism maintain that their children developed normally in the first two years of life—making eye contact, waving goodbye, even saying a few words. Then, these children seemed to abruptly lose these skills.

This autistic regression, reported in about one third of children with the disorder, is baffling researchers. "We haven't found any biological markers to say why this child regressed and another didn't," says pediatrician Michael Davidovitch, chairman of the Israeli Association of Child Development and Rehabilitation. "And, we don't know if their prognosis will be better or worse."

About 20 years ago, researchers began asking whether autistic regression could be a distinct subgroup of autism with its own telltale biological markers. Since then, dozens of contradictory behavioral, physiological, and genetic studies have left the field no closer to finding the answer.

Some researchers are trying to tease out differences between the two groups in specific behavioral skills. So far, they too have failed to find any significant differences. If researchers could find regression to be a distinct phenotype, they might be able to better understand autistic spectrum disorders, and clinicians could make more confident predictions about a child's prospects. But, some experts are skeptical that regressive autism and early-onset autism are distinct types of the disorder. "It's been a very, very hot thing to study," says cognitive scientist Tony Charman of University College London. "Some people are pinning their lots on regression being a good subgroup. But, the evidence for it being a meaningful subgroup is still very equivocal."

## *Studies in Conflict*

Starting in the late 1980s, several studies found that autistic children who had regressed in their first year of life tested between ages three and six with lower intelligence quotients (IQs) and language levels than those who had early-onset autism.[1] But a decade later, some follow-up studies found no difference between the two groups of children.[2] In 1998, British gastroenterologist Andrew Wakefield notoriously suggested a link between the measles-mumps-rubella (MMR) vaccine, gastrointestinal problems, and regressive autism.[3] A slew of epidemiological studies over the following few years showed no causal relationship between MMR and autism. They also showed no difference in intestinal inflammation between children with regressive autism and those with early-onset autism.[4]

Around the same time, other researchers were looking for an association between regressive autism and epilepsy. It was a plausible idea: all children with Landau-Kleffner syndrome—a disorder in which a child suddenly loses the ability to understand and use verbal language—show abnormal electrical patterns in their brain waves, which is similar to what happens in epilepsy.

In 1997, neurologists at Miami Children's Hospital analyzed sleep electroencephalograms (EEGs)—which measure brain activity during sleep using electrodes on the scalp—of about 500 children with autism. Of the children who did not have overt epilepsy, the researchers found epileptic-like EEG readings in 14% who had undergone regression and only 6% of those with early-onset autism.[5] However, when Charman and his colleagues conducted a similar study with 64 children, they found no significant difference between the two groups.[6]

The genetic front is likewise confusing, with different methods garnering different results. If regressive autism were a genetically distinguishable subtype, then it would be likely to run in families. But in 2006, Jeremy Parr of the University of Oxford completed a genetic linkage study showing that multiplex families—those with two or more autistic children—are no more likely than average to share genes that had been previously linked to regression.[7] However, a study published in January by a group at the M.I.N.D. Institute at the University of California, Davis, found that 494 genes are expressed differently in the whole blood of children with regression and those with early-onset autism.[8] So many differences, they wrote, suggest that regressive autism and early-onset autism are "distinct biological disorders."

Newer studies have focused on testing behavioral differences between the two groups. For instance, Sally Rogers' research group at the M.I.N.D. Institute published a study in April that tested 20 children with regressive autism and 16 with early-onset autism for differences in their ability to imitate others. The study found no difference between the two groups.[9] Charman is unsurprised by the results and is critical of this latest wave of research which he says is looking for links between regression and behaviors that are ..."not mechanistically plausible. People who do these studies of subtyping without thinking why they're doing it are probably being rather un-helpful," he says.

## *Defining Regression*

Weighing these conflicting results, some researchers say that all autism could be considered regressive. "The fact that some children have regressive autism depends very much on what people mean by that word," says psychologist Ami Klin of the Yale Child Study Center. Most examples of autistic regression, Klin points out, are based upon a child's loss of a handful of words. Klin says that it's possible that these children were only echoing sounds they heard from their parents, "without necessarily making them an act of true communication"—much like congenitally deaf children sometimes babble even though they do not understand the words.

Regression has also been documented in the rare childhood disin-tegrative disorder, in which children show a dramatic loss of thinking, communication, and language skills after two to four years of normal development. "Now that's a regressive syndrome," Klin says. "Some kind of neurobiological thing is going on inside these children, perhaps the accumulation of some compound, and then there is a tipping point and they regress." But because autistic regression is much less clearly defined, Klin says the same thing is unlikely to be happening in children with regressive autism.

The definitive answer to these lingering questions may lie in pro-spective studies under way on the younger siblings of children with autism. "If we start looking at these children from the first year of life, then maybe we'll see that the proportion who seem to [regress] is higher than we thought it was," Charman says.

Preliminary results from these sibling studies, however, suggest that agreement on the regression issue is still far off. Baby sib research done by speech pathologist Rebecca Landa at the Kennedy Krieger Institute in Baltimore, for instance, suggests that regression might be more com-mon than current published estimates. "Our data show that even if you have early-onset autism, you can still show this worsening of symptoms over time," she says.

But ongoing studies of infant siblings at the M.I.N.D. Institute and at the University of California, Los Angeles, have found the opposite. Rogers reports that of the 185 siblings of children with autism seen so far at both sites, 30 have been diagnosed with autism, and none have shown classic regression. "What exactly that means still lies ahead," she says. "But it sure makes us think differently about it."

## References

1. Luyster R. et al. *Dev. Neuropsychol. 27*, 311–336 (2005) PubMed.

2. Baird G. et al. *J. Autism Dev*. Disord. Epub Ahead of Print (2008) PubMed.

3. Wakefield A.J. et al. *Lancet 28*, 637–641 (1998) PubMed.

4. DeStefano F. and Thompson *W.W. Expert Rev. Vaccines 3*, 19–22 (2004) PubMed.

5. Tuchman R.F. and Rapin I. *Pediatrics 99*, 560–566 (1997) PubMed.

6. Baird G. et al. *Dev. Med. Child Neurol. 48*, 604–608 (2006) PubMed.

7. Parr J.R. et al. *Mol. Psychiatry 11*, 617–619 (2006) PubMed.

8. Gregg J.P. et al. *Genomics 91*, 22–29 (2008) PubMed.

9. Rogers S.J. et al. *J. Child Psychol. Psychiatry 49*, 449–457 (2008) PubMed.

# Section 12.6

# *Challenging Behaviors*

Excerpted from "Adult Autism and Employment: A Guide for Vocational Rehabilitation Professionals," by Scott Standifer, PhD, Office of Disability Policy and Studies, School of Health Professions, University of Missouri. © 2009 University of Missouri. Reprinted with permission.

Some, but not all, persons with autism spectrum disorders (ASD) exhibit challenging behavior on occasion. The term challenging behavior covers a wide range of things, including self-injurious behavior (SIB), aggression towards others, damage to property, inappropriate sexual behavior, and constant screaming among other things. There is very little research on this topic and much concern about stigmatizing particular individuals as problems, but it deserves some attention in planning for employment and independent living.

There are several possible causes of challenging behavior, but there is no research information on which causes are most common or likely. The best way to deal with challenging behaviors is to monitor the behaviors closely, conduct a functional analysis to identify any contributing or associated factors (time of day, time of month, setting, recent activities, events immediately before, events immediately after, and so forth), and then review the possible causes for a likely match.

## *Contingency Plan*

If a person has no current challenging behaviors but does have a history of them (particularly aggression toward others), and if they are in a work situation, it might be useful to talk about a contingency plan with supervisors or coworkers. This plan would cover what to do and whom to contact if the behavior ever happened again.

The problem with making a contingency plan is that it could easily stigmatize the person in the minds of coworkers. It will be important to make sure supervisors and coworkers know that the behavior may never happen again. The behavior should be described as an unusual, unlikely event—a way for the person to express something that they can't express in any other way; and something that is not part of the person's normal behavior. Supervisors and coworkers should also understand that the person knows the behavior is inappropriate and does not want to do it. If the behavior occurs again, it is because the person is experiencing something significant and needs some help.

## Possible Causes of Challenging Behavior

### Communication

Even people with strong communication skills may sometimes have difficulty expressing things in words and resort to behavioral communication.

**Frustration with a situation:** The person may not like an activity, may need something (a tool, a drink of water, a bathroom break, help with something), or may be worried about something.

**Confusion about new aspects of a situation:** The person may not understand the instructions being given to them, changes in a routine, a new situation or activity, changes in the environment, or what others are doing.

**Confusion about goal, purpose, or sequence of activity:** The person may be confused about why they are supposed to do something or about what comes next in the sequence. Even individuals who normally are clear and "anchored" about their regular routine may have an occasional bad day when they don't feel well and lose track of the purpose or sequence of activities. They may become confused and frustrated. If clear, graphic guides are available in the work space, they can reorient themselves.

**Over-stimulation:** The person may be upset about too many new things, new activities, or new people in the environment.

**Under-stimulation:** The person may be bored, may be attracted to certain kinds of stimulation (certain lights, certain sounds, certain textures), or may find certain actions soothing. This can lead to self-stimulating behaviors or self-injuring behaviors, such as licking things, shouting loudly, or pulling his or her own hair.

- **What to look for:** Pay close attention to recent events, actions of others, and settings of the behavior. Notice if the behaviors increase or decrease when the person is engaged in particular activities. Also consider changes in home situations and whether the person is getting some benefit from the behavior.

- **What to do:** The most common approaches for these type of behaviors are "functional communication training" (teaching the person more appropriate ways to communicate their message) and behavior modification techniques. Accommodations might also be useful.

## *Physical/Neurological Issues*

**Gastrointestinal (GI) pain:** The person may be experiencing cramps from diarrhea, constipation, or general intestinal problems. There is a higher incidence of GI problems among people with ASD. It is worth asking about their bowel movements and diet.

**Lack of sleep:** The person may be tired and irritable. There is a higher incidence of sleep disruption among people with ASD.

**Hyper-sensitivity:** The person may find certain kinds of light, sound, or other stimuli very uncomfortable and distracting. These sensitivities are common among people with ASD.

**Migraine:** The person may be experiencing pain and distraction from migraines. There is no evidence of increased incidence of migraines among people with ASD, but migraines are common enough in the general population to consider for people with ASD.

**Pain:** There may be other typical medical issues causing the person pain, including dental problems.

**Seizures:** Individuals showing self-injuring behaviors or periods of being nonresponsive may be experiencing seizures.

**Side effects:** Some research says that more than half of all people with ASD are taking some sort of psychotropic medicine. These medicines can have serious side effects, including nausea, drowsiness/sedation, abdominal pain, fatigue, headaches, and general agitation among other things. It is worth consulting with the person's doctor or medical professional about what medications they are taking.

- **What to look for:** Pay close attention to the person's actions just before and just after the behaviors for signs of pain or distraction. Ask about family medical history and current medications. Issues such as seizures and migraines may be associated with particular settings or activities or may appear random. For seizures, look for confusion and sluggishness after the behaviors.

- **What to do:** Contact a doctor (or other medical professional) for an examination and treatment.

127

## Psychiatric Issues

**Depression:** People with ASD have increased rates of depression and bipolar depression.

**Attention deficit/hyperactivity disorder (ADHD):** The *Diagnostic and Statistical Manual of Mental Disorders, Fourth Edition (DSM-IV)* does not allow a dual diagnosis of ADHD and ASD, but there is anecdotal evidence of ADHD in people with ASD.

**Anxiety disorders:** Individuals with ASD may experience a lot of anxiety from sensory issues, communication issues, and cognition issues. In some cases, the anxiety might become pervasive and require psychiatric treatment.

**Aggressive urges:** A few people with ASD have aggressive urges, emotional outbursts, or extreme self-inuring behavior which they cannot control. The Food and Drug Administration (FDA) has approved one particular anti-psychotic medication for reducing these behaviors in people with ASD. This does not mean these people are experiencing psychosis or schizophrenia, however. This approach should only be used after other strategies have failed.

- **What to look for:** These explanations are a last resort, for situations in which there do not seem to be any connections to other factors or behavior.

- **What to do:** Contact a psychiatrist (or other appropriate medical professional) for an examination.

Chapter 13

# Developmental Screening

## Chapter Contents

# Section 13.1

# *Developmental Milestones*

This section begins with an excerpt from "Screening and Diagnosis: Autism Spectrum Disorders," Centers for Disease Control and Prevention (CDC), May 13, 2010; and continues with text excerpted from "Developmental Milestones," CDC, April 1, 2010.

## Screening and Diagnosis

Diagnosing autism spectrum disorders (ASDs) can be difficult, since there is no medical test, like a blood test, to diagnose the disorders. Doctors look at the child's behavior and development to make a diagnosis. ASDs can sometimes be detected at 18 months or younger. By age two, a diagnosis by an experienced professional can be considered very reliable. However, many children do not receive a final diagnosis until much older. This delay means that children with an ASD might not get the help they need. Diagnosing an ASD takes two steps.

### *Developmental Screening*

Developmental screening is a short test to tell if children are learning basic skills when they should, or if they might have delays. During developmental screening the doctor might ask the parent some questions or talk and play with the child during an exam to see how she learns, speaks, behaves, and moves. A delay in any of these areas could be a sign of a problem.

All children should be screened for developmental delays and disabilities during regular well-child doctor visits. Additional screening might be needed if a child is at high risk for ASDs (such as having a sister, brother, or other family member with an ASD) or if behaviors sometimes associated with ASDs are present. It is important for doctors to screen all children for developmental delays, but especially to monitor those who are at a higher risk for developmental problems due to preterm birth, low birth weight, or having a brother or sister with an ASD. If your child's doctor does not routinely check your child with this type of developmental screening test, ask that it be done. If the doctor sees any signs of a problem, a comprehensive diagnostic evaluation is needed.

## Comprehensive Diagnostic Evaluation

The second step of diagnosis is a comprehensive evaluation. This thorough review may include looking at the child's behavior and development and interviewing the parents. It may also include a hearing and vision screening, genetic testing, neurological testing, and other medical testing. In some cases, the primary care doctor might choose to refer the child and family to a specialist for further assessment and diagnosis. Specialists who can do this type of evaluation include: developmental pediatricians (doctors who have special training in child development and children with special needs), child neurologists (doctors who work on the brain, spine, and nerves), and child psychologists or psychiatrists (doctors who know about the human mind).

## Milestones

Babies develop at their own pace, so it's impossible to tell exactly when your child will learn a given skill. The developmental milestones listed will give you a general idea of the changes you can expect, but don't be alarmed if your own baby's development takes a slightly different course.

### By the End of One Year (12 Months)

*Social and Emotional*

- Shy or anxious with strangers
- Cries when mother or father leaves
- Enjoys imitating people in his play
- Shows specific preferences for certain people and toys
- Tests parental responses to his actions during feedings
- Tests parental responses to his behavior
- May be fearful in some situations
- Prefers mother and/or regular caregiver over all others
- Repeats sounds or gestures for attention
- Finger-feeds himself
- Extends arm or leg to help when being dressed

131

*Cognitive*

- Explores objects in many different ways (shaking, banging, throwing, dropping)
- Finds hidden objects easily
- Looks at correct picture when the image is named
- Imitates gestures
- Begins to use objects correctly (drinking from cup, brushing hair, dialing phone, listening to receiver)

*Language*

- Pays increasing attention to speech
- Responds to simple verbal requests
- Responds to no
- Uses simple gestures, such as shaking head for "no"
- Babbles with inflection (changes in tone)
- Says dada and mama
- Uses exclamations, such as oh-oh!
- Tries to imitate words

*Movement*

- Reaches sitting position without assistance
- Crawls forward on belly
- Assumes hands-and-knees position
- Creeps on hands and knees
- Gets from sitting to crawling or prone (lying on stomach) position
- Pulls him- or herself up to stand
- Walks holding on to furniture
- Stands momentarily without support
- May walk two or three steps without support

*Hand and Finger Skills*

- Uses pincer grasp
- Bangs two objects together
- Puts objects into container
- Takes objects out of container
- Lets objects go voluntarily
- Pokes with index finger
- Tries to imitate scribbling

*Developmental Health Watch*

- Does not crawl
- Drags one side of body while crawling (for over one month)
- Cannot stand when supported
- Does not search for objects that are hidden while he or she watches
- Says no single words (mama or dada)
- Does not learn to use gestures, such as waving or shaking head
- Does not point to objects or pictures
- Experiences a dramatic loss of skills he or she once had.

**Note:** For information about developmental milestones for other preschool ages, visit http://www.cdc.gov/ncbddd/actearly/milestones online.

Section 13.2

# *Recommendations for Routine Health Care Developmental Screening*

Excerpted from "Recommendations and Guidelines, Autism Spectrum Disorders," Centers for Disease Control and Prevention (CDC), May 13, 2010.

The A.L.A.R.M. [**A**utism is prevalent; **L**isten to parents; **A**ct early; **R**efer; **M**oniter] guidelines adapted from key policy statements of the American Academy of Pediatrics (AAP) and American Academy of Neurology, were developed to establish standard practices among physicians, to simplify the screening process, and to ensure that all children receive routine and appropriate screenings and timely interventions.

## *Developmental Surveillance and Screening (American Academy of Pediatrics)*

Early identification of developmental disorders is critical to the well-being of children and their families. It is an integral function of the primary-care medical home and an appropriate responsibility of all pediatric health care professionals.

AAP recommends that developmental surveillance be incorporated at every well-child preventive care visit. Any concerns raised during surveillance should be addressed promptly with standardized developmental screening tests. In addition, screening tests should be administered regularly at the 9-, 18-, and 24- or 30-month visits.

The early identification of developmental problems should lead to further developmental and medical evaluation, diagnosis, and treatment, including early developmental intervention. Children diagnosed with developmental disorders should be identified as children with special health care needs, and chronic-condition management should be initiated. Identification of a developmental disorder and its underlying etiology may also drive a range of treatment planning, from medical treatment of the child to genetic counseling for his or her parents.

# Developmental Surveillance and Screening for Autism Spectrum Disorders (American Academy of Neurology and the Child Neurology Society)

## Clinical Practice Recommendations

1. Developmental surveillance should be performed at all well-child visits from infancy through school age, and at any age thereafter if concerns are raised about social acceptance, learning, or behavior.

2. Recommended developmental screening tools include the *Ages and Stages Questionnaire*, the *BRIGANCE® Screens*, the *Child Development Inventories*, and the *Parents' Evaluations of Developmental Status*.

3. Because of the lack of sensitivity and specificity, the *Denver-II (DDST-II)* and the *Revised Denver Pre-Screening Developmental Questionnaire (R-DPDQ)* are not recommended for appropriate primary-care developmental surveillance.

4. Further developmental evaluation is required whenever a child fails to meet any of the following milestones: babbling by 12 months; gesturing (for example: pointing, waving bye-bye) by 12 months; single words by 16 months; two-word spontaneous (not just echolalic) phrases by 24 months; loss of any language or social skills at any age.

5. Siblings of children with autism should be monitored carefully for acquisition of social, communication, and play skills, and the occurrence of maladaptive behaviors. Screening should be performed not only for autism-related symptoms but also for language delays, learning difficulties, social problems, and anxiety or depressive symptoms.

6. For all children failing routine developmental surveillance procedures, screening specifically for autism should be performed using one of the validated instruments: the *Checklist for Autism in Toddlers (CHAT)* or the *Autism Screening Questionnaire*.

7. Laboratory investigations, including audiologic assessment and lead screening, are recommended for any child with developmental delay and/or autism. Early referral for a formal audiologic assessment should include behavioral audiometric measures, assessment of middle ear function, and

135

electrophysiologic procedures using experienced pediatric audiologists with current audiologic testing methods and technologies. Lead screening should be performed in any child with developmental delay and pica. Additional periodic screening should be considered if the pica persists.

## Section 13.3

# *Screening Tools for Early Identification of Children with ASD*

Excerpted from "Screening and Diagnosis for Healthcare Providers," Centers for Disease Control and Prevention (CDC), May 13, 2010.

Screening tools are designed to help identify children who might have developmental delays. Screening tools can be specific to a disorder (for example, autism) or an area (for example, cognitive development, language, or gross motor skills), or they may be general, encompassing multiple areas of concern. Some screening tools are used primarily in pediatric practices, while others are used by school systems or in other community settings.

Screening tools do not provide conclusive evidence of developmental delays and do not result in diagnoses. A positive screening result should be followed by a thorough assessment. Screening tools do not provide in-depth information about an area of development.

### *Selecting a Screening Tool*

When selecting a developmental screening tool, take the following into consideration:

**Domain(s) the screening tool covers:** What are the questions that need to be answered? What types of delays or conditions do you want to detect?

**Psychometric properties:** These affect the overall ability of the test to do what it is meant to do. The sensitivity of a screening tool is the probability that it will correctly identify children who exhibit developmental delays or disorders. The specificity of a screening tool is the probability that it will correctly identify children who are developing normally.

**Characteristics of the child:** For example, age and presence of risk factors.

**Setting in which the screening tool will be administered:** Will the tool be used in a physician's office, daycare setting, or community setting? Screening can be performed by professionals, such as nurses or teachers, or by trained paraprofessionals.

## Types of Screening Tools

There are many different developmental screening tools. The Centers for Disease Control and Prevention (CDC) does not approve or endorse any specific tools for screening purposes. This list is not exhaustive, and other tests are available. Selected examples of screening tools for general development and ASDs follow:

**Ages and Stages Questionnaires (ASQ):** This is a general developmental screening tool. Parent-completed questionnaire; series of 19 age-specific questionnaires screening communication, gross motor, fine motor, problem-solving, and personal adaptive skills; results in a pass/fail score for domains.

**Communication and Symbolic Behavior Scales (CSBS):** Standardized tool for screening of communication and symbolic abilities up to the 24-month level; the *Infant Toddler Checklist* is a one-page, parent-completed screening tool.

**Parents' Evaluation of Developmental Status (PEDS):** This is a general developmental screening tool. Parent-interview form; screens for developmental and behavioral problems needing further evaluation; single response form used for all ages; may be useful as a surveillance tool.

**Modified Checklist for Autism in Toddlers (M-CHAT):** Parent-completed questionnaire designed to identify children at risk for autism in the general population.

**Screening Tool for Autism in Toddlers and Young Children (STAT):** This is an interactive screening tool designed for children when developmental concerns are suspected. It consists of 12 activities assessing play, communication, and imitation skills and takes 20 minutes to administer.

## Screening for High-Functioning Autism or Asperger Syndrome

Until recently, screening tools often did not identify children with mild ASDs, such as those with high-functioning autism or Asperger syndrome. Today, there are some tools that reliably screen for social and behavioral impairments in children without significant language delay. Selected examples of screening tools for high-functioning autism or Asperger syndrome:

**Autism Spectrum Screening Questionnaire (ASSQ):** A 27-item parent- and teacher-completed checklist; the ASSQ is a useful brief screening device for the identification of Asperger syndrome and other high-functioning ASDs in children and adolescents with normal intelligence or mild mental retardation.

**Australian Scale for Asperger's Syndrome:** Questionnaire designed to identify behaviors and abilities indicative of Asperger syndrome in children during their primary school years.

**Childhood Asperger Syndrome Test (CAST):** Parent-completed questionnaire to screen for autism spectrum conditions.

## Section 13.4

# *Audiological Screening*

When parents and physicians are pursuing concerns about a child's development, one crucial component is the audiological screening. This screening is particularly important for children suspected of having a communication or developmental disorder. Increasingly, routine audiological screenings are recommended for all newborn babies.

"It seems like she doesn't hear me."

"When I call his name, he doesn't respond."

"I can't figure it out: sometimes it seems like he can't hear, sometimes loud noises upset him. What's going on?"

The relationship between a child's hearing, communication, and overall development is complex: A child who appears to have a developmental delay may, in fact, have a hearing impairment. A child with a hearing impairment that goes undiagnosed may experience resulting delays in development and communication. A child with a communication or developmental disorder may also have related issues with sensitivity to sound. For parents, all of this may seem like a puzzle they can't solve.

**The solution is simple:** When addressing concerns about a child, a developmental screening should be followed by audiological testing. The term "audiological" takes its roots from the word "audio," which means sound or hearing. A child's ability to process sound has a profound impact on the child's ability to understand and communicate.

When a child appears to have difficulty seeing, vision testing enables a physician to determine the nature and scope of the problem. Is the child nearsighted? Farsighted? Blind? Colorblind? Or, are there other concerns? Just as it is important to distinguish between different vision impairments, it is crucial to understand what auditory, or hearing and sound-related, issues might be present. This is sometimes referred to as a "differential diagnosis" process. There are many names for disorders of hearing and communication, depending on their cause and their effect. Some of these include: central auditory processing disorder, hearing impairment, deafness, and pervasive developmental disorder.

Audiological testing often takes place at a hospital, and despite the clinical environment, the screening is designed to be child-friendly. Often, a young child will simply sit on his or her parent's lap while a skilled professional will assess hearing through play, toys, and puppets.

Audiological testing can take many different forms, depending on the age of the child. Today, there is increasing interest in having hearing tests made standard for newborns. The American Academy of Pediatrics issued a policy paper stating, "Significant hearing loss is one of the most common major abnormalities present at birth and, if undetected, will impede speech, language, and cognitive development."

When a routine developmental screening raises concerns, or a child is at risk of atypical development or a communication disorder, the following types of audiological tests may be conducted:

- *Otoacoustic emissions:* This non-invasive screening is done with a small probe inserted into the ear canal.

- *Auditory brainstem response:* Electrodes are placed on the head, and brain wave activity in response to sound is recorded.

- *Visual reinforcement audiometry:* This is the method of choice for children between six months and two years of age. The child is trained to look toward (localize) a sound source. When the child gives a correct response, for example, looking to a source of sound when it is presented, the child is rewarded through a visual reinforcement such as a toy that moves or a flashing light.

- *Conditioned play audiometry:* The child is trained to perform an activity each time a sound is heard. The activity may be putting a block in a box, placing pegs in a hole, putting a ring on a cone, and so forth. The child is taught to wait, listen, and respond.

- *Acoustic immittance screening:* This test is often done if an otoacoustic emissions screening raises concerns. This screening may include tympanometry, acoustic reflex, and static acoustic impedance.

# Chapter 14

# *Getting Help for Developmental Delay*

## *Chapter Contents*

## Section 14.1

## *If You Are Concerned, Act Early*

Excerpted from "If You're Concerned, Act Early," Centers for Disease
Control and Prevention (CDC), April 1, 2010.

As a parent, you know your child best. If your child is not meeting the milestones for his or her age, or if you think there could be a problem with the way your child plays, learns, speaks, or acts, talk to your child's doctor and share your concerns. Don't wait.

If you or the doctor thinks there might be a delay, ask the doctor for a referral to a specialist who can do a more in-depth evaluation of your child. Doctors your child might be referred to include developmental pediatricians, child neurologists, or child psychologists or psychiatrists.

At the same time as you ask the doctor for a referral to a specialist, call your state's public early childhood system to request a free evaluation to find out if your child qualifies for intervention services. This is sometimes called a Child Find evaluation. You do not need to wait for a doctor's referral or a medical diagnosis to make this call.

**If your child is younger than three years old,** contact your local early intervention system. To find out the contact for your state, contact the National Dissemination Center for Children with Disabilities (NICHCY) at 1-800-695-0285, or, http://www.nichcy.org/Pages/Home.aspx.

**If your child is three years old or older,** contact your local public school system. Even if your child is not old enough for kindergarten or enrolled in a public school, call your local elementary school or board of education and ask to speak with someone who can help you have your child evaluated.

## Section 14.2

# *Discussing Concerns Parent to Parent*

Many friends, relatives, or caregivers may have concerns about a child's development, but are unsure of how to raise the issue with the parents. It is crucial to pursue any concerns, to ensure early and appropriate interventions; however, it can be difficult to do so.

Drawing on the experience of parents, this section also provides a list of Do's and Don'ts, such as these:

- Listen to the child's parent, start with their observations or concerns.

- Always be supportive, never judgmental.

- Avoid jargon, labels, and terminology.

- Keep it positive, emphasize ruling out anything serious.

No parent wants to hear concerns about a child, particularly regarding a child's development. All parents naturally want to protect their child. But, if a child isn't meeting developmental milestones, or is exhibiting one of the absolute indicators or "red flags," it is crucial that the child be properly screened. In order for this to happen, many friends, grandparents, and clinicians find themselves in the unenviable role of having to discuss developmental screenings with a parent.

Developmental delays and disorders are still poorly understood by much of our society. Few people understand the range of developmental disorders, let alone the opportunities for treatment and intervention. Many of us may recognize the differences in the physical features of children with cerebral palsy or Down syndrome; however, we often aren't aware of more subtle "hidden disorders" such as autism and how they present themselves in babies and toddlers.

The lack of knowledge about developmental disorders is further compounded by stigma. Sadly, what is not understood is often feared. This fear may prevent a parent from pursuing questions or concerns

143

about a child's development. This fear may also prevent those close to the parent—caregivers, grandparents, or friends—from sharing their concerns.

Some caregivers, and even clinicians, may have concern about labeling a child. A diagnosis doesn't have to be a label—an appropriate diagnosis may describe a child's challenges, but should never define a child. If a child is experiencing developmental delays, the specific diagnosis enables that child to have access to the most appropriate educational programs and therapies, such as occupational, speech, and physical therapy.

Early identification and intervention complement the core values of parenting: to seek to understand each child as a unique individual and to meet each child's distinct needs in order to prepare them for adulthood. A child, who is more fully understood, with respect to his/her individual strengths and weaknesses, will have a better quality of life. The goal is simply to help every child reach his or her fullest potential.

If you are concerned about a child's development, and want to bring it to the attention of the child's parent, here are a few Do's and Don'ts:

## *Do*

1. **Set the stage for a successful conversation:** "My mother invited me to go for a long walk to tell me what was concerning her about my child. It confirmed my own suspicions. After, we had a long cry for ourselves over it." Choosing the right time and place for a conversation to share your concerns is very important. Try to speak in person at a time when there will be no interruptions. Arrange to meet in a private setting. Dedicate as much time as you need to have a full conversation. Understand that emotions may be unpredictable. Be ready to offer help.

2. **Start with the observations, questions, or concerns of the child's parent:** "It is critical to respect a parent's perspective; begin with a clear understanding of whether or not they may have concerns, and what those might be." It's important to assess where a parent stands in relation to understanding his/her child's development before sharing your own concerns. The parent may already sense a problem and just not have the words to articulate it. Gently probe and ask questions that will allow a parent to share their own observations, questions, or concerns first. Then share your own observations. By doing so, you will open an exchange and may even validate a parent's hidden concerns and fears.

144

3. **Put yourself in the parent's shoes. Be supportive, not judgmental:** "If you want to talk to a parent, please say it in a loving way. It might be good to begin by making a positive comment about the child's strengths and by reinforcing the parent's skills, love, and dedication to the child." Some of the most memorable conversations that parents of children with special needs report are those that take place at the critical moment a first concern is expressed. An empathetic approach goes much further in establishing trust and understanding than a judgmental or emotionally closed or charged one. Your tone and manner should be open and available. Whatever the outcome, in the long run, the parent will remember and appreciate your discussion if it is framed in a caring way.

4. **Focus on milestones, absolute indicators, and the need to rule out anything serious:** "It is such an emotional subject, with so little that made sense. Milestones made sense to me." Give the parent something positive to read (see a developmental checklist of hallmark milestones and red flags). The checklist gives parents something to think about and consider, but never puts a label on it. It gets the conversation started with the child's physician and provides specific information about strengths and areas of challenge.

5. **Refer parents and caregivers to other resources. Some parents need to come to this understanding on their own:** "I remember seeing a web site that seemed to describe many of my son's unique and, frankly, troubling behaviors. As much as I wanted it to be wrong, the more I read the better I understood that something was going on." Seeing developmental disorders described in writing, whether through literature or on the web, allows a parent to make the match with his/her own child's behaviors and needs. It provides an objective description of common features and allows the parent to come into recognizing developmental concerns at their own pace.

6. **Emphasize the importance of early identification and intervention:** "Early intervention is the key. Tell the parent that the earlier you catch a child, the easier it is to help the child...if you let it go too long, it just takes that much longer for the child to gain ground." One way to look at developmental concerns is that if a child had signs of a serious and persistent physical illness, like asthma, you would want to get it checked out as soon

as possible to rule it out. If there really were a problem, it would only make it worse by not doing so. Developmental delays are no different. By not receiving timely interventions for concerns around language, behavior, and social connectedness, the problems will not go away, but will worsen over time. And what's most hopeful is that early intervention works, improving life in the long and short term for both the child and the family. So life will get better once interventions are underway.

7. **Be confident that sharing your concerns is always the right thing to do. The hardest part is finding the right words and getting started:** "When my son was 18 months old with no language, a friend said that I should march him right down to the pediatrician's office. I have to admit I was a bit offended but when I found out her advice was right, I thanked her. Most people would just sit back on their hands and not say anything. Her delivery lacked some tact, but she got me going." Try role playing what you will say first. Express what you have observed that gives you concern in a caring, supportive way. By doing so, it may lower your own anxiety and give you the confidence to have a heart-to-heart with a positive outcome.

8. **By sharing your concerns, you may help to validate what a parent is afraid or unable to express:** "I felt comfortable in my denial. I just thought 'oh, this too shall pass.' But when my sister expressed her concern, it articulated what I was too afraid to say. Every now and then I need someone to shake me out of my comfort zone and get me moving." Often a parent may have a nagging and persistent subliminal fear that something is indeed wrong developmentally, but they may be afraid to say it out loud. All they may need is to hear the same concern from someone else to confirm their suspicions. These outcomes are usually described by parents as bringing them relief. Now they don't feel so alone. It provides the impetus to take the next step for their child.

## Don't

1. **Don't dismiss a parent's concerns:** "Just listen and observe. Take the time to listen to the parent and observe the child before you do, or say, anything." If a parent shares concerns with you directly, you have a unique opportunity to help them.

Listening is often all that is needed to help parents channel their concerns into words and actions.

2.  **Don't compare one child to another. Each is unique:** "I've heard the story about how a child had no language and then one day, started to speak in volumes, almost miraculously. I've heard about Einstein being a late talker as another way to comfort me. Although well-meaning tales, they did nothing to help me move forward to help my child. They only prolonged my self-doubt." Often family and friends will share a story meant to give comfort to a parent that gives an anecdote of someone else who struggled with early developmental concerns, only to outgrow them in a dramatic or famous way. Instead of having the intended effect of providing comfort and ruling out concerns, parents often sense that they do not address their child's unique concerns and dismiss them. Or they may provide more insecurity to a first time parent who is already experiencing self-doubt. Either way, anecdotes are not useful. It is more important to think about the particular child in question.

3.  **Don't use labels, technical jargon, or loaded terminology:** "When the teacher at my son's preschool said that he 'needed Special Education,' I thought she meant that she thought he was mentally retarded; I just shut down. Similarly, when my doctor told me she'd 'Seen kids like him before,' I stopped listening." It's probably too scary to mention a specific disorder to a parent right out of the gate. Many disorders are misunderstood and just the mention of them can bring up great fear in parents who may shut down. Sometimes giving a parent an article or book to read is enough to make the connection.

4.  **Don't scare a parent, keep it positive:** "I told my doctor that my daughter's daycare provider had some concerns about her, but I disagreed. 'Wasn't it okay for a child to be a little bit different? Why label?' I'll never forget my doctor's simple, steady words: 'Just get it checked out, just rule it out. You have nothing to lose.' She was right. If it hadn't been for the extra help my son got by being identified at such a young age, he—actually, we— would never be doing as well today." If a parent is encouraged to see their pediatrician with developmental concerns about their child, there will be one of two outcomes, but each will have its positive aspects. If concerns are ruled out, parents can rest easy. If there are indeed confirmed concerns, seeking help through

evaluation and referral will eventually get the family back on a healthy developmental path.

No harm can be done by checking out concerns. Things can only get better. This is a positive message that family and friends can share with parents to encourage them to seek help.

## Section 14.3

# *Sharing Concerns with Your Child's Physician*

Each well visit provides an opportunity for your child to receive a routine developmental screening; however, if you don't ask, it may not be offered. Whether or not you have specific concerns about your child's development, it is best to come to the doctor's office prepared.

Physicians rely on parents to provide information about their child. As a parent, you are your child's best advocate and a "resident expert" about your child's health and development. During a well visit, a physician usually sees a child for less than 15 minutes, even less if there has been an emergency that day. It is a challenge, for both the parent and the physician, to cover the wide range of issues related to a child's health within a limited time.

If you have concerns about your child's development, take the following four crucial steps: be prepared, express your concerns clearly, ask questions, and follow up.

1.  **Be prepared:** Before you go to your next well visit, print out a checklist of developmental milestones and note whether your child has met each of the expected milestones. If you have questions or concerns, write down a few concrete examples that might assist your physician:

    - "My child doesn't respond to my voice."

    - "He spends so much time lining up his toys, he has no interest in other children."

- "She hasn't learned a new word in months."

- "He doesn't look at me—he never makes eye contact."

Whether or not you have concerns, ask your doctor for a routine screening.

2. **Express your concerns clearly:** While this issue can be an emotional one, try to focus on your concrete concerns, such as developmental milestones. If your physician doesn't want to perform a screening, or isn't responsive to your concerns, be persistent. Ask why. And remember, "don't worry" or "let's wait and see" are not adequate responses. Schedule a follow up appointment, if necessary, or ask for a referral to a developmental pediatrician. Your child's healthy development is your most important concern.

3. **Ask questions:** If there are terms you don't understand, ask your physician to explain. After the screening, ask what the results show, and what they mean. Inquire about referrals to specialists. Ask what the next step will be.

4. **Follow up:** For most parents, routine screenings indicate that a child is following a typical development pattern. Screenings at well visits in the future will help to confirm that. For other parents, who learn from the screening that their child may be at risk of a developmental delay, follow up is crucial. Children at risk of atypical development are routinely referred to Early Intervention for a closer look by a developmental specialist. You also may want a referral to a developmental pediatrician, a psychologist, a neurologist, a psychiatrist, or a specialist for further evaluation.

Through all four steps, some parents may stumble or falter. Grief and disbelief can prove to be great hurdles. Parents may fear the worst and not move forward. Other parents may feel uncomfortable questioning their physicians. Proceed with confidence, as parents know their child best. Only by pursuing your questions and concerns, forming a sharing relationship with your child's physician and then by following up with him/her, can you ensure the best possible outcome for your child. Be patient with yourself and persistent for your child. Get the help your child needs.

"Pediatricians are the only professionals with knowledge of development who are in routine contact with the families of young children. Parents turn to their pediatrician for information about development, for assessment of whether their children are doing all right or not. If pediatricians don't know or aren't sure or don't have the appropriate tools, the children with delays or disorders are missed." (Frances Page Glascoe, PhD, Professor of Pediatrics)

# Chapter 15

# *Parent's Guide to Assessment of ASD*

## *Chapter Contents*

Section 15.1

# *Defining Assessment*

Excerpted from "Life Journey Through Autism: A Parent's Guide
to Assessment," © 2008 Organization for Autism Research
(www.researchautism.org). Reprinted with permission.

## *What is assessment?*

Assessment is a comprehensive process used to determine your
child's strengths and challenges in multiple areas or types of abilities.
Assessment involves gathering specific information about your child
to inform the treatment and services that your child receives. There
are multiple assessment instruments and methods. As you will learn
in this guide, different types of assessments measure different things.
Which assessment[s] will be used will be based on the questions that
need to be answered about your child. These questions may include:

- Is there something wrong with my child's development?

- Is the current diagnosis or absence of diagnosis accurate?

- For what services are my son or daughter, eligible and which
  ones are most appropriate?

- What should be included in my child's individualized educational program (IEP)?

- What might be the most effective teaching or behavior support
  strategies?

- How should my child's progress be measured?

## *What is an IEP?*

An individualized educational program, or IEP, is a written, legal
contract that identifies the nature and extent of special education
intervention strategies and related services to be provided by your
child's school district. Under the Individuals with Disabilities Education Act (IDEA 2004), an IEP is required by law for all children with
disabilities, including children with autism spectrum disorders. The

IEP sets forth your child's educational program for the coming year in objective and measurable detail. Both formal and informal assessments play a major role in the development, monitoring, and revision of the IEP on an ongoing basis.

## The Assessment Process

The assessment process begins with one of the questions mentioned. Sometimes, it is the parents asking out of concern for perceived developmental or social issues; other times, it might be teachers or medical professionals who raise questions that lead to assessment. Once the assessment decision is reached, the process should involve a multidisciplinary team of professionals to obtain the most accurate and complete picture of your child's functioning. The assessment team may include parents, psychologists, pediatricians, psychiatrists, neurologists, behavior analysts, speech and language pathologists, general and special education teachers, occupational and physical therapists, and other experts who may work with your child, including other family members.

To be most effective, assessment must be a collaborative process between these professionals and you, the parent. The ultimate goal of any assessment is to provide you and the professionals working with your child the specific information they and you require to guide intervention and instructional planning for your child.

Accurate assessment depends on a variety of factors, including:

- a clearly defined goal for the assessment;
- the experience of the professionals conducting the assessment;
- the appropriateness of the assessment instruments;
- the active participation by the child with autism spectrum disorder (ASD) and his or her parents;
- the interpretation of the results by parents, teachers, and other support personnel working with your child.

After the initial diagnostic assessment, it is most useful to think of assessment as a continuous process. First, an assessment will be conducted to provide initial information about your child's current abilities. The professionals who completed the assessment will then review the results with you, and together, you will decide on the most critical skill areas in need of improvement or refinement. You and the involved professionals will then discuss expectations for skill growth and develop an individualized educational or behavioral intervention. After a predetermined period, you and the relevant professionals will review the intervention and determine to what extent it has helped your son or daughter, whether the goals were achieved, or whether the intervention should be revised to maximize skill gains. Another assessment may then be conducted to determine how to revise the intervention. The purpose of this ongoing assessment process is to strengthen your child's skills in multiple areas of functioning.

**Assessment tip:** Throughout any assessment, the parent plays a central role in the process. Your input, insights, and observations about your child, as well as your advocacy on his or her behalf, help to ensure an effective and beneficial process. Do not hesitate to ask questions or to ensure that the information you provided is fully considered in the process. If you are unsure about your role or the process, consider bringing a parent advocate with you to help guide you through the process at least for the initial meetings. By being an informed and active participant in the assessment process, you will help ensure that the results are both accurate and relevant to your child's particular needs.

### Key Terms

The terms assessment, evaluate, and measure appear throughout this chapter. These terms have multiple definitions in general use. Within this chapter, however, the definitions of these words are more specific.

**Assessment:** The process of using instruments (surveys, interviews, questionnaires) or, in some cases, direct observation, to obtain information about a child's performance and behavioral strengths and challenges to inform educational and intervention decision making.

**Evaluate:** To compare the outcomes (or results) of an assessment relative to other children, to a predefined expectation, or to previous outcomes for an individual child.

**Measure:** An instrument used during an assessment (like a survey, interview, or questionnaire).

### Why is assessment important?

There are many benefits to assessment. Assessment can inform you and others about your child's level of functioning across skill areas, giving information on his or her capabilities and challenges. This information will then help to customize treatments and interventions for your child.

Over time, assessments can help you and those who support your child evaluate his or her progress and set new goals for school and home.

Assessment can also provide information about your child's ongoing learning and behavior to educational professionals, who can then better develop, monitor, and evaluate academic and behavioral interventions that have been implemented.

In addition, an assessment provides valuable information that can be used to assist your child's IEP team in developing the IEP and identifying appropriate support services. Assessment should identify present levels of performance across a number of skill areas, as well as highlight strengths and identify specific areas of concern that can be incorporated into the IEP. By using the results of an assessment, appropriate interventions and necessary services can be identified based on your child's specific needs, abilities, and interests.

## Benefits of an Assessment

An assessment offers an important insight into your child's abilities and helps measure his/her strengths and weaknesses. More specifically, it helps you and your child's teachers, IEP team, and other caregivers by the following:

- Measuring the level of functioning across skill areas
- Providing comparative information on your child's performance
- Evaluating your child's progress at home and school
- Setting outcome-oriented goals for your child
- Suggesting objectives to be included in your child's IEP
- Guiding the planning and development of interventions for your child
- Communicating measurable results to professionals working with your child in terms they can best understand
- Determining your child's strengths and challenges in a variety of skill areas

"Our assessments provided information that was critical to developing an IEP that addressed the unique needs of our son. We were able to develop meaningful and measurable objectives and have mechanisms in place to track his progress. We were also able to establish accommodations that would allow him to be productive and comfortable in the classroom."—Parent of young child with autism

## Section 15.2

# *Types of ASD Assessment*

Excerpted from "Life Journey Through Autism: A Parent's Guide
to Assessment," © 2008 Organization for Autism Research
(www.researchautism.org). Reprinted with permission.

This section provides an overview of the skills and abilities that are most frequently evaluated. An evaluation in any of these areas could take place during an initial diagnostic assessment, a re-evaluation, or an assessment of specific skills.

## *Diagnosis*

A diagnostic assessment for autism spectrum disorder (ASD) is a comprehensive, multidimensional process. Various types of assessment tools will be used, including standardized measures, interviews, checklists, and direct observations, to give an accurate diagnosis of your child.

At the beginning of the diagnostic assessment process, you will be asked to provide a developmental history of your child. This history will review your child's communication skills, social skills, and behavioral development. Often, to document this information, the professional conducting the assessment will use standardized measures developed to assist with the diagnosis of ASD, such as a semi-structured interview or self-report measure. The answers to some of the questions asked may be a bit difficult to recall so having ready access to calendars, journals, e-mails, photos, or videos can help provide as accurate a history as possible. With your permission, the professional will often review information from medical or educational records to consider additional medical and psychiatric issues that may be affecting your child.

In addition to using standardized interviews and self-report measures in the diagnostic assessment, a professional may informally observe your child in several settings, such as the classroom, play area, or lunchroom. It is essential that the professional get to know your child and interact with him or her to understand your child's capabilities and to effectively and accurately provide a diagnosis.

Other aspects to consider during a diagnostic assessment include your child's cognitive abilities, language skills, and adaptive behavior. Cognitive abilities are assessed by looking at your child's cognitive strengths in areas such as attention, memory, and problem solving, which will help to plan for your child's educational and service needs. Language skills are assessed through a variety of techniques, as discussed in the Speech and Language Assessment area of this section. The methods used to assess adaptive behavior are described in the Adaptive Behavior Assessment section. Lastly, as part of the initial evaluation for diagnosis, a thorough medical examination should be completed to ensure an accurate diagnosis.

A professional or team of professionals with experience diagnosing and developing interventions should conduct the diagnostic assessment for children with ASDs. Professionals may include a developmental pediatrician, pediatric neurologist, child psychologist, or child psychiatrist. In addition, speech and language pathologists, occupational therapists, and physical therapists may be part of the assessment. After completing the comprehensive diagnostic assessment process, the professional will review the collected information and make a judgment on the diagnosis based on the classification system outlined in the *Diagnostic and Statistical Manual of Mental Disorders, Fourth Edition, Text Revision (DSM-IV-TR)*.

**Autism Diagnostic Observation Schedule:** Sometimes referred to as the gold standard in assessment for diagnosis, the Autism Diagnostic Observation Schedule (ADOS) (Lord, et al., 2000) is a standardized measure that uses a combination of structured and unstructured activities to assess the following areas: communication, social interaction, play, imagination, stereotyped behaviors, and restricted interests. This measure uses four different modules that are each individually designed for a particular developmental age and language ability level. Module 1 is used with children who do not consistently use phrase speech. Module 2 is used with those who use phrase speech but are not verbally fluent. Module 3 is used with fluent children, and Module 4 is used with fluent adults. The one group that ADOS does not address is nonverbal adolescents and adults.

## Cognitive Assessment

Because cognitive abilities affect your child's social, psychological, and developmental world and deficits in this area are often prevalent in children with ASDs, an accurate cognitive assessment is important and often revealing in terms of your child's particular areas of strength or difficulty. A thorough cognitive assessment consists of a series of tasks designed to evaluate a wide range of your child's abilities, including attention/concentration, memory, problem solving, and verbal skills. The results of a cognitive assessment can provide you and your child's teachers and related support personnel with some of the information needed to better understand your child's current capabilities.

It is important to keep in mind that many commonly used intelligence quotient (IQ) tests may not be appropriate or accurate for children with ASDs because they have not been proven reliable or valid for this population. Because IQ tests are standardized, the manner in which they are administered is critical. Variations to strict procedure may cause the results to be inaccurate or invalid. In addition, the social interaction and communication problems that many children with ASDs display can influence the accuracy of the results. For example, while a child with Asperger syndrome may have an above-average IQ, his heavy reliance on social gesturing and unfamiliarity with social norms can create difficulties in testing situations and give inaccurate assessment results. Further, standardized tests do not take into account learning differences or preferences. Many children with ASD are reportedly more visual than auditory learners. Given these difficulties, it is sometimes helpful to view the outcomes of cognitive assessment as basals, rather than maximals. In other words, the results may represent the worst your child can do under difficult conditions, rather than the best your child can do under ideal conditions.

To decrease the heavy reliance on communication and social skills (specifically receptive language, expressive language, and auditory processing) in test instructions, a small group of cognitive assessments exists that require little to no verbal instructions or responses on the part of the child. These assessments are called tests of nonverbal intelligence. For children with little to no verbal responding abilities, these tests can be helpful. It is important to note one potential drawback: During the administration of these tests, children are still required to attend to the test administrator and demonstrate some basic social skills (such as motor imitation), which may be a challenge for some younger children with ASDs.

The cognitive assessment, like other forms of assessment, is a complex and comprehensive process. Multiple areas of functioning will be evaluated to provide you with an understanding of your child's cognitive capabilities. It is important to have a professional who is knowledgeable about ASD and experienced in a variety of cognitive assessments to conduct the tests administered to your child. Typically, cognitive tests are only administered and interpreted by psychologists or psychometricians.

## Speech and Language Assessment

Central to a diagnosis of an ASD are deficits in: (1) verbal and nonverbal communication, and (2) social interaction. Although a speech language pathologist (SLP) cannot diagnose a child with ASD, he or she does play a significant role in the diagnostic process and educational planning of your child's speech and language skills. Generally, an SLP evaluates how your child communicates with words, gestures, and symbols. A speech and language assessment also looks at your child's ability to understand language, initiate and use language, and communicate with others. Ideally, the results of a speech and language assessment are used to develop interventions to increase your child's ability to communicate.

A speech and language skills assessment will usually involve observing your child interacting with others in a variety of contexts, such as at home or in school. An SLP may observe you and your child together and work directly with your child on a variety of tasks. Depending on your child's verbal language skills, some standardized tests may be appropriate. For a nonverbal child, however, more direct observations should be done to assess speech and language.

Given the challenges children with ASDs have in understanding and communicating with others, a speech and language assessment is key to determining how to support and guide your child. Like other areas of assessment, a comprehensive speech and language assessment will yield specific information to assist with the development of educational planning.

## Adaptive Behavior Assessment

An adaptive behavior assessment looks at real-life skills, such as caring for self or independent functioning. Personal skills, home-related skills, and community living skills are assessed. Adaptive behavior skills often vary, depending on the age of the child. For example, in young children, certain self-help skills would include dressing, eating, and toileting. For older children, it would include skills like selecting and caring for appropriate clothing, and eating without parental supervision in the cafeteria and at restaurants. An adaptive behavior assessment gives you and the professionals working with your child information regarding (1) the extent to which your child can function independently; (2) the level of direct supervision they might require; and (3) specific areas of deficit that should be targeted for improvement.

Adaptive behavior refers to age-appropriate typical performance of daily activities based on social standards and expectations. Unlike their typical peers, children with ASDs do not learn well by simply watching and imitating others. Thus, they often have challenges in the area of adaptive behavior, which tend to become more apparent as your child gets older. The adaptive behavior assessment will examine your child's range of adaptive behavior skills and help identify areas that will require more direct and intensive instruction. The information from an adaptive behavior assessment can help you and the professionals who work with your child set goals for both school and home during treatment planning, and map out a course to promote your child's greatest degree of independence across environments.

Unlike traditional assessments or standardized tests, adaptive behavior assessments rely primarily on information provided by someone who is familiar with your child's performance in real-life settings, typically either you or a teacher. Adaptive behavior is examined in this indirect manner because the assessment considers performance over time and in real-life situations that do not lend themselves to practical observation. Adaptive behavior assessments are often administered within a structured or semi-structured interview format (for example, the evaluator asks you a series of questions) or as a self-report measure (you answer the questions on your own).

## Social Functioning

Social functioning is a common area of assessment for children with ASDs as they typically display a wide variety of deficits and challenges in social functioning that, similar to adaptive behavior skills, may become more evident as they grow older. Usually, a social functioning assessment will be conducted as part of an adaptive behavior assessment or a speech and language assessment, but it can sometimes be completed as a separate assessment.

It is important to understand, however, that to assess the many factors associated with social functioning, it is helpful to employ several measurement approaches as opposed to only one. For example, rating scales can be effective in identifying specific social behavior excesses and deficits, but they do not address context variables, such as with whom your son or daughter is interacting or where the interaction is taking place. Conversely, behavioral observation may not identify the full range of social behavior necessary for programming in all areas that are important to the individual. Therefore, to best assess social functioning, a multi-modal approach involving rating scales, behavioral observation, and functional assessment offers the most complete picture of your child.

## Academic Assessment

Sometimes social and behavioral aspects of autism in the school setting overshadow the primary reason children go to school—to learn. Academic functioning or academic achievement assessment refers to the skills your child has learned through direct instruction, independent study, or life experience. In addition to highlighting how your child learns, an assessment of academic functioning will tell you what your child has learned. Achievement tests are designed to assess proficiency in various learned skills, such as reading, math, spelling, writing, vocabulary, or subject-specific knowledge like science and social studies. This information can then be used to inform educational instruction, planning, and monitoring of your child's progress in an academic environment.

The purpose of an academic assessment is to determine your child's strengths and deficits in relation to his or her educational setting. This assessment can include both formal and informal assessment methods. A formal academic assessment usually involves having your child take norm-referenced, standardized tests. These types of tests allow professionals to compare your child's performance to other, same-age children; assess your child's individual academic levels; and begin planning individually determined academic interventions. School-wide, state academic tests are examples of formal academic assessments. There are no formal, norm-referenced assessments designed specifically for children with ASD.

Informal academic assessment then becomes the tool for looking at how your child learns in a nonstandardized way. It may include interviews, reviews of your child's school records, or a curriculum-based assessment—small, focused assessments of specific topic areas or abilities (such as a classroom test or quiz). Unlike formal assessment, informal assessment is more flexible to administer and can be changed to accommodate different learners. While the person using an informal assessment must be skilled, this type of assessment can be created to meet the needs of your child. Informal assessments are typically conducted by certified special or regular education teachers, as well as other classroom- or school-based educational specialists. Informal academic assessment is needed to receive ongoing information about your child's progress in an academic setting.

The ultimate goal of an academic assessment is to determine your child's learning strengths and weaknesses, and what educational methods are most appropriate for your child. Academic assessment results can then be used to develop educational plans and inform his or her

IEP. These assessments also help to evaluate how well a particular intervention has worked in a school setting. Academic assessments should be administered on a regular basis to provide up-to-date information on how well your child is doing educationally, and what other challenges may need to be addressed.

## Curriculum-Based Assessment

In a curriculum-based assessment (CBA), the assessment items are developed from your child's own school curriculum; thus, it evaluates specifically what your child has learned using his or her own school programs. CBAs are useful to track whether your child is learning at school, and to determine his or her progress in learning the school's materials. This assessment only looks at whether your child knows the information taught or can perform a skill following instruction; it does not assess how your child approaches a task. Of particular note: a CBA cannot be used as a basis for determining your child's diagnosis or eligibility for services.

**Academic assessment example:** At the beginning of fourth grade, Zach's IEP will need to be updated. To evaluate his progress in school and set new goals, an educational specialist conducts an academic assessment. In addition to re-administering the Wechsler Individualized Achievement Test, his teachers develop a curriculum-based assessment encompassing the skills and lessons taught previously to Zach. The assessment focuses on Zach's abilities in reading, math, and written language. The results reveal that Zach is at the same level as his classmates in math; however, his reading comprehension skills are below average. Thus, Zach's IEP is updated to include additional goals and proposed interventions to target his reading comprehension skills.

## Functional Behavioral Assessment

If your son or daughter engages in challenging (for example, aggressive) or inappropriate (such as screaming) behavior, a functional behavior assessment (FBA) may be called for. An FBA gathers a significant amount of information about a child's specific behavior or group of behaviors. As such, the central purpose of an FBA is to determine the function or purpose of this challenging or unwanted behavior. Once the function of the behavior is determined, trained behavior specialists working with other professionals and family members can develop interventions to decrease the occurrence of these challenging behaviors and increase the number of more appropriate or adaptive behaviors.

During an FBA, the professional conducting the assessment directly observes your child at different times and in different settings over a period of time. During these observations, he or she systematically records information on the environment, the actual behavior, and what your child achieved as a result of the behavior. The results of an FBA allow professionals to identify the challenging behavior and the circumstances leading up to the behavior, and then to create a behavior intervention plan for your child that has specific goals and methods for changing challenging behaviors. An FBA is a comprehensive process that may involve interviews, records review, rating scales, direct observation, and data collection and analysis. Whatever indirect measures are used (interview, records review, or rating scale), a comprehensive FBA should always include direct observation and data collection and analysis.

**Functional behavioral assessment example:** To inform the development of Jake's IEP, his school recommends a functional behavioral assessment (FBA). A behavior analyst first completes several questionnaires and behavior rating scales with Jake's teacher and parents, while also reviewing his school records. Then, this evaluator observes Jake in several environments at school (classroom, cafeteria, recess) to assess any challenging behaviors or situations. When the evaluator observes challenging behaviors, he collects data on any number of factors preceding the behavior, as well as the apparent consequences of the behavior (e.g., removed from the area). The evaluator then summarizes the results of the FBA in a comprehensive document that is used to guide the development of a behavior intervention plan.

## Occupational Therapy/Physical Therapy Assessment

Children with autism often have difficulties with motor skills, such as hand/eye coordination, which are important for daily life. Occupational therapy (OT) and physical therapy (PT) assessments are used to help identify skill deficits that have a direct and negative impact on your child's ability to function independently in his or her daily routines. The goals of OT and PT generally focus on increasing physical strength and improving visual perceptual skills (for example: the ability to recognize and identify shapes, objects, and colors), fine and gross motor skills (handwriting, jumping, and skipping), sensory modulation (processing information from the environment more effectively), and cognition (understanding the steps involved to complete a specific task).

An OT and/or PT assessment looks at your child's skills in the areas showcased in the list on the next page. Both standardized and nonstandardized assessment tools, as well as parent interviews and direct observation of your child, will be used to assess his or her performance.

The results from an OT and/or PT assessment can help you and your child's teacher implement individualized strategies to promote greater levels of independence and structure the environment to both minimize sensory distracters or challenges and increase individual tolerance to such distracters. OT and/or PT assessments can also help you and your child's teachers develop strategies to develop your child's skills at home, offer suggestions on how to break down a task into manageable steps for your child, and facilitate transitions from home to school while developing your child's skills.

*Areas Evaluated during OT and/or PT Assessment*

- Fine motor skills: Movement and dexterity of the small muscles in the hands and fingers

- Gross motor skills: Movement of the large muscles in the arms and legs

- Visual motor skills: Movement based on the perception of visual information

- Oral motor skills: Movement of muscles in the mouth, lips, tongue, and jaw, including sucking, biting, chewing, and licking

- Self-care skills: Daily dressing, feeding, and toilet tasks

- Motor planning skills: Ability to plan, implement, and sequence motor tasks

- Sensory deficits/excesses: Ability to interpret and organize various sensory experiences, including sight, sound, smell, touch, movement, body awareness, and the pull of gravity

## Social-Emotional Assessment

At different times in their lives, children with ASDs may experience emotional difficulties in the form of anxiety and other mood disorders, such as depression or bipolar disorder. For that reason, the assessment process may include measures of social-emotional well-being. This type of assessment can add valuable information in support of an FBA and the subsequent development of an appropriate behavior support plan. Such assessments are most helpful when they target specific symptomatology (symptoms or difficulties that they experience).

For example, if the school psychologist suspects clinical depression, she could work to assess changes in sleep patterns or appetite, along with measures of changes in affect/mood or increased lethargy (tiredness), to either rule in or out a mood disorder. Particularly for individuals who may not have the language capabilities and are unable to accurately self-report, such a direct assessment of student behavior may be very useful and appropriate.

## Educational Placement Evaluations

A distinct, yet critically important, type of assessment is the educational placement evaluation. An educational placement evaluation is the process by which you and your child's IEP team work to determine the extent to which a particular educational program is likely to be effective for your child. The educational placement evaluation looks at the chain of events that begins with the identification of a student's unique strengths and areas of need, and ends with an informed opinion on the potential of the IEP, as implemented by the program, to address your child's unique educational and behavioral needs.

There are a variety of reasons why an educational placement evaluation might be conducted. Many school programs conduct periodic self-evaluations to ensure that their program is operating in accordance with their own educational guidelines or to evaluate the appropriateness of a placement for a particular student. In some instances, specific evaluation procedures are required by outside state or funding agencies. As part of a placement evaluation, you will generally observe classrooms, review data or progress notes, and evaluate the fit between your child's needs and the school program in preparation for a placement team meeting.

In the event of a disagreement between you and your school district, a hearing officer may be called on to evaluate the appropriateness of a school program for your child. In each of these situations, it is often helpful to have an independent expert conduct a thorough assessment of your child's unique needs in relation to both the child's IEP and the actual implementation of that IEP.

In some respects, an educational placement is similar to a diagnostic evaluation. Evaluations should be conducted by experienced professionals working in the field of autism treatment and could include those with professional training in a variety of disciplines, including psychology, behavior analysis, and special education at the master's or doctoral level. Evaluators should not only be knowledgeable practitioners in the field of autism education, but also have training and experience that would qualify them as experts in program design and implementation. In particular, evaluators should have experience that is relevant to your child.

For example, those who work primarily in an academic setting may not have the clinical expertise to provide a detailed description of educational protocols, or those working primarily with adults may not be best suited to assess a very young child. Similarly, those with experience with young children may not be ideal evaluators of a program for a young adult. Because there are currently no state or national standards to regulate the administration of this kind of evaluation, it is important to learn about an evaluator's credentials, check references, and request sample reports before engaging the services of an evaluator.

Once the evaluator has gathered all of the information and conducted his own direct observations of your child, he prepares a report. The report generally summarizes what specific activities the evaluator has conducted, key information provided by those interviewed, and results of any additional testing conducted. It also offers specific educational recommendations that describe if and how the educational environment and educational programming is, or is not, appropriate to meet the needs of your son or daughter.

Should the evaluator identify areas where your child's needs are not being met, then he should offer further specific recommendations about how, when, where, and by whom different educational strategies should be implemented to help the parents and educational team make an effective change. Although written reports are helpful, evaluators will often meet with parents and/or have a dialogue with school personnel to ensure that everyone understands what the findings and recommendations are, and how to make meaningful changes to instructional settings to help the child achieve greater success.

## *Reference*

Lord, C., Risi, S., Lambrecht, L., Cook, E. H., Leventhal, B. L., et al. (2000). The autism diagnostic observation schedule-generic: A standard measure of social and communication deficits associated with the spectrum of autism. *Journal of Autism and Developmental Disorders, 30*, 205–223.

# Section 15.3

# *Assessment Process*

Excerpted from "Life Journey Through Autism: A Parent's Guide
to Assessment," © 2008 Organization for Autism Research
(www.researchautism.org). Reprinted with permission.

We have covered a significant amount of information about what
types of assessments may be conducted and the purpose of each assessment. This section will cover the process or the steps that you and
your family will take from the initial referral for a diagnosis through
to the assessment.

## *Referral Process*

The referral process can differ from one family to the next, and the
referral can come from a number of sources. You may approach your
family physician out of concern for your child. Conversely, your pediatrician may approach you and your family regarding developmental
concerns and recommend that your child receive an assessment. Finally, the school may recommend that your child be evaluated due to
concerns about his or her behavior or rate of educational progress.

As the parent of a child with an autism spectrum disorder (ASD),
you do not need to be reminded that the responsibility is often on you.
If you have significant concerns about your child's development or progress, do not wait for a professional to second your concerns. Follow your
instincts and actively seek a referral for a diagnostic assessment.

During the referral process, be sure you understand the reason
behind the referral and, in particular, what questions you expect to
have answered about your child as a result of the assessment. At this
point, one of the most important preliminary steps you can take is
to ensure the individual conducting the assessment has experience
working with and assessing children with ASDs. This will facilitate
accurate and reliable assessment results.

If you are interested in finding professionals on your own to obtain
an assessment of your child, you can begin by soliciting recommendations from your pediatrician, neurologist, other involved professionals, or

other parents of children with ASDs. In addition, many autism-related websites offer searchable databases of professionals in your area.

"Whenever an assessment is done, parents need to make certain that clinicians are aware of previous testing that has recently been done. Some tests are not valid if repeated within a specified time frame. This is particularly true with outside or independent evaluations completed during the 12 months prior to a school-based re-evaluation."—Parent of child with autism

### Who conducts assessments?

Only qualified professionals with experience working with children with ASDs should conduct assessments with your child. The purpose of the assessment will determine what type of professional will conduct it. For example, a neurological assessment would be conducted by a trained pediatric neurologist or psychiatrist and should not be done by professionals without qualifications or experience doing a neurological assessment. The next section provides more information on who should conduct particular types of assessments.

When you receive a referral for an assessment, it is important for you to learn about the professional's expertise and credentials. Be sure to check references and research them to learn about his or her level of experience and manner in working with children with ASDs. You want to find the most appropriate professional to work with you and your child. By researching this additional information, you will be more confident in your decision.

### Who conducts what type of assessment?

Different professionals perform different types of assessments. Again, the who depends on the specific referral question, as well as the individual's expertise. Table 15.1 provides a general picture of which professionals conduct which assessments. This is an illustration only, not an all-inclusive list.

### What happens during an assessment?

What occurs during an assessment depends on the type of assessment being completed. Initially, there may be an interview with you, the parent. Sometimes, a single member of the evaluation team will interview you; other times, each member of the team may wish to speak with you. The interviews will generally focus on your child's developmental and medical history in addition to family medical history and

**Table 15.1**. Professionals That Conduct ASD Assessments

| Assessment Type | Who Can Conduct |
| --- | --- |
| Diagnostic | Developmental pediatrician<br>Psychologist<br>Psychiatrist<br>Neurologist |
| Cognitive | Neurologist<br>Psychologist<br>Psychiatrist |
| Speech and Language | Speech and language pathologist |
| Adaptive Behavior | Psychologist<br>Behavior Analyst<br>Clinical Social Worker |
| Social Functioning | Psychologist<br>Psychiatrist |
| Academic Functioning | School district evaluator<br>Psychologist<br>Special education teacher |
| Occupational Therapy (OT) and/or Physical Therapy (PT) | Occupational therapist<br>Physical therapist |
| Functional Behavior | Psychologist<br>Behavior analyst |
| Emotional/Psychological | Psychologist<br>Psychiatrist |

day-to-day functioning. Depending on the professional and the primary focus of the assessment, the interview may extend to other topics (such as, current social skills).

As part of the assessment, the evaluation team may ask you and your child to complete some tasks together. At other times the team may ask you to complete some standardized measures and/or checklists designed to give the professional additional, often necessary, information. These checklists and measures frequently relate to your child's adaptive behavior, emotional status, or social functioning. In addition, the team may ask you to provide a release for medical records or records from a previous school.

Assessments vary in length. Some may take a few hours; others may last a few days, depending on the complexity and amount of information being gathered. After the assessment is complete, the professional will create a written report of the results and observations from the assessment. Clinical assessments should include a discussion of treatment recommendations relevant to the assessment outcomes.

Once the evaluation team's report is written, the team should meet with you to review the assessment results and recommendations. If a meeting does not occur, then it is your responsibility to ask for one. At this meeting you will have the opportunity to ask questions and get any clarifications you feel necessary. A specific goal of this meeting should be for you to receive both accurate assessment results and, equally important, information on the next steps and services for your child based on the assessment.

If the assessment was specifically completed as part of the individual education program (IEP) process, the review may occur in the context of an IEP meeting. No matter what the setting, take the time to understand the assessment results and how they relate to your child's development. Feel free to ask each member of the IEP or assessment team to clarify any information that you do not understand. The team, with your input, then must decide what the educational and behavioral goals will be and the most appropriate interventions and services to support your child and your family.

**Assessment tip:** Ask to receive the report for any assessment before any meetings with the evaluation or IEP teams. In this way, you will have time to review the information beforehand, prepare for the meeting, and formulate questions. It is also important to keep a record of your child's assessment results to monitor his or her progress. Please make several photocopies and/or write your child's assessment results after each assessment. You can use these documents to monitor their development in various skill areas.

## *Limitations of Assessment*

Assessment is a means of gathering specific information about your child's functioning across different domains. It is not without its limitations. Assessment can be a subjective process, the outcome of which is contingent on the skill of the individual conducting the assessment, the measures used, and their interpretation.

Assessment captures your child's functioning at a specific point in time. Because children with ASDs do grow and change over time, it is important to have re-evaluations completed at periodic intervals (usually a minimum of three years). Remember to keep copies of previous assessments to gauge your child's progress over time.

Each type of assessment measure has its own strengths and weaknesses. Therefore, assessment results need to be interpreted with some caution, taking into account the specific type of measure used, its potential limitations, and the implications for the results.

## A Final Word of Advice

Assessment for whatever purpose results in a snapshot of your child's strengths, deficits, challenges, and abilities at a given point in time. As such, assessment results can provide valuable information regarding the development of both long-term goals and short-term objectives for your child. These goals and objectives can both build on your child's documented strengths or target specific areas of deficit in need of more direct intervention. It is important to work closely and collaboratively with all of the professionals who work with your child. Collaboration should begin with the assessment process and extend throughout your child's academic career to ensure that you help shape the goals and expectations for your child and his or her future.

# Chapter 16

# *Diagnostic Criteria for ASD*

### *What is a diagnosis?*

A diagnosis is a categorical term that describes a group of behaviors or characteristics that, in most cases, are linked with a particular disease or disorder through cause, trajectory, and effective treatments.

### *How is a diagnosis of an autism spectrum disorder (ASD) different from other diagnoses?*

Because we do not know the causes, autism spectrum disorder (ASD) diagnoses are based purely on observations or reports of behaviors. Unlike many medical syndromes, ASDs are not diseases. They are not contagious and are not yet treatable through medication (though medicine can help some symptoms). They are developmental disorders that reflect differences in the way that children develop from very early on (from infancy and toddlerhood) and that usually continue to affect development into adulthood. The primary treatments are educational (for example, teaching individuals with ASDs ways to do things that may not come as easily for them) and compensatory (helping individuals learn to use their strengths to make up for areas that are more difficult), as well as behavioral (helping individuals and families to minimize behaviors that interfere with daily living, such as tantrums or self-injury).

"FAQ about Autism Spectrum Diagnoses," by Catherine Lord, PhD. Reprinted with permission from the Interactive Autism Network (IAN) Community (www.iancommunity.org), © 2007 Kennedy Krieger Institute.

## How are autism spectrum disorders defined?

ASDs are defined by difficulty in three areas of behaviors: 1) reciprocal social interaction, 2) communication, and 3) repetition and insistence on sameness. Exactly how an individual is impacted across these three areas varies greatly. There is no one behavior that is present in all individuals with ASDs or that would rule out ASDs in every person. Many, but not all, individuals with ASD have language delays. Some individuals with ASD, but not all, have lifelong language disorders. Some, but not all, individuals with ASD also have mental retardation that affects development of nonverbal problem-solving, everyday self-care (such as dressing, academics) and language.

## Are there different types of ASDs? Are some cases of ASD more severe than others?

Within the category of autism spectrum disorder (sometimes known as pervasive developmental disorders or PDD), there are a number of subtypes that are associated with different levels of severity in different areas.

Autism is the disorder that has received the most study and has been recognized for the longest time. It is defined by the presence of difficulties in each of the three areas listed (social deficits, communication problems, and repetitive or restricted behaviors), with onset in at least one area by age three years. It may or may not be associated with language delays or mental retardation.

Asperger syndrome is a form of ASD that is often identified later (after age three, usually after age five) and is associated with the social symptoms of autism and some repetitive interests or behaviors, but not with language delay or mental retardation. Many parents and professionals use this term with older and/or more verbally fluent individuals with autism because they feel it is less stigmatizing.

Rett syndrome and child disintegrative disorder are both very rare, severe forms of ASD that have particular patterns of onset, and, in the case of Rett syndrome, a specific genetic basis.

Pervasive developmental disorder not otherwise specified (PDD-NOS) is a form of ASD used to describe individuals who meet criteria for autism in terms of social difficulties but not in both communication and restricted, repetitive behaviors. It can also be used for children who do not have clearly defined difficulties under age three or later. This term is often used by professionals when they are not quite sure of a diagnosis or when the symptoms are mild. Several epidemiological studies have reported that as many or more children have PDDNOS or less clear symptoms as have classic autism. The difficulties of children and adults with Asperger syndrome or PDDNOS are similar, and milder than those of individuals with autism, suggesting that these distinctions are fairly arbitrary and should not be used to limit services or benefits.

## What benefit is a diagnosis of ASD?

A diagnosis should go beyond a description of defining features of a disorder to provide important information about other aspects of behavior or development. For example, where ASDs are concerned, it is essential to know that families with one child with ASD are at greater risk for having another child with ASD, though this risk is probably less than one in five. Also important is the fact that adolescents with ASD are more likely to have a seizure or develop epilepsy than other children their age. Most important of all, a diagnosis often provides children access to services through school systems and early intervention networks. It can also provide adults access to services through vocational programs. A diagnosis can give parents and family members a way to start acquiring information about other children with similar difficulties and ways to find support through local, national, and international organizations.

A diagnosis should provide information about effective and ineffective treatments. Though there is no one-size fits all treatment for ASDs, it is clear that low intensity interventions that are not built on engaging a child in social interaction and communication, and that do not involve parents, are not appropriate programs for young children with ASDs. In ASD, many children's behavior problems (such as tantrums) are linked to not being able to communicate. Providing the child with a way to let others know what he or she wants (for example, through words or signs or pictures), and helping the child understand what others are saying (also through pictures or objects or gestures) can decrease problem behaviors greatly. Medications may help treat additional symptoms in ASD, such as hyperactivity, but are often less effective in children with ASD than other children.

A diagnosis is necessary for doing research to find the causes and to improve treatments for ASDs, so that scientists can know who they are studying and can compare findings across different research projects. Because there are probably many subtypes of ASD, researchers need to work with large numbers of children and families in order to have adequate numbers of similar children. This means that researchers need to merge samples, which requires that they agree on common diagnostic procedures (or else they will not know what differences across samples mean if they occur).

## What are the differences among screening, diagnosis, and a full assessment of ASD?

A screening involves determining if a child or adult is at risk for having an ASD and should have a more detailed assessment. This screening may be specific to autism or may be part of a more general screening for developmental disorders such as language delay. Screenings are intended to be brief, easy to use (by parents and professionals), and inexpensive. A positive screening should be followed up by a diagnostic assessment. The biggest difficulty in autism screenings to date is that, at least with young children, children later determined to have autism are often found to have been missed by earlier screenings. Thus, if parents are concerned, they should be wary of quick screenings and reassurances that everything will be all right without careful attention to their concerns.

## What makes a good diagnostic assessment?

Because children and adults with ASDs have such varying profiles, most good diagnostic assessments provide a description of strengths and weaknesses, including attention to children's language, cognitive, and other skills. These factors are often as important as the actual diagnosis of an ASD in setting appropriate goals and intervention plans. In the end, the most important factors in a diagnosis are the experience and care of the diagnostician. Many different healthcare professionals can diagnose autism including a child psychiatrist, clinical psychologist, developmental pediatrician, or a speech-language pathologist. In most cases, more than one discipline should be involved, if not at the same visit, at least in communicating their perspectives with each other.

A diagnostic assessment for ASD should involve both a history and a description of current behavior by a caregiver, as well as direct observation of the behavior of the child or adult suspected of having ASD by an experienced clinician. These observations require sufficient knowledge that having a less experienced person (such as a clinical assistant, a resident) do the assessment and then consult with the more experienced supervisor is generally not appropriate.

The most well-known diagnostic instruments for ASD are the *Autism Diagnostic Interview – Revised (ADI-R)* and the *Autism Diagnostic*

*Observation Schedule (ADOS)*. The ADI-R is a caregiver interview that takes about two hours; the ADOS is a series of play-based tasks administered to the child, usually with the parent(s) present. These instruments require training to administer and require more specialist hours than most health insurance is willing to reimburse. Many centers may use different combinations of these instruments and other, quicker measures (parent questionnaires) in a diagnostic assessment. What is important is not so much the specific instruments, as the combination of information from the caregivers and from an expert working with and observing the child. Also vital is the assessing clinician's experience with ASD.

In almost all cases, interpreting diagnostic information also requires knowledge about the child's receptive and expressive language and nonverbal functioning. A child who is very far behind in all areas (for example, a three-year-old who has the abilities of a nine-month-old) may score in the range of autism, not because he or she has ASD, but because there are so many things he or she cannot do, that scores will be high on any instrument. A very bright verbal three-year-old with ASD will not have the same behaviors as a child with ASD with a severe language delay in comprehension and expressive language. Other pieces of information (such as ensuring the child can hear and that there are no contributing medical conditions, talking to the child's current teachers, if he or she is in preschool) are also important to a diagnosis of ASD. With increasing media awareness, many professionals who are not experts in ASD can recognize some symptoms of ASD and suggest possible diagnoses. Because of the variation in ASDs, however, experts in these disorders often can provide information beyond a diagnostic term that can help parents in making decisions about treatments.

### How young can a child be to receive a diagnosis of ASD?

Some children have such clear symptoms that they can be reliably diagnosed with ASD at 12–15 months, but most clinicians will want to wait until a child is 18–24 months before giving a diagnosis. Diagnoses made under age three are less reliable (less predictive of stable diagnoses over time) than diagnoses made in older children, so it is important for children who receive diagnoses when they are very young to be re-evaluated each year, including measurement of changes in cognitive and language skills. In later years, re-evaluations usually focus more on how behaviors and skills have changed more than on diagnosis.

## What is the relationship between getting a diagnosis and getting services?

Legally, in the United States, a child is supposed to receive educational and early childhood services according to his or her needs, not according to a diagnosis, but many states and school systems do differentially allocate services to children with autism diagnoses. Some states do not provide the same services to children with a diagnosis of PDDNOS or Asperger syndrome as they do to children with a diagnosis of autism. This is not scientifically or educationally justifiable, but it means that families may feel pressed to get a clear diagnosis of autism in order for their child to receive the services he or she needs, even though they, and professionals, may prefer the more ambiguous classifications (PDDNOS, Asperger syndrome) because they imply milder symptoms. While sometimes service providers may treat autism (and scores on autism diagnostic instruments) as all or none, this is not correct. This is one reason to be sure that a child's evaluation is done by someone experienced and knowledgeable about ASD.

## Are there ways to get the most out of a diagnostic assessment for ASD?

The more prepared parents are for a diagnostic assessment, the more they will usually get out of it. If at all possible, both parents should attend the assessment so that both can see what was done and be able to ask questions. If this is not possible, having a relative or friend come along can be very helpful, too. Preparing a list of questions to ask the clinician both before the assessment and after can be very helpful. Making copies of these lists to give to the clinicians may help the clinician remember to address what is most important to the caregiver. Taking a list of people who already work with the child, their phone numbers, and good times to reach them can also save tracking information down later. In addition, taking copies of any previous assessments and reports is a very good idea. Even if the parents want an independent assessment, being able to tell the examiner what tests their child has already had can save time and money.

Whether it is the child's pediatrician or a local autism society or a friend, asking the person making the referral for the assessment to describe what to expect and how to prepare can be useful. Taking snacks and small toys that a child likes is often helpful. (Sometimes, rather than giving them to the child right away, it is best to ask the clinician if he or she would like to use them.) If the child can understand, rehearsing with him or her where they are going, who they will see, and what they may do (play with toys), is usually a good idea as well. With a young child, a parent or parents should almost always be present during the evaluation, unless the child is so distracted by the parent's presence that the examiner cannot get a fair assessment. Reviewing the child's baby book and talking to other people who knew the child when he or she was younger can also be helpful in refreshing a parent's memory in order to provide a more accurate history.

If parents feel that they have not had enough time to process the information they are getting, they should ask to come back in a week or two and review the results after they have had time to think about it. Or, if this is only an assessment clinic, they might ask the clinician to refer them to someone who does follow-up. The value of an assessment is not in the assessment process, but in what the family learns and is able to take back to the community in terms of being better able to understand and advocate for the child.

# Chapter 17

# *Medical Tests and Evaluations Used to Diagnose ASD*

Autism and related disabilities, such as PDDNOS (pervasive developmental disorder not otherwise specified), Asperger syndrome, and Rett syndrome, are difficult to diagnose, especially in young children where speech and reasoning skills are still developing. A child may be three years old before the full characteristics of these disabilities are apparent.

Typically, medical professionals are not trained extensively in diagnosing and evaluating autism and related disabilities. Doctors will usually rule out other possibilities before mentioning autism.

Although autism is considered a neurological disability, no specific medical test or procedure can confirm a diagnosis of autism. To gather more information that will accurately profile an individual's strengths and needs, a variety of tests, assessments, and evaluations should be administered.

This chapter includes brief descriptions of some medical tests and evaluations that may be ordered for children suspected of having autism or a related disability.

## *Medical Tests*

Given the variety of theories about the causes of autism and related disabilities doctors may use various medical tests and procedures to help with diagnosis. There is not always a clinical need to do medical tests. Your doctor(s) can recommend when, or if, a test should be done.

"Diagnosing and Evaluating Autism: Part I," © 2005 Center for Autism and Related Disabilities (CARD)–University of Central Florida. Reprinted with permission. Reviewed in October 2010 by David A. Cooke, MD, FACP.

The following medical tests may help with diagnosis and possibly suggest changes in an intervention or treatment strategy.

**Hearing:** Various tests such as an audiogram, tympanogram, and the brainstem evoked response can indicate whether a person has a hearing impairment. Audiologists, or hearing specialists, have methods to test the hearing of any individual by measuring responses such as turning their head, blinking, or staring when a sound is presented. If a hearing impairment is detected, treatment could involve minor surgery, use of hearing aids, or antibiotics.

**Electroencephalogram (EEG):** An EEG measures brain waves that can show seizure disorders. In addition, an EEG may indicate tumors or other brain abnormalities. Additional tests will be needed to make an accurate diagnosis of these conditions. During an EEG, sixteen small sensors are placed at various locations on the scalp to record brain waves that a neurologist interprets. An EEG may take one to 24 hours depending on the doctor's goals when ordering the test. If seizure activity is detected, additional testing may be required and various medications could be prescribed.

**Metabolic screening:** Blood and urine lab tests measure how a person metabolizes food and its impact on growth and development. Some autism spectrum disorders can be treated with special diets.

The following medical tests may help locate neurological factors that can affect typical development and could possibly identify or rule out a cause. Results will probably not change intervention or treatment.

**Magnetic resonance imaging (MRI):** An MRI involves using magnetic sensing equipment to create an image of the brain in extremely fine detail. The patient lies on a sliding table inside a cylinder shaped magnetic machine and must be still during the procedure. Sometimes patients are sedated in order to complete the MRI.

**Computer-assisted axial tomography (CAT scan):** An x-ray tube rotates around the patient taking thousands of exposures that are sent to a computer where the section of the body that is x- rayed is reconstructed in great detail. CAT scans are helpful in diagnosing structural problems with the brain.

**Genetic testing:** Blood tests look for abnormalities in the genes which could cause a developmental disability.

## Therapy Evaluations

Many individuals with autism and related disabilities require some form of special therapy at some point during their lives. Therapeutic evaluations can help determine if therapy is required to help an individual fulfill their potential.

**Speech-language therapy:** People with autism usually have delays in communication. The most obvious is when they are nonverbal. Yet people who are verbal may also have serious difficulties. Some individuals can repeat words but can't use language in a meaningful way which is called echolalia. A speech pathologist who specializes in the diagnosis and treatment of language problems and speech disorders can help a person learn how to effectively communicate. Speech therapists look for a system of communication that will work for an individual with autism and may consider alternatives to the spoken word such as signing, typing, or a picture board with words.

**Occupational therapy:** Commonly focuses on improving fine motor skills, such as brushing teeth, feeding, and writing, or sensory motor skills that include balance (vestibular system), awareness of body position (proprioceptive system), and touch (tactile system). After the therapist identifies a specific problem, therapy may include sensory integration activities such as: massage, firm touch, swinging, and bouncing.

**Physical therapy:** Specializes in developing strength, coordination, and movement. Therapists work on improving gross motor skills, such as running, reaching, and lifting. This therapy is concerned with improving function of the body's larger muscles through physical activities including exercise and massage.

## Interpreting the Results

Medical tests look for a physical cause of a disability. Autism and related disabilities are not commonly caused by a physical problem. It is important to work with medical professionals that look at your whole child, which includes their medical condition as well as their behavior, communication, and school environment.

# Chapter 18

# *Genetic Test for Autism*

A newer type of genetic test is better at detecting abnormalities that predispose a child to autism than standard genetic tests, new research has determined. Researchers offered about 933 people aged 13 months to 22 years who had been diagnosed with an autism spectrum disorder three genetic tests: G-banded karyotype testing, fragile X testing, or chromosomal microarray analysis (CMA) which has been available only for the past few years.

Karyotype tests identified chromosomal aberrations associated with autism in about 2% of patients, while the fragile X genetic mutation was found in about 0.5% of patients.

CMA detected chromosomal abnormalities in slightly more than 7% of patients, making it the best available genetic test for autism spectrum disorders, the study authors said. "The CMA test alone has triple the detection rate of karyotyping or fragile X," said co-senior author Bai-Lin Wu, director of the Genetics Diagnostic Laboratory at Children's Hospital Boston. "CMA should be added to first-tier genetic testing for autism spectrum disorders." The study appeared online March 15, 2010 and will be published in the April print issue of *Pediatrics*.

"When parents have a child diagnosed with an autism spectrum disorder, one of the first questions they often ask is 'how did this happen?'" said Dr. Robert Marion, a pediatric geneticist at Children's Hospital at Montefiore Medical Center in New York City. "In the vast majority of cases, we believe there is at least a genetic predisposition to autism, but the ability to identify a specific genetic cause has been very elusive," Marion said. "Part of that is because of the technology that's been available. A larger part is at this point, we just don't fully understand what the genetic mechanism that leads to autism is."

Standard practice is to offer children with autism two tests as a first-line genetic work-up: karyotype and fragile X testing, the researchers said. In karyotyping, forms of which have been around since the 1960s, geneticists use a microscope to look for chromosomal abnormalities that are associated with autism, explained Dr. David Miller, a clinical geneticist and assistant director of the Genetics Diagnostic Laboratory at Children's Hospital Boston, which conducted the new research along with Boston's Autism Consortium. Like karyotyping, CMA also looks for chromosomal abnormalities, but does so at 100 times the resolution of the earlier test, Miller said. CMA, a genome-wide test, can identify sub-microscopic deletions of duplications of deoxyribonucleic acid (DNA) sequences, called copy-number variants, known to be associated with autism, he said. "Think of chromosomes as a library full of books and each book as a gene," Miller said. "What we look for are shelves of books that have gone missing, which represent a missing fragment of a chromosome, or extra fragments of chromosome, that could contain genes related to autism."

While both Children's Hospital Boston and Montefiore have offered CMA testing for several years, not all hospitals do, nor does all insurance pay for it, the researchers noted. The main purpose of genetic testing of children with autism is to help parents determine if they're at a higher risk of having another child with autism, Marion said. If tests pinpoint an autism-related chromosomal abnormality in the child, the parents are then offered testing. If a parent is also found to have the abnormality, geneticists conclude that the couple is at higher risk of having a child with autism. (The precise risk depends on what the variant is.) But if the parents don't have the abnormality, geneticists conclude that the deletion or duplication happened by chance, and the parents are probably not at any greater risk of having another child with autism than the general population, Marion said.

Still, there is much geneticists can't tell parents. Between 10% and 15% of autism cases can be traced to a known genetic cause, the researchers noted. Of that, CMA alone can detect 7% of those. There are a few other genetic tests that can explain another few percentage points of autism cases. But that leaves 85% or more families with little explanation for the disorder, Marion said. "CMA is better, but it's not great," Marion said. "The vast majority of children who have autism have no identifiable genetic markers that will help in genetic counseling for future pregnancies. That is very frustrating."

# Chapter 19

# *Language in Children with ASD*

## *Introduction*

Autism is a neurodevelopmental disorder characterized by primary impairments in social interactions, communication, and repetitive and stereotyped behaviors (American Psychiatric Association, 2000). In addition, autism often results in significant disability, including intellectual deficits, language and adaptive behavior deficits, as well as problem behaviors. It is now recognized that classic autism is part of a spectrum of related disorders that includes pervasive developmental disorder-not otherwise specified (PDD-NOS) and Asperger syndrome; this set of diagnoses, collectively, is referred to here as autism spectrum disorders (ASD). Outcomes for children with ASD represent a broad continuum, with only a small percentage achieving independence and full employment as adults (Howlin, Goode, Hutton, and Rutter, 2004). ASDs are no longer thought to be rare disorders. Current reports indicate that one in every 150 children in the United States will receive an ASD diagnosis (Bertrand, Mars, Byle, Bove, 2001; Kuehn, 2007; Yeargin-Allsopp, Rice, Karapurka, Doernberg, Boyle, Murphy, 2003).

Children with ASD have long been known to respond to interventions that target specific skills and behaviors (NRC, 2001), and numerous

"Defining Spoken Language Benchmarks and Selecting Measures of Expressive Language Development for Young Children with Autism Spectrum Disorders," by Helen Tager-Flusberg, et al. *Journal of Speech, Language, and Hearing Research Volume 52*, pp 643–52, June 2009. © 2009 American Speech-Language-Hearing Association. Reprinted with permission.

studies have demonstrated the positive effects of early intervention on language development for the majority of children with ASD (Dawson and Osterling, 1997; Koegel and Koegel, 1988; Lovaas, 1987; Rogers, 2005; Rogers and Vismara, 2008), with some, though sparse, evidence of long-lasting benefit. The fact that language development can be positively affected by early treatment has tremendous potential significance because the emergence of spoken language is one of the most important variables predicting better outcomes in later childhood and adulthood (Gillberg and Steffenburg, 1987; Howlin et al., 2004; Venter, Lord, and Schopler, 1992). Thus, given the role of language acquisition in shaping long-term outcomes, it has become important to identify the most successful strategies for facilitating language acquisition in young children with ASD, who uniformly demonstrate significant delays in at least some aspects of language and communicative development, especially in the domain of pragmatics (Tager-Flusberg, Paul and Lord, 2005).

While various intervention approaches teach and measure language acquisition in different ways, depending on the philosophy and underlying theory of the approach (see Rogers 2005 for a review), consumers of this literature must be able to compare language outcomes from different treatment approaches. Despite the numerous published language outcome studies of early intervention in ASD (Rogers, 2005), it is not possible to compare language outcomes across reports because of the lack of uniform measurement approaches to assessing language skills, and the lack of uniform terminology for describing language outcomes in ASD. Many intervention programs for children with ASD aim to facilitate the development of functional speech. However, because there has never been consensus on the definition of functional speech it is impossible to compare the longer term efficacy of different treatment programs. In this paper, we offer an alternative framework for describing spoken language acquisition in children with ASD. The proposal described here replaces the arbitrary singular categorical distinction encompassed by the terminology of functional speech with a framework that captures the continuous developmental processes that underlie language acquisition.

## Goals

In December 2006, the National Institute on Deafness and Other Communication Disorders (NIDCD) assembled a group of experts in language disorders and language acquisition in young children with ASD to address these issues. Over the next year, the group worked together through a series of conference calls and correspondence culminating in a meeting held in December 2007. This paper summarizes the group's recommendations relating to our primary goal of providing benchmarks for defining the acquisition of spoken language in the expressive modality in young children with ASD.

The working group set two major objectives:

1. To develop a set of recommended measures that can be used for evaluating the efficacy of interventions that target spoken language acquisition as part of treatment research studies or for use in applied settings.

2. To propose and define a common terminology for describing levels of spoken language ability and set benchmarks for determining a child's spoken language level in order to establish a framework for comparing outcomes across intervention studies.

As such, this chapter is addressed primarily to researchers; however, practitioners and other consumers are also relevant audiences. For researchers in early autism intervention who may come from a wide range of theoretical backgrounds and practices, our goal is to provide common terminology and a suggested approach to defining language abilities before, during, and after treatment. The varying measurement approaches used in language intervention research require different levels of financial and human resources and expertise. In addition, researchers have differing aims and hypotheses that may require specialized descriptions of language acquisition of their participants. Thus, we propose a measurement approach that may be applied in a "bare bones" fashion (for example, relying on direct assessments and parent reports), as well as a more elaborated measurement system (such as, adding in measures derived from natural language samples), covering the full range of language domains that could be included in treatment programs. By proposing these guidelines we hope to move beyond the ambiguously defined treatment goal of functional speech to a more standardized approach, using common measures and common definitions that will allow comparison of outcomes across studies.

For practitioners, the proposed measures and benchmarks presented here provide a framework for describing the language progress of their clients during treatment. By providing a common framework we hope to facilitate the assessment process for clinicians allowing them to measure their clients' language gains in relation to the research literature. Thus, we aim to enhance the relationship between treatment research and clinical practice in the field of language intervention in ASD.

Our final target group of readers includes parents, early intervention professionals, and others who work to extract evidence of progress, whether research effectiveness or clinical efficacy, from clinical reports and research papers that use language measures to chart change in children with ASD. Clearly defined benchmarks of speech and language development will aid families, early childhood educators, and others who turn to the language research literature to understand language growth in young children with ASD.

Some additional comments are in order. First, we focus here exclusively on the development of spoken language through the preschool years, omitting consideration of measures and benchmarks for defining preverbal communicative skills. While the working group recognizes that sophisticated language skills take many forms, including both verbal and non-verbal means for effective communication, and that children with ASD continue to make important advances in language well into the school years, we selected these constraints because outcome studies are uniform in the predictive power of spoken language (for example, speaking in sentences that serve a variety of functions; Paul and Cohen, 1984) by age five for individuals with ASD (for example, Howlin et al., 2004; Venter et al., 1992). Second, we limited our focus to the development of expressive language skills in children with ASD because most intervention studies target expressive language as the primary outcome and also because expressive language is more reliably assessed, especially in children with ASD (compare Tager-Flusberg, 2000). Third, we have limited our recommendations for measures and benchmarks to English, in part because almost all current studies have focused on English-speaking children with ASD. We hope, however, that the overall framework and guidelines presented here can be readily translated into other languages with some modifications.

## Recommendations for Measuring Expressive Language

In order to capture the spoken language and communicative abilities of young children with ASD and to avoid sampling effects, assessments in this domain should include measures derived from multiple sources. These sources should ideally include (1) natural language samples, (2) parent report, and (3) direct standardized assessment.

### Natural Language Sample (NLS)

Natural language samples that are collected in different communicative contexts provide excellent measures of a child's expressive language abilities, including phonological repertoire, lexical and grammatical knowledge, and pragmatic/communicative skills; the latter are especially difficult to measure using other types of assessment. A NLS may be collected during either experimenter/clinician-child or mother-child interactions. Contexts during which a NLS may be collected include the administration of the Autism Diagnostic Observation Schedule (ADOS; Lord et al., 2000), the Communication and Symbolic Behavior Scales (CSBS; Wetherby and Prizant, 2002), the Early Social and Communication Scales (ESCS; Mundy et al. 1996; Siebert et al., 1982), or equivalent contexts that include social communicative presses. The specific context should be determined based on the goals of the assessment. For example, if a primary outcome measure of a treatment program includes the functional use of specifically targeted forms, then adequate sampling of a range of different communicative contexts (such as, contexts for requesting, protesting, sharing) would be needed.

Typically, natural language samples will be at least 30 minutes in length to provide adequate time and opportunity to sample a sufficient number and range of utterances. For children with ASD, one may need to concatenate several short language samples to obtain 30 minutes of language behavior. Following the collection of a NLS (see Miller and Chapman, 2000 for discussion of methods), the data must be transcribed and coded to derive useful measures of the child's language. The particular level of transcription (for example: phonetic, lexical, inclusion of adult language) will again depend on the specific focus of the assessment. Transcription and analyses can be supported by computer-based software, including the widely used Systematic Analysis of Language Transcripts (SALT; Miller and Chapman, 2008), Child Language Data Exchange System (CHILDES; MacWhinney, 2000), Lingquest (Mordecai and Palin, 1982), or Computerized Profiling (Long and Fey, 2004).

### Parent Report

Parent report measures, administered in questionnaire or interview format, can provide useful information about a child's language skills that may not be observed in a laboratory or clinic setting. The most widely used measure is the MacArthur-Bates Communicative Development Inventory (MCDI; Fenson et al., 1993; 2007). The MCDI can be used to assess children's expressive vocabulary and grammatical knowledge between the ages of 8–42 months. Although there are concerns that some parents may over- or under-report their child's language repertoire, parent report instruments have generally been shown to provide valid assessments of young children's language as measured by evidence that early predictors of language also predict MCDI productive raw scores in children with ASD (Charman, Baron-Cohen, Swettenham, Baird, Drew, and Cox, 2003; Luyster, Qui, Lopez and Lord, 2007). There is also evidence that MDCI scores are highly correlated with other measures of language in children with autism (Luyster, Kadlec, Connolly, Carter and Tager-Flusberg, 2008).

### Direct Assessment/Standardized Tests

Direct assessment of a child's language skills should be accomplished using standardized tests that have good psychometric properties with particular attention paid to the reliability and validity of the measures that are derived from such tests for children with ASD. Standardized tests can be used to assess expressive language skills in phonological, lexical, grammatical, and pragmatic domains of language. We note, however, that few standardized assessment instruments provide opportunities for assessing language skills aside from basic naming ability in children younger than 24 months of age. In addition, most elicited production tests have very few items during this early language period, which means that age equivalency or standard scores can change dramatically with a difference of only one or two raw score points.

### Imitation/Echolalia

Many children in the process of acquiring language use imitation and repetition of spoken language, especially during the early stages, to serve some functional communicative goals. Echolalia and stereotyped language, consisting of scripts heard in previous contexts repeated in a non-communicative way, are atypical imitation behaviors that are part of the symptom pattern of ASDs (Kanner, 1946; Prizant, 1983). During the early stages of language acquisition, it may be difficult to discriminate typical from atypical verbal repetition in young children, and there are no clear criteria for defining delayed echolalia (Prizant and Duchan, 1981). Nevertheless, when characterizing the complexity of children's language, we recommend that echolalic (and imitative) language should be omitted from analyses and from speech samples used to classify children according to the benchmarks described in the following pages.

192

## Framework for Describing Spoken Language Acquisition in ASD

We take as our starting point a developmental approach in which we benchmark criteria for the acquisition of spoken language and recommend measures for expressive language at different development levels. For each level, we provide approximate age ranges though these should be viewed as overlapping and not necessarily definitive. A developmental perspective provides a conceptual framework to guide intervention and evaluation of children with ASD, ensuring that researchers and clinicians strategically plan to target key language milestones within language intervention programs for children with ASD. Within a developmental framework, we identify five key phases of expressive language acquisition:

1. **Preverbal communication:** Children in this phase communicate using preverbal intentional communication through vocal (babble) and gestural means. This phase generally covers the age range of 6–12 months in typically developing children. As noted earlier, we have not included measures or benchmarks for this developmental phase as it is outside the scope of our goals.

2. **First words:** Children in this phase use non-imitated spontaneous single words referentially and symbolically to communicate about objects and events, including those outside the immediate context. At least some of their speech is intelligible and incorporates the most frequent consonant sounds heard in typical babble (Oller, 2000; Stoel-Gammon, 1998). Children in this phase use speech with a variety of people in different settings to serve several functions, including, but not limited to, labeling, requesting, and commenting on (directing joint attention) some objects or activities. This phase generally covers the age range of 12–18 months in typically developing children.

3. **Word combinations:** Children in this phase have a vocabulary that is rapidly increasing in size and includes a variety of parts of speech (nouns, verbs, descriptors). They are able to combine words creatively to refer to objects and events. Two- and three-word combinations are used for several different communicative functions. This phase generally covers the age range of 18–30 months in typically developing children.

4. **Sentences:** Children in this phase combine words into clausal structures, or sentences, and use some morphological

193

markers such as plurals, prepositions, and some verb endings. Their vocabulary is sufficiently large to serve their communicative needs in everyday situations. They communicate a wide range of functions in different settings with both familiar and unfamiliar people. The portion of this phase relevant for the proposed benchmarks defined here corresponds to typically developing children between the ages of 30–48 months.

5. **Complex language:** By the end of the preschool years, typically developing children have large and rich vocabularies that they use to communicate a wide range of topics (including abstract or hypothetical ideas) using complex grammatical constructions (for example: relative clauses, sentential complements, anaphora) in different discourse contexts (such as conversation, narrative). We do not include either measures or benchmarks for this developmental phase (excluding measures not designed for children below the age of 48 months) as our focus is primarily on younger children with ASD. (For further reading, see Hoff and Shatz, 2007; Menn and Bernstein Ratner, 2000).

## Language Benchmarks

Table 19.1 provides a summary of our proposed benchmarks that define the key developmental phases for spoken language expression (first words, word combinations; sentences) across the different domains of language, with examples of how each type of measure can be used to assess children's level of language use. As noted earlier, our objective in presenting this framework of benchmarks in each language domain at different developmental phases is explicitly designed to move away from the commonly used term functional speech as the outcome goal for intervention studies.

The benchmarks presented in Table 19.1 can be used for multiple purposes: (1) evaluating whether a child meets criteria for achieving the various language phases in the context of treatment research; (2) as measures to be incorporated into intervention studies; or (3) as a means for monitoring a child's progress in ongoing community treatment. Although we present our benchmarks in each of the developing phases of language, it is important to keep in mind that these phases are dynamic and overlapping periods that, in reality, have no clear boundaries.

194

## *Criteria for Defining a Child's Language Level*

Some treatment studies include goals to advance a child's language to a particular level. For example, in studies that begin with very young or preverbal children (for example, children who do not meet the criteria for being in the first words phase), the goal might be to provide interventions that lead the child into becoming verbal—which might then be defined as the first words level. Other studies might have a more flexible goal of advancing children to the next level within a prescribed treatment period, or to chart language gains based on continuous measures (such as, number of different consonants, words, or communication functions). Across all intervention studies, criteria for defining each language phase will facilitate the comparison of different treatment studies that may have different designs or measures.

For each language phase we defined the minimum criteria for evaluating a child's language level: In order for a child to be considered to be at a particular level of expressive language functioning, the child's measured language must meet at least one of the defined minimum benchmarks in every language domain that defines that phase. This stringent approach recognizes the comprehensive developmental approach to language acquisition in children with ASD that we have proposed, one which encompasses all aspects of language used to communicate effectively with others in everyday life.

Though each phase contains benchmarks for all language domains based on how language develops in typically developing children, we recognize that particularly in children with ASD there is likely to be asynchrony across different language domains (for example, vocabulary development may be significantly more advanced than pragmatics). This will result in a mixed phase profile for many children. A child might meet minimum criteria for one phase in all domains and also meet criteria for the more advanced level in one or two domains assessed. Researchers or clinicians may choose to describe a child's language separately for each language domain in place of the criteria defining the language phase.

### *First Words*

This phase represents the emergence of spoken language covering the age range of 12–18 months in typically developing children. The benchmarks targeting this phase are placed at the 15 month age-equivalent level. To conclude that a child has reached the first words phase, he or she must meet the following criteria within each of the following domains:

- *Phonology:* Meets one of the two phonological criteria presented in Table 19.1 based on a NLS.

- *Vocabulary:* Meets criterion for number of different words used on the NLS, or the age-equivalent criterion on a parent report measure, or the age-equivalent criterion on a direct assessment measure.

- *Pragmatics:* Meets criterion of a minimum of two communicative functions, including use of spoken language to comment.

## Word Combinations

The phase covers the age range of 18–30 months in typically developing children. The benchmarks targeting this phase are placed at the 24-month age-equivalent level. The following criteria define meeting the benchmarks for this phase:

- *Phonology:* Meets one of the four phonological criteria presented in Table 19.1 based on a NLS.

- *Vocabulary:* Meets criterion for number of different words used on the NLS or the age-equivalent criterion on a parent report measure, or the age-equivalent criterion on a direct assessment measure. The table lists one measure that focuses exclusively on vocabulary at this age range; in addition a number of direct assessment tests, for example the Mullen Scales for Early Learning (Mullen, 1995), Reynell Developmental Language Scales (Reynell and Gruber, 1990), or Preschool Language Scale-4 (Zimmerman, Steiner and Pond, 2002) all provide measures of expressive language that combine vocabulary and word combination/grammar items. These measures may be used as an alternative to cover the vocabulary and grammar domains for this phase.

- *Grammar:* Meets the criteria on the NLS, parent report, or direct assessment measures (see previous) listed.

- *Pragmatics:* Meets criterion for one of the three measures based on the NLS or the age-equivalent score on a parent report measure.

## Sentences

This phase covers the broad age range from 30–48 months in typically developing children. The benchmarks are targeted to the 36-month age-equivalent level. The following criteria need to be met for this phase:

196

- *Phonology:* Meets criterion of 75% intelligible in a NLS, or a 36-month level on a direct assessment measure.

- *Vocabulary:* Meets criterion for number of different words used on the NLS or the age-equivalent criterion on a direct assessment measure.

- *Grammar:* Meets criterion for a 36-month age-equivalent score on a direct assessment measure or the MLU criterion on a NLS. By this phase it is strongly preferred that the NLS include a minimum of 100 spontaneous (non-imitative/echolalic) child utterances, for obtaining a more reliable MLU estimate.

- *Pragmatics:* Meets criterion based on an elicited narrative, or the criterion for a conversational NLS, or a 36-month age-equivalent on parent report or direct assessment measures.

## Conclusions

This report represents the consensus of our working group based on discussions carried out over the course of 18 months. We offer here the following summary and conclusions.

We recommend a move away from using the term functional speech as a goal for intervention research and practice, replacing it with a developmental framework. We recognize that the impetus for the use of the term came from studies suggesting that achieving functional speech by age five is an important prognostic indicator in children with ASD. Nevertheless, it is not clear from the literature what definitions earlier studies relied on, though the descriptions in these studies suggest that children with optimal outcomes were able to speak in full sentences serving a range of communicative functions (Paul and Cohen, 1984). In our view, given the significant changes in the age of diagnosis and the increased access to early intensive intervention, it is time to re-open the question of the timing and role of language acquisition as key prognostic indicators in ASD.

In evaluating treatment outcomes, we depend on objective measures, but we recognize that the measures available to us are imperfect. This is particularly evident when assessing the earliest phases of language in the emergence of words, grammatical combinations or the pragmatic uses of communication for which few if any standardized direct assessments are available for children under the age of two. To address these limitations, we encourage the use of measures derived from natural language samples and parent report. We recognize that the collection, transcription, and coding of natural language samples

197

**Table 19.1.** Proposed Benchmarks That Define the Key Developmental Phases for Spoken Language Expression (continued on next page)

| Language Phase | Language Domain | Measures | Variables | Range in Typical Development | Example | Minimum Criteria |
|---|---|---|---|---|---|---|
| First Words 12–18 months | Phonology | NLS<br>NLS | CV combinations or<br>Consonant inventory | CV-CVC<br>2–8 different consonants | hi, Mommy<br>m, b, y, n, w, d, p, h (Early 8) | CV, or<br>4 consonants |
| | Vocabulary | NLS | # different words used referentially in 20 mins. or | 2–15 words | more, bubble, go, open, ball | 5 types and 20 tokens, or |
| | | Parent Report | # different word roots or | (range for 13–18 mo.) | MCDI | AE for 15 months, or |
| | | Direct Assessment | Confrontation naming | (range for 13–18 mo.) | Mullen, Reynell | AE for 15 months |
| | Pragmatics | NLS | # different communicative functions or | 2–5 functions | comments, request | Comments + 1 other or |
| | | Direct Assessment | # communication functions | (range for 13–18 mo.) | CSBS | AE for 15 months. |
| Word Combinations 18–30 months | Phonology | NLS | CV combinations or<br>Word structures or<br>% fully intelligible or<br># consonants | CV-CCVCC<br>1–3 syllable words<br>40–80%<br>8–18 consonants | go, drink<br>Early 8 + t, ng, k, g, f, v, ch, j | Closed syllables or<br>Syllable words, or<br>50% intelligible, or<br>10 consonants |
| | Vocabulary | NLS | # different words used referentially in 20 min. or | 10–50 words | MCDI, LDS EOWVT | 30 words, or |
| | | Parent Report | # different words or | (range for 21–27 mo.) | | 24 mo. AE, or |
| | | Direct Assessment | Confrontation naming | 21–27 mo. age range | | 24 mo. AE |
| | Grammar | NLS | mean length of utterance or | MLU: 1.1–2.4 (in morphemes) | MCDI See text | MLU=1.8, or |
| | | Parent Report | mean length in words of 3 longest utterances or | (ranges for 21–27 mo.; on MCDI:2.6–5.5) | | MCDI: 3.8, or |
| | | Direct Assessment | | | | 24 mo. AE |
| | Pragmatics | NLS | # different communicative functions or<br>Proportional JA + Social/Total Comm. Acts or<br>Conversational functions or | 3–6 functions<br>.3–.7<br>responds and initiates | comments, request, turn-taking<br>answer/ask question | comments, requests, or<br>0.5, or<br>2 initiations+2 responses |
| | | Parent Report | Inventory of child's communicative use | 21–27 mo. age range | LUI | 24 mo. AE |

Table 19.1, *continued*

| Sentences 30–48 months | | | | | |
|---|---|---|---|---|---|
| Phonology | NLS | % fully intelligible or | 70–100% | | 75% intelligible, or |
| | NLS | Consonant Inventory or | 16–24 different C; 75% correct | Previous Ca+ sh, th, s, z, l, zh | |
| | Direct Assessment | AE score | | GFTA-2 | 36 mo. AE |
| Vocabulary | NLS | # different word roots or | 70–136 in 65 utterances (range for 30–48 mo.) | SALT norms | 92 in 65 utterances |
| | Direct Assessment | AE score | | | 36 mo. AE |
| Grammar | NLS | MLU in morphemes or | 2.7–4.0 MLU | | MLU=3.0, or |
| | Direct Assessment | AE score | | TEGI; SPELT-3 | 36 mo. AE |
| Pragmatics | Elicited NLS | Discourses functions or | narration | pretense; talk about past/future | 1 narrative, or |
| | NLS | Conversational topic-related turn taking or | | | 2 full turns on same topic, or |
| | Parent Report | Inventory of child's communicative use or | 30–48 mo. age range | LUI | 36 mo. AE, or |
| | Direct Assessment | Communicative functions | 30–48 mo. age range | CASL | 36 mo. AE on Pragmatic subtest |

**Key**

**Tests:**

Mullen: Mullen Scales of Early Learning (Mullen, 1995)
Reynell: Reynell Developmental Language Scales (Reynell and Gruber, 1990)
CSBS: Communication and Symbolic Behavior Scales (Wetherby and Prizant, 2002)
MCDI: MacArthur-Bates Communicative Development Inventory (Fenson et al., 2007)
LDS: Language Development Survey (Rescorla, 1989)
EOWVT: Expressive One Word Vocabulary Test-Revised (Gardner, 1990)
LUI: Language Use Inventory (O'Neil, 2007)
GFTA-2: Goldman-Fristoe Test of Articulation-2 (Goldman and Fristoe, 2000)
SALT norms: Miller and Chapman (1981)
TEGI: Test of Early Grammatical Impairment (Rice and Wexler, 2001)
SPELT 3: Structured Photographic Expressive Language Test 3 (Dawson and Stout, 2003)
CASL: Comprehensive Assessment of Spoken Language (Carrow-Woolfolk, 1999)

**Other Abbreviations:**

NLS: Natural Language Sample
AE: Age equivalent
MLU: Mean Length of Utterance
C: Consonant
V: Vowel

involves increased labor costs in research and clinical settings. However, we believe this cost cannot be avoided if we are to ensure that the data gathered have the highest degree of validity possible.

We provide objective criteria for defining children's expressive language development in order to provide guidance to researchers and clinicians who assess language in young children with ASD. These may be used to guide intervention research as well as treatment offered in clinical settings. The use of benchmarks based on typical development for charting children's progress reflects findings that language development in early ASD generally follows a similar developmental pathway as in other children (Tager-Flusberg et al., 2005). Using benchmarks from typical development also draws attention to those typical language milestones that should be targeted by early intervention programs. These definitions and benchmarks will allow comparisons of outcomes across different studies.

Finally, we set ourselves a practical goal: to provide a common vocabulary for discussing language acquisition to a wide interdisciplinary professional and lay audience. The terms selected for the benchmarks are intended to be transparent, reflecting important language features that define them. For each benchmark, we have provided definitions for behavior that can be objectively assessed by a broad range of early intervention professionals.

The framework we have developed here should be expanded in several ways: (1) incorporating benchmarks for identifying a range of preverbal communication skills; (2) development of valid and reliable measures of language comprehension for children with ASD; (3) adaptation of the framework for assessing children who communicate using AAC systems; and (4) evaluating the relative merits of different types of measures for children with ASD. Further research is needed to address these important issues, nevertheless, we hope that the concepts and recommendations presented in this paper will enhance early intervention research targeting spoken language development in ASD and will provide clinical professionals the ability to extract and clearly define important information about treatment effectiveness in their work.

## *Notes*

The group was co-chaired by Helen Tager-Flusberg, Sally Rogers and Judith Cooper (NIH). Members included Rebecca Landa, Catherine Lord, Rhea Paul, Mabel Rice, Carol Stoel-Gammon, Amy Wetherby and Paul Yoder.

We have limited our recommendations on measures and benchmarks to spoken language, although we recognize that many children with ASD who do not speak can successfully acquire some expressive language skills using augmentative or alternative communication (AAC) systems such as vocal-output devices or manual signing. We have not included a detailed presentation of how our framework might apply to interventions that target AAC systems as there are no clear guidelines available for how to measure non-spoken language skills that are comparable to those available for spoken language.

Children with ASD will often have a very small spoken vocabulary used primarily to regulate others' behavior, however, unless the criteria for the definition of the first words phase as specified in Table 19.1 are met, they should be considered to be in the preverbal communication phase.

## References

American Psychiatric Association (2000). *Diagnostic and statistical manual of mental disorders. Fourth Edition, Text Revision*. Washington, DC: Author.

Bertrand, J., Mars, A., Byle, C., Bove, F., Yeargin-Allsopp, M., and Decoufle, P. (2001). Prevalence of autism in a United States population: The Brick Township, New Jersey, investigation. *Pediatrics, 108*, 1155–1161.

Carrow-Woolfolk, E. (1999). *Comprehensive Assessment of Spoken Language*. Bloomington, MN: Pearson Assessments.

Charman, T., Baron-Cohen, S., Swettenham, J., Baird, G., Drew, A., and Cox, A. (2003). Predicting language outcome in infants with autism and pervasive developmental disorder. *International Journal of Language and Communication Disorders, 38*, 265–285.

Dawson, G., and Osterling, J. (1997). Early intervention in autism: Effectiveness and common elements of current approaches. In M.J.Guralnick (Ed.), *The effectiveness of early intervention: Second generation research*. (pp. 307–326). Baltimore, MD: Brookes Publishing Co.

Dawson, J. and Stout, C. (2003). *The Structured Photographic Expressive Language Test–Third Edition*. DeKalb, IL: Janelle Publications.

Fenson, L., Dale, P. S., Reznick, S., Thal, D., Bates, E., Hartung, J. P., Pethick, S., and Reilly, J. S. (1993). *MacArthur Communicative Development*

*Inventories: User's guide and technical manual.* Baltimore, MD: Paul H. Brookes.

Fenson, L., Marchman, V., Thal, D., Reznick, S., and Bates, E. (2007). *MacArthur-Bates Communicative Development Inventories: User's guide and technical manual–Second edition.* Baltimore, MD: Paul H. Brookes.

Gardner, M. F. (1990). *Expressive One Word Vocabulary Test–Revised.* Los Angeles, CA: Western Psychological Services

Gillberg, C., and Steffenburg, S. (1987). Outcome and prognostic factors in infantile autism and similar conditions: A population-based study of 46 cases followed through puberty. *Journal of Autism and Developmental Disorders, 17,* 273–287.

Goldman, R. and Fristoe, M. (2000). *Goldman-Fristoe Test of Articulation–2.* Cicle Pines, MN: American Guidance Service.

Hoff, E. and Schatz, M. (Eds.), (2007). *Handbook of language development.* Oxford: Blackwell.

Howlin, P., Goode, S., Hutton, J. and Rutter, M. (2004). Adult outcome for children with autism. *Journal of Child Psychology and Psychiatry, 45,* 212–229.

Kanner, L. (1946). Irrelevant and metaphorical language. *American Journal of Psychiatry, 103,* 242–246.

Koegel, R., and Koegel, L. K. (1988). Generalized responsivity and pivotal behavior. In R. H. Horner, G. Dunlap, and R. L. Koegel (Eds.), *Generalization and maintenance: Lifestyle changes in applied settings,* (pp. 41–66). Baltimore: Paul H. Brookes Publishing Co.

Kuehn, B. M. (2007). CDC: Autism Spectrum Disorders Common. *Journal of the American Medical Association, 297,* 940

Lovaas, O. I. (1987). Behavioral treatment and normal educational and intellectual functioning in young autistic children. *Journal of Consulting and Clinical Psychology, 55,* 3–9.

Long, S. and Fey, M. (2004). *Computerized profiling* (Computer program version 6.9). Milwaukee, WI: Marquette University.

Lord, C., Risi, S., Lambrecht, L., Cook, E. H., Leventhal, B. L., DiLavore, P. S., Pickles, A., and Rutter, M. (2000). The Autism Diagnostic Observation Schedule–Generic: A standard measure of social and communication deficits associated with the spectrum of Autism. *Journal of Autism and Developmental Disorders, 30,* 205–223.

Luyster, R. Qui, S., Lopez, K., and Lord, C. (2007). Predicting outcomes of children referred for autism using the MacArthur-Bates Communicative Development Inventory. *Journal of Speech, Language, and Hearing Research, 50*, 667–681.

Luyster, R., Kadlec, M. B., Connolly, C., Carter, A., and Tager–Flusberg, H. (2008). Language assessment and development in toddlers with autism spectrum disorders. *Journal of Autism and Developmental Disorders, 38*, 1426–1438.

MacWhinney, B. (2000). *The CHILDES Project: Tools for Analyzing Talk (Third Edition)*. Mahwah, NJ: Lawrence Erlbaum Associates.

Menn, L. and Bernstein Ratner, N. (Eds). (2000). *Methods for studying language production*. Mahwah, NJ: Lawrence Erlbaum Associates.

Miller, J. and Chapman, R. (1981). The relation between age and mean length of utterance in morphemes. *Journal of Speech and Hearing Research, 24*, 154–161.

Miller, J. and Chapman, R. (2000). *Systematic Analysis of Language Transcripts (SALT)*. Madison, WI: Language Analysis Lab.

Miller, J. and Chapman, R. (2008). *Systematic Analysis of Language Transcripts* (SALT Software). Madison, WI: Language Analysis Lab.

Mordecai, D. and Palin, M. (1982). *Lingquest 1 and 2* (Computer Program). East Moline, IL: Lingquest Software.

Mullen, E. (1995). *Mullen Scales of Early Learning*. Circle Pines, MN: American Guidance Service.

Mundy, P., Hogan, A., and Doehring, P. (1996). *A preliminary manual for the abridged Early Social Communication Scales (ESCS)*. Coral Gables, FL: University of Miami.

National Research Council. (2001). *Educating children with autism*. Washington, DC: National Academy Press.

O'Neill, D. (2007). The Language Use Inventory for young children: A parent–report measure of pragmatic language development for 18- to 47-month-old children. *Journal of Speech, Language and Hearing Research, 50*, 214–228.

Oller, K. (2000). *The emergence of the speech capacity*. Mahwah, NJ: Lawrence Erlbaum Associates.

Paul, R., and Cohen, D. J. (1984). Outcomes of severe disorders of language acquisition. *Journal of Autism and Developmental Disorders, 14*, 405–422.

Prizant, B.M. (1983). Echolalia in autism: Assessment and intervention. *Seminars in Speech and Language, 4,* 63–77.

Prizant, B., and Duchan, J. (1981). The functions of immediate echolalia in autistic children. *Journal of Speech and Hearing Disorders, 46,* 241–249.

Rescorla, L. (1989). The Language Development Survey. A screening tool for delayed language in toddlers. *Journal of Speech Language and Hearing Research, 54,* 587–599.

Reynell, J. K. and Gruber, C. P. (1990). *Reynell Developmental Language Scales.* Western Psychological Services.

Rice, M. L. and Wexler, K. (2001). *Rice / Wexler Test of Early Grammatical Impairment.* San Antonio TX: Pearson Education Inc.

Rogers, S. J. (2005). Evidence-based practices for language development in young children with autism. In T. Charman and W. Stone (Eds), *Social and Communication development in autism spectrum disorders* (pp. 143–179) New York: Guilford.

Rogers, S. J., and Vismara, L. A. (2008). Evidence-based comprehensive treatments for early autism. *Journal of Clinical Child and Adolescent Psychology, 37,* 8–38.

Seibert, J., Hogan, A., and Mundy, P. (1982). Assessing social interactional competencies: The early social-communication scales. *Infant Mental Health Journal, 3,* 244–258.

Stoel-Gammon, C. (1998). Sounds and words in early language acquisition: The relations between lexical and phonological development. In R. Paul (Ed.). *Exploring the speech-language connection* (pp. 25–52). Baltimore, MD: Paul H. Brookes.

Tager-Flusberg, H. (2000). The challenge of studying language development in autism. In L. Menn and N. Bernstein Ratner (Eds.) *Methods for studying language production* (pp. 313–332). Mahwah, NJ: Lawrence Erlbaum Associates.

Tager-Flusberg, H., Paul, R., and Lord, C.E. (2005). Language and communication in autism. In F. Volkmar, R. Paul, A. Klin and D. J. Cohen (Eds.) *Handbook of autism and pervasive developmental disorder, Third Edition, Volume 1* (pp. 335–364). New York: Wiley.

Venter, A., Lord, C., and Schopler, E. (1992). A follow-up study of high-functioning autistic children. *Journal of Child Psychology and Psychiatry, 33,* 489–507.

Wetherby, A. and Prizant, B. (2002). *Communication and Symbolic Behavior Scales*. Baltimore, MD: Paul H. Brookes.

Yeargin-Allsopp, M., Rice, C., Karapurkar, T., Doernberg, N., Boyle, C., and Murphy, C. (2003). Prevalence of autism in a U.S. metropolitan area. *Journal of the American Medical Association, 28*, 249–255.

Zimmerman, I. L., Steiner, V. G., and Pond, R. E. (2002). *Preschool Language Scale, Fourth Edition (PLS–4)*. Harcourt Assessment.

# Chapter 20

# *Measuring*
# *Autistic Intelligence*

There are frequent claims in the literature that a majority of children with autism are mentally retarded (MR). The present study examined the evidence used as the basis for these claims, reviewing 215 articles published between 1937 and 2003. Results indicated 74% of the claims came from nonempirical sources, 53% of which never traced back to empirical data. Most empirical evidence for the claims was published 25 to 45 years ago and was often obtained utilizing developmental or adaptive scales rather than measures of intelligence. Furthermore, significantly higher prevalence rates of MR were reported when these measures were used. Overall, the findings indicate that more empirical evidence is needed before conclusions can be made about the percentages of children with autism who are mentally retarded.

To be diagnosed with autism in the United States, a child must meet criteria as defined in the *Diagnostic and Statistical Manual of Mental Disorders (DSM)*. The child's cognitive ability has never been part of the diagnostic criteria for autism in any of the versions of the DSM in which autism has appeared (American Psychiatric Association [APA], 1980, 1987, 1994, 2000). However, the authors of the current manual, *DSM-IV Text Revision (TR)*, note that "in most cases, there is an associated diagnosis of mental retardation, which can range from mild to profound" (APA, 2000, p. 71). In fact, in each version of the *DSM*, mental retardation (MR) has been considered an associated condition of autism, and in some versions of the manual, it is noted that 70% to 75% of children with autism are also mentally retarded (APA, 1980, 1994).

Autism was first described by Kanner (1943), who maintained that children with autism had normal intellectual functioning; he stated that "even though most of these children were at one time or another looked upon as feebleminded, they are all unquestionably endowed with good cognitive potentialities" (p. 247; Kanner's emphasis). Kanner never systematically nor empirically assessed the intelligence of individuals with autism; his statements were made based on observations of 11 children. There were, however, early studies that did obtain empirical evidence regarding the intelligence of children with autism; rates of MR in samples of children with autism were typically between 30% and 40% in these reports (Pollack, 1958), much lower than the rates cited today. Questions arise as to when the assumptions about the rates of MR in children with autism changed and, more importantly, upon what evidence they changed.

Creak (1961) was the first author to make a claim that children with autism were likely to have MR. As part of a working group for establishing diagnostic criteria for autism in Great Britain, Creak described nine criteria for schizophrenic syndrome of childhood, one of which was "a background of serious retardation in which islets of normal, near normal, or exceptional functioning or skill may appear" (Creak, 1961, p. 818). In a subsequent paper, Creak (1963) again claimed that the psychotic child "is the most ineducable of any" (p. 88). The empirical evidence at the time, while scant, did not support Creak's assertions that there was generally a "background of serious retardation," and Creak herself never cited any evidence for her claims. However, shortly after Creak's publications, researchers began finding much higher rates of MR in children with autism, and this seemed to follow other nonempirical claims that could be traced back to Creak (for example: Lockyer and Rutter, 1970; Rutter, 1974). Since then, hundreds of additional claims have been made, and currently it is commonly reported that between 67% and 90% of children with autism also have MR.

To date, no systematic examination of the evidence for the claims regarding the rates of MR in children with autism has been conducted. In view of this, the purpose of the present study was to examine the origin of the statistics regarding the high prevalence rates of MR in children with autism to ascertain the nature of the support for these statistics. Before this examination can take place, it is important first to understand how a diagnosis of MR is made and how intelligence level is typically assessed. A diagnosis of MR is based on three criteria: cognitive impairments defined by IQ scores less than 70, adaptive skills deficits, and age of onset prior to 18 years (APA, 2000). Children who have autism will meet the latter two criteria as part of meeting the diagnostic criteria for autism (APA, 2000). However, because intelligence level is independent of a diagnosis of autism, the focus of the present examination is specifically on intelligence determination in children with autism.

In children without autism, standard measures of intelligence, such as the *Wechsler Intelligence Scale for Children—Third edition* (WISC-III; Wechsler, 1991) or the *Stanford-Binet* (Thorndike, Hagen, and Sattler, 1986), are frequently used. Although these and other intelligence tests were frequently used with children with autism in the 1960s and 1970s, this practice has been largely discontinued because of the acknowledgment that there are often language difficulties (see Tager-Flusberg, 1989; Rutter, 1978), attention deficits (see Burack, Enns, Stauder, Mottron, and Randolph, 1997; Dawson and Lewy, 1989), and processing delays and dysfunction (see Burack et al., 1997) that may make customary measures of intelligence challenging to use and, in some cases, inappropriate for children with autism. Language deficits, for example, may be independent of intelligence (Lord and Paul, 1997; Rutter, 1978), which may make verbal measures particularly troublesome for this population. For these reasons, some researchers, even in the early days of autism research, relied on subtests of intelligence tests or used alternative methods to assess the intelligence of children with autism.

Historically, alternative methods used to assess intelligence in children with autism included developmental measures such as the *Bayley Scales* (Bayley, 1969) or adaptive skills measures such as the *Vineland Social Maturity Scale* (Doll, 1965) or the AAMD *Adaptive Behavior Scale* (Fogelman, 1975). Although the use of these measures avoided some of the difficulties highlighted, it is important to note that these are not measures of intelligence and do not provide the same kind of information as do intelligence tests. Developmental scales provide developmental quotient (DQ) scores, a reflection of the attainment of developmental milestones relative to same-age peers. Adaptive and social maturity scales provide social quotient (SQ) scores, a measure of the acquisition of social and adaptive behaviors also relative to one's cohort.

Research has shown that low scores on developmental scales do not predict subsequent development in children with autism as well as they predict development in typical children (Rogers, 2001) and that adaptive scales can underestimate the intelligence of children with autism (Fombonne, Siddons, Achard, Frith, and Happé, 1994). Developmental and adaptive scales may be particularly problematic for higher functioning children with autism, who may have a large discrepancy between their intelligence and what adaptive or developmental measures would predict (Liss et al., 2001). Therefore, the alternative methods used by some researchers to assess the intelligence of children with autism may also be problematic and should be examined systematically.

When evaluating the evidence supporting the claims regarding the rates of MR in children with autism, one must examine the source of the claims, the time when the studies were published, and the specific methods by which intelligence level was determined. The fact that the diagnostic criteria for autism have evolved since Kanner first identified the disorder cannot be ignored in the evaluation of the existing evidence. Because of this, the nature of the children comprising the samples in research has shifted over the years, and thus it could be argued that comparing prevalence rates across time may not make sense. It might also be argued that children with autism used in earlier studies may have had more severe autism than those assessed more recently. These issues are important to acknowledge. However, prevalence rates reported in the current literature cite past articles, often transcending periods during which various definitions of autism as well as diverse samples of children were used. Because of the use of prior research to support claims regarding the rates of MR in individuals with autism at the present, it is important to examine literature published across time frames regardless of the definition of autism or the nature of the sample utilized.

In the examination of the prevalence rates of MR in children with autism, three issues are important: (a) Do the prevalence rates reported in the literature derive from empirical sources? (b) Can nonempirical sources of these statistics be traced historically to valid empirical studies? and (c) When empirical studies have been conducted, are the methods by which intelligence is assessed appropriate?

## Method

Attempts were made to obtain all articles written in English published through December 2003 that made claims or provided data in support of the claims concerning the rates of MR in children with autism. The initial step in the process of locating appropriate articles

210

for review involved an online search of the literature from 1943 (when autism was first coined by Kanner) through December 2003 using the PsycINFO database. Because of the early use of the terms childhood schizophrenia and early infantile autism for what is now called autism, the search included all three terms. A total of 6,876 articles were found as a result of the search for autism, early infantile autism, or childhood schizophrenia; 27,985 articles were found as a result of the search for mental retardation. There were 842 articles that included the key terms autism, early infantile autism, or childhood schizophrenia, and mental retardation. It should be noted that in the context of the present study, the term article refers to any published source, whether journal article, book, or chapter in an edited book.

Articles that (a) investigated levels of intelligence in children with autism; (b) discussed, in detail, the cognitive abilities of children with autism; or (c) cited a claim about the comorbidity between autism and MR served as the starting point for the present review. I examined the abstracts of the 842 articles to determine whether they met any of the criteria. If they did, they were considered for further review. Of the 842 reviewed, 145 met at least one of the three criteria.

Of these 145 articles, those that made specific claims about the prevalence of MR in children with autism or that provided data regarding the intelligence of children with autism that could be used to determine prevalence rates of MR were included in the present review. Also, a sample of recent child psychopathology, abnormal psychology, and general textbooks on autism was examined to determine if they made statements regarding the intelligence of children with autism. Any of these sources that made claims or provided data regarding the intelligence of children with autism were also included. Articles that provided support for any statistics or claims cited in articles already in the review were additionally examined and included if they met any of the three criteria outlined. Finally, any additional articles of which the researcher was aware that made claims regarding the prevalence of MR in children with autism were included.

Once an article was chosen for inclusion in the present review, every reference cited by the authors of that article that was used to support the claim of MR was obtained and examined to determine the support for the original claim. These articles were then also included in the review if the reference also made specific statements concerning the prevalence of MR in children with autism or provided data in support of a claim. This practice of following a citation trail historically continued until the citation trail ended. Both peer-reviewed journal articles and non-peer-reviewed publications (for example, chapters in edited books, claims in textbooks) were included in the sample, as both types of sources were frequently referenced by those making claims. It is recognized that, given the vast literature on autism, some articles making claims about the prevalence of MR in children with autism will have been missed, despite the measures taken to identify all such articles. However, given the size and scope of the sample of articles, it is believed that the sample is representative of the articles in the relevant literature.

After examination, only articles that either made specific claims concerning the occurrence of MR in children with autism or that reported data that could be used by others as support for claims were included in the final sample. Some articles screened for inclusion in the present review ultimately were not included. For example, some articles implied a relationship between intelligence level and autism. The title of one of these articles illustrates this occurrence: "Long-Term Follow-up of 100 'Atypical' Children of Normal Intelligence" (Brown, 1978). These articles were not included in the final sample because they made no explicit prevalence claims. Some articles reported prevalence rates of children with autism who scored above and below an IQ of 50 (such as, Lewis, 2003; Sponheim and Skjeldal, 1998). These articles distinguished what the authors often termed low-functioning children with autism (those scoring in the severe and profound categories of MR) from high-functioning children with autism (those scoring in the moderate range of MR or above). Because it was not possible to tease apart the percentages of children scoring above and below the actual cutoff for MR, an IQ of 70, these studies also were not included in the present review. Finally, articles including children with Asperger syndrome or other autism spectrum disorders (ASD) were specifically excluded from the review, as the purpose of the current research was to examine the evidence for MR claims specifically in individuals with autism.

The final sample consisted of 215 articles that were classified into two types: (a) those that provided data regarding the prevalence rates of children with autism who also had MR (labeled empirical articles) and (b) those that made claims in the absence of empirical evidence (labeled nonempirical articles). Articles that both provided empirical data and made nonempirical claims were considered in both categories. Whether an article was classified as empirical or nonempirical was determined solely with regard to the claim made about the prevalence of children with autism who had MR, not whether the article reported the results of an empirical study. Of the 215 articles in the final sample, 58 made empirically based claims, and 165 made nonempirical claims; 8 of the 215 articles were considered in both the empirical and nonempirical article categories. Thus, 223 total claims were evaluated spanning 1937 to 2003. The one article published prior to Kanner's label of autism in 1943 (Piotrowski, 1937) was obtained when following the citation trail of another article (Pollack, 1958).

Separate examinations of the empirical and nonempirical articles were conducted. Specific findings will be discussed, and some of the articles reviewed will be used as illustrations of particular results. However, due to the amount of data collected for each article, it is not possible to discuss in detail each article included in the review. The interested reader is referred to the author's website, which offers detailed tables summarizing the information about each nonempirical and empirical article reviewed (www.willamette.edu/~medelson).

## Results

Because the vast majority of the claims regarding the prevalence of MR in children with autism originated from nonempirical sources, these results will be presented first.

### Results from Nonempirical Articles

Seventy-four percent of the claims about the prevalence of MR in individuals with autism came from nonempirical articles; 26% derived from empirical studies. Of the nonempirical articles, 36% never provided a citation in support of the claim. Of the 106 nonempirical articles that did make citations, 8% of the citations failed to provide supporting evidence for the claim, and 21% reported higher prevalence rates than those reported in the articles that the authors cited. Finally, of the 165 nonempirical articles that made claims about the prevalence of MR in individuals with autism, 88 (53%) of the citations never traced back to empirical data when the reference trail was followed historically.

Of the nonempirical articles, 104 cited specific percentages of individuals with autism who had MR. The remainder of the nonempirical articles made such statements as "a majority of children with autism are also mentally retarded" (for example: Gillberg and Coleman, 2000, p. 10). For analysis purposes, if an article cited a percentage range, the highest end of the range was considered, as the current review determined that this was most likely the percentage to be cited by subsequent authors. The average prevalence rate reported in the 104 articles citing specific rates was 77.83%, the median prevalence rate reported was 75% MR, and the modal prevalence rate of MR in individuals with autism that was reported was also 75% (reported 45 times); the second most frequently reported prevalence rate was 80% (reported 23 times).

Prevalence rates reported in the nonempirical articles varied by decade of publication. The average rates reported in the nonempirical articles were 40% for the one article published prior to 1960; 75% for the one article published between 1960 and 1969; 79.39% for the 13 articles published between 1970 and 1979; 75.56% for the 27 articles published between 1980 and 1989; and 79.15% for the 62 articles published since 1990. A one-way analysis of variance (ANOVA) and subsequent Bonferroni post hoc analysis indicated that there was a significant difference between the prevalence rate reported in the one article published prior to 1960 and the average prevalence rates reported since then, $F(4, 99) = 8.683$, $p < .001$. However, this finding should be interpreted with caution as only one nonempirical article reported a specific prevalence rate of MR in children with autism prior to 1960.

When all of the nonempirical articles are considered together, not just those reporting specific prevalence rates, a consistent increase is evident over the years in the number of articles making claims that a majority of children with autism have MR. Of all 165 nonempirical articles reviewed, one article made this claim prior to 1960 (1% of the nonempirical articles); four articles made claims between 1960 and 1969 (2.5% of the articles); 32 articles made claims between 1970 and 1979 (19% of the articles); 47 articsles made claims between 1980 and 1989 (28.5% of the articles); and 81 articles have made claims since 1990 (49% of the articles). A chi-square analysis indicated that the number of nonempirical articles claiming that children with autism have MR differed across decades, $x^2(4) = 132.30$, $p < .001$.

One hundred seventeen empirical citations were offered as direct evidence by the authors of the 106 nonempirical articles that made citations for their claims, and they were examined to determine when the empirical data used in support of the nonempirical claims were obtained. For this analysis, only the original empirical citations were considered; nonempirical citation trails were not followed historically as it would be expected that the more the citation trail is traced back, the less recent the studies would be.

None of the empirical citations were to studies published prior to 1960. Forty-four citations (38%) were to empirical articles published from 1960 to 1969; 32 citations (27%) were to empirical articles published from 1970–1979; 26 citations (22%) were to empirical articles published from 1980 to 1989; and 15 citations (13%) were to empirical articles published between 1990 and 2003. A chi-square analysis indicated that there were significant differences in the number of citations across decades, $x^2(3) =$

14.885, p < .01. Overall, nearly two thirds of the empirical citations were to articles published 25–45 years ago. Figure 20.1 presents a comparison of the dates of publication of the articles making nonempirical claims that a majority of children with autism are MR and the dates of publication of the empirical data used to support these claims.

## Results from Empirical Articles

Of the 58 empirical articles included in the current review, 53 had data for which prevalence rates of MR could be determined (the remaining five were included because they were cited by nonempirical articles as empirical support for their claims). The average prevalence rate for these 53 empirical articles was 75.28%, similar to the median and modal prevalence rates reported in the nonempirical articles.

Of these 53 empirical articles, three articles (6%) were published prior to 1950; ten articles (19%) were published from 1960 to 1969; nine articles (17%) were published from 1970 to 1979; 14 articles (26%) were published from 1980 to 1989; and 17 articles (32%) were published from 1990 to 2003. There was a significant difference in the numbers of empirical articles published across decades, $x^2(4) = 4.0$, $p < .05$. The results suggest a slight increase in data speaking to the prevalence rates of MR in children with autism over the years, which is interesting given that the authors of most nonempirical articles cited less recent empirical studies as support for their claims.

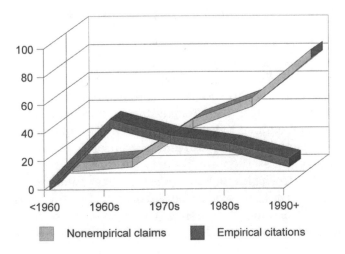

*Figure 20.1.* Numbers of nonempirical claims and direct empirical citations in support of the claims by decade of publication.

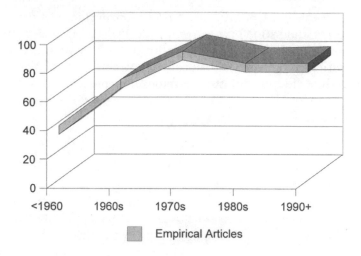

Empirical Articles

*Figure 20.2.* Mean prevalence rates of MR reported for children with autism in empirical articles by decade of publication.

The average prevalence rates were also calculated separately by the decade in which they were published, and a one-way ANOVA was conducted to determine whether the percentages differed across the decades. As can be seen in Figure 20.2, there was a significant difference in prevalence rates across the years, $F(4.48) = 7.231, p < .001$. The average prevalence rates reported were 34.33% for the three studies conducted prior to 1960; 66.9% for the ten studies conducted from 1960 to 1969; 86.78% for the nine studies conducted from 1970 to 1979; 78.29% for the 14 studies conducted from 1980 to 1989; and 78.88% for the 17 studies conducted since 1990.

Bonferroni post hoc comparisons determined that the results were due to significant differences in prevalence rates reported between studies published prior to 1960 and studies published later. Thus, the empirical data show that the reported prevalence rates of individuals with autism determined to be MR increased from prior to 1960 to the 1970s, where peak prevalence rates were reported (averaging approximately 86%), and have remained fairly consistent since then.

Of the 53 empirical articles providing data regarding prevalence rates of MR, 51 could be evaluated with regard to the methodologies they used to determine intelligence (two articles were reviews of epidemiological surveys previously conducted; see Fombonne, 1998; Wing, 1993). Thirty-five of these 51 articles described the specific methodologies by which the researchers determined intelligence in their samples of children with autism. Thus, of the 223 total claims evaluated, only

35 (15.7%) were both empirical and of such a design that they allowed for an examination of the specific methods used to determine the prevalence rates of MR in children with autism. Although there was not a statistically significant difference between rates of MR reported in articles that did and did not describe their methodology, the mean prevalence rate of MR in the studies that described their methodology was 71.89% compared with 82.88% for the studies that did not describe how intelligence was assessed, t(49) = 1.88, ns.

## Analyzing the Effects of Individual Methods Used to Determine Intelligence

The types of methods described in the 35 articles varied, and most articles reported utilizing more than one type of measure. T tests were utilized to assess differences between empirical studies that did and did not rely on specific methodologies to determine intelligence. When the standard deviations of the two groups were similar, the t tests were based on pooled variances; otherwise, separate variances were used.

Two types of measures of intelligence were used: verbal measures or timed (performance) measures. There were no significant differences in prevalence rates depending on whether the study employed one of these methods or not, and the majority of studies that described their methodology employed both of these measures. Furthermore, most studies that used these measures of intelligence used subtests rather than the full scales. The average prevalence rate of the eight studies not utilizing verbal measures was 77.25%, compared with a mean prevalence rate of 70.3% for the 27 studies that did use these measures, t(9.3) = .486, ns. The average prevalence rate of the five studies that did not use timed measures was 73.4%, compared with an average prevalence rate of 71.63% for the 30 studies that did use this method, t(4.4) = .121, ns.

Many studies used developmental scales, adaptive scales, or other alternative measures of intelligence. Developmental scales were used in 16 studies, and the average reported prevalence rate of MR in individuals with autism for these studies was 80.25%, compared with an average rate of 64.68% for the 19 studies not utilizing developmental scales, t(33) = 2.495, p < .05. A similar finding was obtained for the use of adaptive scales as measures of intelligence. For the 13 studies using adaptive scales as measures of intelligence, the average prevalence rate reported was 79.46%, compared with the mean prevalence rate of 67.27% for the 22 studies that did not use adaptive scales; this difference, however, was not statistically significant, t(33) = 1.824, ns.

Finally, there was a nonsignificant difference in the prevalence rates of MR reported in studies that used estimates or observations of intelligence (average rate for the seven studies was 77.71%) compared with those that did not (average rate for the 28 studies was 70.43%, $t(11.7) = 1.013$, ns).

In the 1960s and 1970s, some researchers assumed that children who were "untestable" had MR. These researchers assigned untestable children to the severe or profound MR category and then reported prevalence rates incorporating the data from these children (for example, Kolvin, Humphrey, and McNay, 1971; Rutter, 1966a; Rutter and Lockyer, 1967). Although not statistically significant, there were higher prevalence rates of MR reported for studies that equated untestability with MR. The average prevalence rate for the eight studies utilizing this practice was 80.5%, compared with the average prevalence rate of 69.33% for the 27 studies that did not utilize this practice, $t(23.4) = 1.971$, ns.

## *Analyzing the Effects of the Combined Use of Alternative Measures of Intelligence*

Most studies utilized at least one alternative measure of intelligence, and the majority of these used more than one such measure. Table 20.1 presents the findings for the combined use of methods other than true measures of intelligence. It should be noted that the total number of empirical studies included in these analyses exceeds 35 because if an article did not describe a specific method used to determine intelligence but made general statements that allowed for a classification regarding whether a general type of method was employed, the article was included.

As can be seen in Table 20.1, when studies used either developmental or adaptive measures of intelligence, higher average prevalence rates of MR were obtained; there was a mean prevalence rate of 79.85% for the 20 studies using at least one of these methods, compared with an average rate of 63.75% for the 16 studies that used neither method, $t(34) = 2.576$, $p < .05$. The 28 studies that used developmental or adaptive scales or that relied on observations or estimates of intelligence reported an average prevalence rate of MR of 80.96%, compared with a rate of 57.17% for the 12 studies that did not utilize any of these methods, $t(38) = 4.274$, $p < .001$. Finally, the 30 studies that used at least one of these three methods or that assigned untestable children to the MR category had an average prevalence rate of MR of 80.53%, compared with an average rate of 55.91% for the 11 studies that did not utilize any of these four methods, $t(39) = 4.101$, $p < .001$.

## An Examination of DeMyer et al. (1974)

Only one study used an unstandardized measure of intelligence, a study conducted by DeMyer et al. (1974), who used the Vineland Social Maturity Scale or the DeMyer Profile Test as measures of performance IQ in children with autism. The Vineland is an adaptive behavior scale, and a Social Quotient (SQ), not an IQ, is obtained. The DeMyer Profile Test is an unstandardized test created by the authors and for which there is no normative or psychometric data. DeMyer et al. measured verbal IQ either by "estimating" verbal age through an interview with their 115 participants, 78 of whom had no speech or echolalic speech only, or by again using the DeMyer Profile Test. In most cases, general IQ was obtained by averaging the performance and verbal IQs. Thus, this study used an unstandardized measure of intelligence with no psychometric data speaking to its reliability or validity, a measure of adaptive skills, and an interview of predominantly nonverbal participants. DeMyer et al. reported that 94% of their sample had MR. Despite the poor methodology and the fact that the article is 30 years old, this study is still being cited as direct evidence that a majority of children with autism have MR in sources as recent as the late 1990s and the early 21st century (for example: deBildt et al., 2003; Erickson, 1998; Prior and Ozonoff, 1998; Sigman, Dissanayake, Arbelle, and Ruskin, 1997; Zelazo, Burack, Boseovski, Jacques, and Frye, 2001). Furthermore, of the 77 nonempirical articles that traced to empirical data, 26 (34%) of these traced either directly or indirectly to this one study.

## Discussion

### An Examination of the Three Issues

The results from the analyses of nonempirical and empirical articles are considered together to address the three issues put forth at the beginning of the paper.

### Did the prevalence rates reported derive from empirical sources?

Seventy-four percent of the articles making claims about the prevalence of MR in children with autism came from nonempirical articles; only 26% derived from empirical studies. Of the 165 nonempirical claims made, 36% never gave a citation in support of the claim; an additional 8% gave a citation that did not provide evidence to support the claim; and a surprising number of nonempirical articles (21%)

claimed that a higher percentage of children with autism had MR than was claimed in the citation used to support the percentage (for example: Asarnow, Tanguay, Bott, and Freeman, 1987; Burack, 1992, 1994; Burack and Volkmar, 1992; DeMyer, 1979; Gillberg, 1993; Myers, 1989; Prior and Werry, 1986; Rutter, 1974; Rutter, Bartak, and Newman, 1971; Seligman, Walker, and Rosenhan, 2001; Volkmar and Cohen, 1988; Wing, 1974, 1976). This latter finding indicates a practice of inflating the prevalence rates, which in turn can result in these higher percentages being cited by subsequent authors.

**Table 20.1.** Differences in the Reported Prevalence Rates of Mental Retardation in Children with Autism in Empirical Articles: A Combined Examination of the Use of Alternative Measures of Intelligence

| | Mean prevalence rate | | | | |
| | Studies using methods | | Studies not using methods | | |
| Method | % | n | % | n | p value of difference (using t test) |
| --- | --- | --- | --- | --- | --- |
| Developmental or adaptive skills measures | 79.85 | 20 | 63.75 | 16 | < .05 |
| Developmental or adaptive skills measures or estimates of intelligence | 80.96 | 28 | 57.17 | 12 | < .001 |
| Developmental or adaptive skills measures, estimates of intelligence, or assuming untestable children are mentally retarded | 80.53 | 30 | 55.91 | 11 | < .001 |

Note: The total number of studies for these analyses exceeds 35 because some empirical articles that did not describe specific methodologies did make general statements about the types of measures used. Therefore, if it could be determined whether a particular article did or did not use one of the general combined methods being analyzed, it was included in the analysis.

### Could nonempirical sources of the prevalence rates of MR in children with autism be traced historically to valid empirical studies?

A total of 53% of the nonempirical articles making claims about the prevalence of MR in children with autism never traced back to an empirical source when the citation trail was followed historically. However, some authors making nonempirical claims made specific reference

220

to data supporting their claims even though their claims never traced back to empirical evidence. For example, Schreibman (1988) stated that "the data acquired to date indicate that the majority of autistic children are mentally retarded" (p. 25). Yet, the citation Schreibman provided in support of this statement was a nonempirical article (Ritvo and Freeman, 1978). Although Ritvo and Freeman (1978) claimed that 80% of children with autism were MR, they did not provide a citation in support of their own claim. Thus, neither Schreibman's citation nor the citation trail derived from it provided the "data" she asserted in her claim. The practice of using nonempirical citations to support nonempirical claims was fairly widespread, but most readers would not be cognizant of the fact that, over half the time, the citation trail ended before leading to empirical data.

## *Were the methods by which intelligence was assessed in the empirical studies valid given the interference of autism on the process of intellectual assessment?*

Empirical evidence for the high prevalence of MR in children with autism came from two sources: epidemiological studies and empirical investigations. A significant number of the recent empirical articles were epidemiological studies investigating the prevalence of autism in various communities (for example: Arvidsson, Danielsson, Forsberg, Gillberg, Johansson, and Kjellgren, 1997; Fombonne and du Mazaubrun, 1992; Fombonne, du Mazaubrun, Cans, and Grandjean, 1997; Gillberg, Steffenburg, and Schaumann, 1991; Honda, Shimizu, Misumi, Niimi, and Ohashi, 1996; Magnússon and Sæmundsen, 2001; Wignyosumarto, Mukhlas, and Shirataki, 1992). These studies frequently reported prevalence rates of MR based on intelligence assessments that were obtained prior to the study by individuals other than the researchers. Because of this, there was little detail reported about the specific measures of intelligence and methods of administration used in these studies. Only 8% of the empirical articles published prior to 1980 were epidemiological studies compared with 60% of the empirical articles published since 1980, $x^2(1) = 6.96$, $p < .01$.

The first empirical study of the intelligence of children with autism was conducted by Piotrowski (1937), who found that 30% of individuals with "childhood schizophrenia" had MR. Other early reports describe similar prevalence rates (see Pollack, 1958). The first reports that a majority of children with autism also had MR occurred in the mid to late 1960s (for example: Gibson, 1968; Gillies, 1965; Gittelman and Birch, 1967; Lotter, 1966a, 1966b; Rutter, 1966a; Rutter and Lockyer,

1967; Wing, 1969). These studies reported prevalence rates of MR in children with autism ranging from 56% to 100%. High prevalence rates of MR in children with autism continued to be reported in the 1970s, where the average prevalence rates of MR in children with autism peaked at over 86%, and the prevalence rates reported since then seem to have stabilized at approximately 78%.

## Where the Empirical Support Originated and the Quality of the Data

Most (65%) of the empirical citations provided for nonempirical claims came from studies conducted in the 1960s and 1970s, and 87% were prior to 1990. Of the sample of empirical articles reviewed, 55% of the empirical studies were conducted prior to 1980; 75% were conducted prior to 1990. Thus, most of the empirical data used in support of the prevalence claims are not recent.

In all likelihood, early empirical studies followed the established standards of practice for testing at the time. However, less was known about autism and the possible interfering effects of autism on the assessment of intelligence. Because of this, few if any modifications were made in determining the intelligence of children with autism; only a handful of authors acknowledged the possible interference of autistic symptomatology on the assessment process (for example: Lotter, 1966a; Mittler, 1966; Viitamaki, 1964; Vorster, 1960). Moreover, there was little or no discussion of whether the examiners administering the measures of intelligence even had experience in working with children with autism.

Mittler (1966) was one of the first authors to acknowledge the possible adverse effects of autistic symptomatology on intelligence testing. He noted that intelligence scores of individuals with autism may be inaccurate, especially when refused items are counted as failures, as they are on most performance scales. Mittler also stated that verbal measures of intelligence may be inappropriate because of the language deficits often present in children with autism. Other early researchers agreed on this latter point, including Rutter (1966b), who stated that many commonly used measures of intelligence are "usually unsuitable" (p. 91) for children with autism given their reliance on verbal subtests. However, in another chapter in the same book, Rutter (1966a) reported that 71% of children with autism in his sample had MR, a statistic obtained in a study that utilized the Wechsler Intelligence Scale for Children, a commonly used measure of intelligence with many verbal subtests (see Rutter and Lockyer, 1967, which is a report of the same study). Thus, despite the recognition that certain methods of intelligence determination were inappropriate for children with autism, they were still used; and data from these studies were then cited by subsequent authors.

The current standards of practice for testing suggest that modifications need to be made in the assessment of individuals with a disability; the standards state that (a) testers must select appropriate tests and make test accommodations when necessary given the disability; (b) testers must recognize the effects of the environment in which the person is assessed and the demands of the tests themselves on the performance of individuals with disabilities; and (c) testers must ensure that test scores are accurate indicators of the construct being measured rather than reflecting "construct-irrelevant characteristics associated with the disability" (Turner, DeMers, Roberts Fox, and Reed, 2001, p. 1104).

It is important to recognize that most of the empirical articles reporting rates of MR in children with autism made no mention of the experience of the examiner in working with individuals with autism or whether any modifications were made in the testing given the interference of autistic symptoms on the process of assessment. Freeman and Ritvo (1976) noted that the particular test used to assess intelligence and the skill of the examiner are important contributors to test outcome. Ironically, it was DeMyer (1979) who acknowledged that "few clinicians, even psychologists, are familiar with the techniques of reliably estimating the intelligence of an autistic child" (p. 133).

Because the early empirical research "establishing" the prevalence of MR in children with autism did not take into account these issues when using standard measures of intelligence with children with autism, the validity of the data obtained from these early studies is called into question. However, perhaps a greater concern is that researchers frequently utilized methods to determine intelligence level that were not actual measures of intelligence.

The most commonly used alternative methods of determining intelligence were developmental and adaptive scales. Developmental scale scores are not meant to reflect the intelligence of children but rather whether children have obtained skills normative for their chronological age (Goldman et al., 1983). Adaptive scale scores reflect the attainment of social milestones and adaptive behaviors. Both types of scores are based on observer reports of a child's behavior and are not comparable to IQ scores, which require responses from the person being assessed (Goldman et al., 1983). Moreover, recent research has indicated that these measures may be particularly poor substitutes for measures of intelligence in samples of children with autism (Fombonne et al.,1994; Rogers, 2001).

The results from the analyses of the empirical articles demonstrated that significantly higher prevalence rates of MR were found in children with autism when developmental or adaptive scales were used as measures of intelligence than when these scales were not utilized. In fact, there was a difference of nearly 25% in reported average prevalence rates of MR if studies used developmental measures, used adaptive skills measures, made estimates of intelligence, or assumed that untestable children had MR. Thus, much of the data supporting the high prevalence rates of MR in children with autism was obtained using measures that were not designed to assess intelligence and that were likely to inflate these percentages.

It is important to note that nearly all of the empirical studies utilized more than one method of determining intelligence. Therefore, even if some measures of intelligence were used that were appropriate given the symptoms of autism, it was not possible to determine which scores of intelligence were obtained on which measures. An example of this occurred in a study by Rutter and Lockyer (1967). Only three of the 63 children in their study were administered the *Leiter International Performance Scale* (Leiter), a nonverbal measure of intelligence. Research has indicated that the same children with autism have been shown to score significantly better on the Leiter than on the *Wechsler Intelligence Scale for Children—Revised (WISC-R*; see Shah and Holmes, 1985). In Rutter and Lockyer's study, ten of the children were deemed untestable and were arbitrarily assigned an IQ of 25, and the remainder were assessed using verbal measures of intelligence, adaptive scales, or projective measures of personality. The way in which Rutter and Lockyer (1967) reported their data does not allow the reader to know how rates of MR varied depending on the measure used, and this was true of virtually all empirical studies reviewed. Thus, the fact that nearly all studies employed at least some inappropriate measures may account for why the prevalence rates were generally high across all studies even when individual methods were considered separately.

## Acceptance in the Field That a Majority of Children with Autism Have MR

According to Rutter (1999), researchers in the field of autism research long ago determined that most children with autism were, in fact, mentally retarded. In a lecture on the evolution of research and clinical practice related to autism from the 1950s through 1998, Rutter (1999) discussed the focus of autism research across four time frames.

He stated that in the 1950s and 1960s, there were many comparative studies focusing on the differentiation of autism from MR. By the 1970s, Rutter noted that it was already believed to be the case the most children with autism had MR. In the 1970s through mid-1980s, the cognition research shifted to understanding the particulars of reported cognitive deficits in individuals with autism. According to Rutter's report, after the mid-1980s, few research studies focused on determining the intelligence level of children with autism; this might, in part, explain why a greater percentage of recent empirical articles were epidemiological surveys of the prevalence of autism rather than empirical studies assessing the intelligence of children with autism.

Historically, our knowledge of autism, as reflected in what is cited in the literature, has transformed slowly. For example, Bettleheim (1967) asserted that autism was caused by psychogenic factors, specifically "refrigerator mothers" who coldly rejected their children. It took many years before authors stopped citing Bettleheim's theory as fact, even in the absence of supporting data and even after there was ample evidence refuting his theory. The unfortunate consequences of this slow transition in the literature was that there was a continued practice of blaming mothers of children with autism long after it was clear that they were not the cause of their child's condition.

Similarly, authors may continue to cite high prevalence rates of MR in these children long after it has been shown that the data are not present to support these claims. An unfortunate consequence of this may be the failure to provide the most effective interventions due to incorrect assumptions about the intelligence of these children. Yet, it is likely that most individuals reading the high prevalence claims in the literature are unaware of the state of the evidence used to support the claims. Most readers of the research likely accept the citations given for a claim without checking the strength of the evidence provided by the citation. Moreover, given the frequency with which claims of MR are made, it seems probable that readers of the literature assume that it is an established fact that children with autism have MR. This may also explain why many nonempirical claims about the prevalence of MR in individuals with autism do not have a supporting citation.

## Conclusions and Implications

In view of the present findings on these three issues, the conclusion that the majority of children with autism also have MR does not seem warranted. Most of the claims originate from nonempirical sources that (a) do not trace to empirical data, (b) cite empirical research that is 25 to 45 years old, (c) used inappropriate measures, or (d) typically failed to acknowledge the possible interference of autism on the assessment of intelligence. Furthermore, only 15.7% of all claims made actually traced to empirical data that were obtained from studies whose authors described specific methods used to assess intelligence. Thus, only a small percentage of studies reported methods that could be evaluated with regard to their validity.

Although recent data have shown that some children with autism do, in fact, have MR, the rates are much lower than the high prevalence rates cited in the past. Recent epidemiological surveys have shown that the prevalence rates of MR in children with autism are between 40% and 55% (for example: Chakrabarti and Fombonne, 2001), much lower than the typical rates cited in the literature. Recent empirical studies indicate that when appropriate measures of intelligence are used— those that take into account the interference of autism—a significantly lower prevalence rate of MR is found relative to the rates typically reported in the literature (see Edelson, Schubert, and Edelson, 1998; Koegel, Koegel, and Smith, 1997).

However, the practice of claiming that a majority of children with autism are mentally retarded continues largely unabated. These claims can be found in recent journal articles (such as: Bodfish, Symons, Parker, and Lewis, 2000; Dennis, Lockyer, Lazenby, Donnelly, Wilkinson, and Schoonheyt, 1999; Happé, 1999; Ruble and Dalrymple, 2003); chapters on autism in edited books, many of which are still in books on MR (for example: Kasari, Freeman, and Paparella, 2001; Minshew, Johnson, and Luna, 2001; Volkmar and Klin, 2001); chapters on autism from child psychopathology textbooks (such as: Mash and Wolfe, 2002; Wicks-Nelson and Israel, 2000); chapters in abnormal psychology textbooks (for example: Davison and Neale, 2003; Seligman, Walker, and Rosenhan, 2001); "ask the editor" columns in journals on autism (Volkmar, 2003); and in the most recent edition of the *Diagnostic and Statistical Manual of Mental Disorders* (American Psychiatric Association, 2000).

Given the present results, it seems prudent to obtain additional empirical evidence before making any definitive conclusions regarding the prevalence rates of MR in children with autism. Empirical studies need to be conducted in which measures of intelligence take into account the interfering symptoms of autism on the process of assessment, examiners are knowledgeable about and have experience in assessing children with autism, and modifications to the testing situation are made to minimize the "construct-irrelevant" error in test outcome. Until that time, researchers in the autism field should use caution when making assumptions or citing claims about the rates of MR in children with autism.

**About the author:** Meredyth Goldberg Edelson, PhD, is a professor of psychology at Willamette University in Salem, Oregon. Her teaching and research interests include the intellectual functioning of children with autism, legal outcomes and other variables related to the sexual abuse of children, and the effects of domestic violence on women and children. Address: Meredyth Goldberg Edleson, Willamette University, Department of Psychology, 900 State Street, Salem, OR 97301; e-mail: medelson@willamette.edu

## Notes

1. The author would like to acknowledge the help of Steve Edelson and Jim Friedrich, who provided comments on an earlier version of this article.

2. This research was supported by a Faculty Study Time Leave and Atkinson Grant awarded to the author by Willamette University.

3. A portion of this research was presented at the Western Psychological Association Annual conference, May 2003.

## References

American Psychiatric Association. (1980). *Diagnostic and statistical manual of mental disorders (3rd ed.)*. Washington, DC: Author.

American Psychiatric Association. (1987). *Diagnostic and statistical manual of mental disorders (3rd ed., rev.)*. Washington, DC: Author.

American Psychiatric Association. (1994). *Diagnostic and statistical manual of mental disorders (4th ed.)*. Washington, DC: Author.

American Psychiatric Association. (2000). *Diagnostic and statistical manual of mental disorders* (4th ed., text rev.). Washington, DC: Author.

Arvidsson, T., Danielsson, B., Forsberg, P., Gillberg, C., Johansson, M., and Kjellgren, G. (1997). Autism in 3–6 year old children in a suburb of Göteborg, Sweden. *Autism, 1*, 163–173.

Asarnow, R. F., Tanguay, P. E., Bott, L., and Freeman, B. J. (1987). Patterns of intellectual functioning in non-retarded autistic and schizophrenic children. *Journal of Child Psychology and Psychiatry, and Allied Disciplines, 28*, 273–280.

Bayley, N. (1969). *Manual: Bayley Scales of Infant Development*. New York: Psychological Corp.

Bettleheim, B. (1967). *The empty fortress: Infantile autism and the birth of the self*. New York: The Free Press.

Bodfish, J. W., Symons, F. J., Parker, D. E., and Lewis, M. H. (2000). Varieties of repetitive behavior in autism: Comparison to mental retardation. *Journal of Autism and Developmental Disorders, 30*, 237–243.

Brown, J. L. (1978). Long-term follow-up of 100 "atypical" children of normal intelligence. In M. Rutter and E. Schopler (Eds.), *Autism* (pp. 463–474). New York: Plenum Press.

Burack, J. A. (1992). Debate and argument: Clarifying developmental issues in the study of autism. *Journal of Child Psychology and Psychiatry and Allied Disciplines, 33*, 617–621.

Burack, J. A. (1994). Selective attention deficits in persons with autism: Preliminary evidence of an inefficient attentional lens. *Journal of Abnormal Psychology, 103*, 535–543.

Burack, J. A., Enns, J. T., Stauder, J. E. A., Mottron, L., and Randolph, B. (1997). Attention and autism: Behavioral and electrophysiological evidence. In D. J. Cohen and F. R. Volkmar (Eds.), *Handbook of autism and pervasive developmental disorders (2nd ed.*, pp. 226–247). New York: Wiley.

Burack, J. A., and Volkmar, F. R. (1992). Development of low- and high-functioning autistic children. *Journal of Child Psychology and Psychiatry and Allied Disciplines, 33*, 607–616.

Chakrabarti, S., and Fombonne, E. (2001). Pervasive developmental disorders in preschool children. *Journal of the American Medical Association, 285*, 3093–3099.

Creak, M. (1961). Schizophrenic syndrome in childhood. *Lancet, 2*, 818.

Creak, E. M. (1963). Childhood psychosis: A review of 100 cases. *The British Journal of Psychiatry, 109*, 84–89.

Davison, G. C., and Neale, J. M. (2003). *Abnormal psychology (8th ed.)*. New York: Wiley.

Dawson, G., and Lewy, A. (1989). Arousal, attention, and the socioemotional impairments of individuals with autism. In G. Dawson (Ed.), *Autism: Nature, diagnosis, and treatment* (pp. 49–74). New York: Guilford Press.

deBildt, A., Sytema, S., Ketelaars, C., Kraijer, D., Volkmar, F., and Minderaa, R. (2003). Measuring pervasive developmental disorders in children and adolescents with mental retardation: A comparison of two screening instruments used in a study of the total mentally retarded population from a designated area. *Journal of Autism and Developmental Disorders, 33*, 595–605.

DeMyer, M. K. (1979). *Parents and children in autism.* Washington, DC: V. H. Winston and Sons.

DeMyer, M. K., Barton, S., Alpern, G. D., Kimberlin, C., Allen, J., and Steele, R. (1974). The measured intelligence of autistic children. *Journal of Autism and Childhood Schizophrenia, 4*, 42–60.

Dennis, M., Lockyer, L., Lazenby, A. L., Donnelly, R. E., Wilkinson, M., and Schoonheyt, W. (1999). Intelligence patterns among children with high-functioning autism, phenylketonuria, and childhood head injury. *Journal of Autism and Developmental Disorders, 29*, 5–16.

Doll, E. E. (1965). *Vineland Social Maturity Scale, condensed revised edition. Manual of direction.* Minneapolis, MN: American Guidance Service.

Edelson, M. G., Schubert, D. T., and Edelson, S. M. (1998). Factors predicting intelligence scores on the TONI in individuals with autism. *Focus on Autism and Other Developmental Disabilities, 13*, 17–26.

Erickson, M. T. (1998). *Behavior disorders of children and adolescents: Assessment, etiology and intervention.* Upper Saddle River, NJ: Prentice Hall.

Fogelman, C. J. (1975). *American Association on Mental Deficiency (AAMD) Adaptive Behavior Scale, revision.* Washington, DC: AAMD.

Fombonne, E., and du Mazaubrun, C. (1992). Prevalence of infantile autism in four French regions. *Social Psychiatry and Psychiatric Epidemiology, 27*, 203–210.

Fombonne, E., du Mazaubrun, C., Cans, C., and Grandjean, H. (1997). Autism and associated medical disorders in a French epidemiological survey. *Journal of the American Academy of Child and Adolescent Psychiatry, 36*, 1561–1569.

Fombonne, E., Siddons, F., Achard, S., Frith, U., and Happé, F. (1994). Adaptive behavior and theory of mind in autism. *European Child and Adolescent Psychiatry, 3*, 176–186.

Freeman, B. J., and Ritvo, E. R. (1976). Cognitive assessment. In E. R. Ritvo, B. J. Freeman, E. M. Ornitz, and P. E. Tanguay (Eds.), *Autism: Diagnosis, current research, and management* (pp. 27–39). New York: Spectrum.

Gibson, D. (1968). Early infantile autism: Symptom and syndrome. *Canadian Psychology, 9*, 36–39.

Gillberg, C. (1993). Autism and related behaviours. *Journal of Intellectual Disability Research, 37*, 343–372.

Gillberg, C., and Coleman, M. (2000). *The biology of the autistic syndromes*. London: Mac Keith Press.

Gillberg, C., Steffenburg, S., and Schaumann, H. (1991). Is autism more common now than 10 years ago? *The British Journal of Psychiatry, 158*, 403–409.

Gillies, S. (1965). Some abilities of psychotic children and subnormal controls. *Journal of Mental Deficiency Research, 9*, 89–101.

Gittelman, M., and Birch, H. G. (1967). Childhood schizophrenia: Intellect, neurologic status, perinatal risk, prognosis, and family pathology. *Archives of General Psychiatry, 17*, 16–25.

Goldman, J., L'Engle Stein, C., and Guerry, S. (1983). *Psychological methods of child assessment*. New York: Bruner/Mazel.

Happé, F. (1999). Autism: Cognitive deficit or cognitive style? *Trends in Cognitive Sciences, 3*, 216–222.

Honda, H., Shimizu, Y., Misumi, K., Niimi, M., and Ohashi, Y. (1996). Cumulative incidence and prevalence of childhood autism in children in Japan. *The British Journal of Psychiatry, 169*, 228–235.

Kanner, L. (1943). Autistic disturbances of affective contact. *Nervous, 2*, 217–250.

Kasari, C., Freeman, S. F. N., and Paparella, T. (2001). Early intervention in autism: Joint attention and symbolic play. In L. M. Glidden (Ed.), *International review of research in mental retardation: Vol. 23. Autism* (pp. 207–237). San Diego: Academic Press.

Koegel, L. K., Koegel, R. L., and Smith, A. (1997). Variables related to differences in standardized test outcomes for children with autism. *Journal of Autism and Developmental Disorders, 27*, 233–244.

Kolvin, I., Humphrey, M., and McNay, A. (1971). VI. Cognitive factors in childhood psychoses. *The British Journal of Psychiatry, 118*, 415–419.

Lewis, V. (2003). Disorders of development. In A. Slater and G. Bremner (Eds.), *An introduction to developmental psychology* (pp. 456– 475). Malden, MA: Blackwell.

Liss, M., Harel, B., Fein, D., Allen, D., Dunn, M., Feinstein, C., et al. (2001). Predictors and correlates of adaptive functioning in children with developmental disorders. *Journal of Autism and Developmental Disorders, 31*, 219–230.

Lockyer, L., and Rutter, M. (1970). A five- to fifteen-year follow-up study of infantile psychosis: IV. Patterns of cognitive ability. *The British Journal of Social and Clinical Psychology, 9*, 152–163.

Lord, C., and Paul, R. (1997). Language and communication in autism. In D. J. Cohen and F. R. Volkmar (Eds.), *Handbook of autism and pervasive developmental disorders (2nd ed.*, pp. 195–225). New York: Wiley.

Lotter, V. (1966a). Epidemiology of autistic conditions in young children: I. Prevalence. Social Psychiatry. *Sozialpsychiatrie. Psychiatrie Sociale, 1*, 124–137.

Lotter, V. (1966b). Services for a group of autistic children in Middlesex. In L. Wing (Ed.), *Early childhood autism: Clinical, educational and social aspects* (pp. 241–255). Oxford: Pergamon Press.

Magnússon, P., and Sæmundsen, E. (2001). Prevalence of autism in Iceland. *Journal of Autism and Developmental Disorders, 31*, 153–163.

Mash, E. J., and Wolfe, D. A. (2002). *Abnormal child psychology*. Belmont, CA: Wadsworth.

Minshew, N. J., Johnson, C., and Luna, B. (2001). The cognitive and neural basis of autism: A disorder of complex information processing and dysfunction of neocortical systems. In L. M. Glidden (Ed.), *International review of research in mental retardation: Vol. 23. Autism* (pp. 111–138). San Diego: Academic Press.

Mittler, P. (1966). The psychological assessment of autistic children. In L. Wing (Ed.), *Early childhood autism: Clinical, educational and social aspects* (pp. 145–158). Oxford: Pergamon Press.

Myers, B. A. (1989). Misleading cues in the diagnosis of mental retardation and infantile autism in the preschool child. *Mental Retardation, 27*, 85–90.

Piotrowski, Z. A. (1937). A comparison of congenitally defective children with schizophrenic children in regard to personality structure and intelligence type. *Proceedings of the American Association on Mental Deficiency, 42*, 78–90.

Pollack, M. (1958). Brain damage, mental retardation, and childhood schizophrenia. *The American Journal of Psychiatry, 115*, 422–428.

Prior, M., and Ozonoff, S. (1998). Psychological factors in autism. In F. R. Volkmar (Ed.), *Autism and pervasive developmental disorders* (pp. 64–108). Cambridge: Cambridge University Press.

Prior, M., and Werry, J. S. (1986). Autism, schizophrenia, and allied disorders. In H. C. Quay and J. S. Werry (Eds.), *Psychopathological disorders of childhood* (pp. 156–210). New York: Wiley.

Ritvo, E. R., and Freeman, B. J. (1978). Current research on the syndrome of autism. *Journal of the American Academy of Child Psychiatry, 17,* 565–575.

Rogers, S. J. (2001). Diagnosis of autism before the age of 3. In L. M. Glidden (Ed.), *International review of research in mental retardation: Vol. 23. Autism* (pp. 1–31). San Diego: Academic Press.

Ruble, L. A., and Dalrymple, N. J. (2003). Social/sexual awareness of persons with autism: A parental perspective. *Archives of Sexual Behavior, 22,* 229–240.

Rutter, M. (1966a). Behavioural and cognitive characteristics of a series of psychotic children. In L. Wing (Ed.), *Early childhood autism: Clinical, educational and social aspects* (pp. 51–81). Oxford: Pergamon Press.

Rutter, M. (1966b). Prognosis: Psychotic children in adolescence and early adult life. In L. Wing (Ed.), *Early childhood autism: Clinical, educational and social aspects* (pp. 83–99). Oxford: Pergamon Press.

Rutter, M. (1978). Language disorder and infantile autism. In M. Rutter and E. Schopler (Eds.), *Autism* (pp. 85–104). New York: Plenum Press.

Rutter, M. (1974). The development of infantile autism. *Psychological Medicine, 4,* 147–163.

Rutter, M. (1999). The Emanuel Miller Memorial Lecture 1998: Autism: Two-way interplay between research and clinical work. *Journal of Child Psychology and Psychiatry and Allied Disciplines, 40,* 169–188.

Rutter, M., Bartak, L., and Newman, S. (1971). Autism—A central disorder of cognition and language? In M. Rutter (Ed.), *Infantile autism: Concepts, characteristics, and treatment* (pp. 148–171). Edinburgh: Churchill Livingstone.

Rutter, M., and Lockyer, L. (1967). A five- to fifteen-year follow-up study of infantile psychosis. I. Description of sample. *The British Journal of Psychiatry, 113,* 1169–1182.

Schreibman, L. (1988). Autism. Newbury Park, CA: Sage. Seligman, M. E. P., Walker, E. F., and Rosenhan, D. L. (2001). *Abnormal psychology (4th ed.)*. New York: Norton.

Shah, A., and Holmes, N. (1985). Brief report: The use of the Leiter International Performance Scale with autistic children. *Journal of Autism and Developmental Disorders, 15*, 195–203.

Sigman, M., Dissanayake, C., Arbelle, S., and Ruskin, E. (1997). Cognition and emotion in children and adolescents with autism. In D. J. Cohen and F. R. Volkmar (Eds.), *Handbook of autism and pervasive developmental disorders (2nd ed.*, pp. 248–265). New York: Wiley.

Sponheim, E., and Skjeldal, O. (1998). Autism and related disorders: Epidemiological findings in a Norwegian study using ICD-10 diagnostic criteria. *Journal of Autism and Developmental Disorders, 28*, 217–227.

Tager-Flusberg, H. (1989). A psycholinguistic perspective on language development in the autistic child. In G. Dawson (Ed.), *Autism: Nature, diagnosis, and treatment* (pp. 92–115). New York: Guilford Press.

Thorndike, R. L., Hagen, E. P., and Sattler, J. M. (1986). *Technical manual: Stanford-Binet Intelligence Scale: Fourth edition*. Chicago: Riverside.

Turner, S. M., DeMers, S. T., Roberts Fox, H., and Reed, G. M. (2001). APA's guidelines for test user qualifications: An executive summary. *The American Psychologist, 56*, 1099–1113.

Viitamaki, R. O. (1964). II. Psychoses in childhood: A psychological follow-up study. *Acta Psychiatrica Scandinavica, 40*(Suppl. 174), 35–73.

Volkmar, F. R. (2003). Ask the editor. *Journal of Autism and Developmental Disorders, 33*, 109–110.

Volkmar, F. R., and Cohen, D. J. (1988). Classification and diagnosis of childhood autism. In E. Schopler and G. B. Mesibov (Eds.), *Diagnosis and assessment in autism* (pp. 71–89). New York: Plenum Press.

Volkmar, F. R., and Klin, A. (2001). Asperger's disorder and higher functioning autism: Same or different? In L. M. Glidden (Ed.), *International review of research in mental retardation: Vol. 23. Autism* (pp. 83–110). San Diego: Academic Press.

Vorster, D. (1960). An investigation into the part played by organic factors in childhood schizophrenia. *Journal of Mental Science, 106*, 494–522.

Wechsler, D. (1991). *Manual for the Wechsler Intelligence Scale for Children–Third edition*. New York: Psychological Corp.

Wicks-Nelson, R., and Israel, A. C. (2000). *Behavior disorders of childhood*. Upper Saddle River, NJ: Prentice Hall.

Wignyosumarto, S., Mukhlas, M., and Shirataki, S. (1992). Epidemiological and clinical study of autistic children in Yogyakarta, Indonesia. *The Kobe Journal of Medical Sciences, 38*, 1–19.

Wing, L. (1969). The handicaps of autistic children—A comparative study. *Journal of Child Psychology and Psychiatry, and Allied Disciplines, 10*, 1–40.

Wing, L. (1974). Language development and autistic behavior in severely mentally retarded children. *Proceedings of the Royal Society of Medicine, 67*, 1031–1032.

Wing, L. (1976). Epidemiology and theories of aetiology. In L. Wing (Ed.), *Early childhood autism* (pp. 65–92). Oxford: Pergamon Press.

Zelazo, P. D., Burack, J. A., Boseovski, J. J., Jacques, S., and Frye, D. (2001). A cognitive complexity and control framework for the study of autism. In J. A. Burack, T. Charman, N. Yirmiya, and P. R. Zelazo (Eds.), *The development of autism: Perspectives from theory and research* (pp. 195–217). Mahwah, NJ: Erlbaum.

# Chapter 21

# *Moving Forward after a Child Is Diagnosed with ASD*

## *How will I deal with this diagnosis?*

It's not easy to hear the news that your child has autism, and realize that your life will be utterly different than you had expected it to be. Daily life with a special-needs child presents many unique challenges. How do you come to terms with the fact that your child has autism? How do you cope once you get over the initial shock? We aim to help you by providing regular features on topics ranging from how autism affects your family to day-to-day survival strategies.

You are never prepared for a diagnosis of autism. It is likely that you will experience a range of emotions. It is painful to love so much, to want something so much, and not quite get it. You want your child to get better so much you may feel some of the stages commonly associated with grieving. You may revisit these feelings from time to time in the future. Part of moving forward, is dealing with your own needs and emotions along the way.

## *Stages Associated with Grieving*

**Shock:** Immediately after the diagnosis you may feel stunned or confused. The reality of the diagnosis may be so overwhelming that you're not ready to accept it or you initially ignore it. You may also question the diagnosis or search for another doctor who will tell you something different.

---

"Your Family and Autism." Reprinted with the permission of Autism Speaks, www.autismspeaks.org, © 2010.

**Sadness or grief:** Many parents must mourn some of the hopes and dreams they held for their child before they can move on. There will probably be many times when you feel extremely sad. Friends may refer to this as being depressed which can sound frightening.

There is, however, a difference between sadness and depression. Depression often stands in the way of moving forward. Allowing yourself to feel sadness can help you grow. You have every right to feel sad and to express it in ways that are comfortable. Crying can help release some of the tension that builds up when you try to hold in sadness. A good cry can get you over one hurdle and help you face the next.

**Anger:** With time, your sadness may give way to anger. Although anger is a natural part of the process, you may find that it's directed at those closest to you—your child, your spouse, your friend, or at the world in general. You may also feel resentment toward parents of typical children. Your anger may come out in different ways—snapping at people, overreacting at small things, even screaming and yelling. Anger is normal. It is a healthy and expected reaction to feelings of loss and stress that come with this diagnosis. Expressing your anger releases tension. It's an attempt to tell the people around you that you hurt, that you are outraged that this diagnosis has happened to your child.

**Denial:** You may go through periods of refusing to believe what is happening to your child. You don't consciously choose this reaction; like anger, it just happens. During this time, you may not be able to hear the facts as they relate to your child's diagnosis. Don't be critical of yourself for reacting this way. Denial is a way of coping. It may be what gets you through a particularly difficult period. You must, however, be aware of that you may be experiencing denial so that it doesn't cause you to lose focus on your child's treatment.

Try not to "shoot the messenger." When someone, a professional, a therapist, or a teacher, tells you something that is hard to hear about your child, consider that they are trying to help you so that you can address the problem. It is important not to alienate people who can give you helpful feedback and monitoring of your child's progress. Whether you agree or not, try to thank them for the information. If you are upset, try considering their information when you have had a chance to calm down.

**Loneliness:** You may feel isolated and lonely. These feelings may have many causes. Loneliness may also come from the fact that in your new situation you simply don't feel you have the time to contact friends or family for company or that, if you did reach out, they wouldn't understand or be supportive. In the pages that follow, we have some suggestions for taking care of yourself and for getting the support you need.

**Acceptance:** Ultimately, you may feel a sense of acceptance. It's helpful to distinguish between accepting that your child has been diagnosed with autism and accepting autism. Accepting the diagnosis simply means that you are ready to advocate for your child.

The period following an autism diagnosis can be very challenging, even for the most harmonious families. Although the child affected by autism may never experience the negative emotions associated with the diagnosis, parents, siblings, and extended family members may each process the diagnosis in different ways, and at different rates.

**Give yourself time to adjust:** Be patient with yourself. It will take some time to understand your child's disorder and the impact it has on you and your family. Difficult emotions may resurface from time to time. There may be times when you feel helpless and angry that autism has resulted in a life that is much different than you had planned. But you will also experience feelings of hope as your child begins to make progress.

## *Caring for the Caregiver*

Changing the course of your child's life with autism can be a very rewarding experience. You are making an enormous difference in his or her life. To make it happen, you need to take care of yourself. Take a moment to answer these questions: Where does your support and strength come from? How are you really doing? Do you need to cry? Complain? Scream? Would you like some help but don't know who to ask?

"Remember that if you want to take the best possible care of your child, you must first take the best possible care of yourself."

Parents often fail to evaluate their own sources of strength, coping skills, or emotional attitudes. You may be so busy meeting the needs of your child that you don't allow yourself time to relax, cry, or simply think. You may wait until you are so exhausted or stressed out that you can barely carry on before you consider your own needs. Reaching this point is bad for you and for your family.

You may feel that your child needs you right now, more than ever. Your to do list may be what is driving you forward right now. Or, you may feel completely overwhelmed and not know here to start. There is no single way to cope. Each family is unique and deals with stressful situations differently. Getting your child started in treatment will help you feel better.

Acknowledging the emotional impact of autism and taking care of yourself during this stressful period will help prepare you for the challenges ahead. Autism is a pervasive, multi-faceted disorder. It will not only change the way that you look at your child, it will change the way you look at the world. As some parents may tell you, you may be a better person for it. The love and hope that you have for your child is probably stronger than you realize.

Here are some tips from parents who have experienced what you are going through:

**Get going:** Getting your child started in treatment will help. There are many details you will be managing in an intensive treatment program, especially if it is based in your home. If you know your child is engaged in meaningful activities, you will be more able to focus on moving forward. It may also free up some of your time so you can educate yourself, advocate for your child, and take care of yourself so that you can keep going.

**Ask for help:** Asking for help can be very difficult, especially at first. Don't hesitate to use whatever support is available to you. People around you may want to help, but may not know how. Is there someone who can take your other kids somewhere for an afternoon? Or, cook dinner for your family one night so that you can spend the time learning? Can they pick a few things up for you at the store or do a load of laundry? Can they let other people know you are going through a difficult time and could use a hand?

**Talk to someone:** Everyone needs someone to talk to. Let someone know what you are going through and how you feel. Someone who just listens can be a great source of strength. If you can't get out of the house, use the phone to call a friend. "At my support group I met a group of women who were juggling the same things I am. It felt so good not to feel like I was from another planet!"

**Consider joining a support group:** It may be helpful to listen or talk to people who have been or are going through a similar experience. Support groups can be great sources for information about what services are available in your area and who provides them. You may have to try more than one to find a group that feels right to you. You may find you aren't a support group kind of person. For many parents in your situation, support groups provide valuable hope, comfort, and encouragement.

**Try to take a break:** If you can, allow yourself to take some time away, even if it is only a few minutes to take a walk. If it's possible, getting out to a movie, going shopping, or visiting a friend can make a world of difference. If you feel guilty about taking a break, try to remind yourself that it will help you to be renewed for the things you need to do when you get back.

**Try to get some rest:** If you are getting regular sleep, you will be better prepared to make good decisions, be more patient with your child, and deal with the stress in your life.

**Consider keeping a journal:** Louise DeSalvo, in *Writing as a Way of Healing*, notes that studies have shown that "writing that describes traumatic events and our deepest thoughts and feelings about them is linked with improved immune function, improved emotional and physical health," and positive behavioral changes. Some parents have found journaling a helpful tool for keeping track of their children's progress, what's working and what isn't.

**Be mindful of the time you spend on the internet:** The internet will be one of the most important tools you have for learning what you need to know about autism and how to help your child. Unfortunately, there is more information on the web than any of us have time to read in a lifetime. There may also be a lot of misinformation. Right now, while you are trying to make the most of every minute, keep an eye on the clock and frequently ask yourself these important questions:

- Is what I'm reading right now very likely to be relevant to my child?
- Is it new information?
- Is it helpful?
- Is it from a reliable source?

Sometimes, the time you spend on the internet will be incredibly valuable. Other times, it may be better for you and your child if you use that time to take care of yourself.

## *Fifteen Tips for Your Family*

As a result of her work with many families who deal so gracefully with the challenges of autism, family therapist Kathryn Smerling, PhD, offers these—five tips for parents, five for siblings, and five for extended family members:

## *Five Tips for Parents*

Learn to be the best advocate you can be for your child. Be informed. Take advantage of all the services that are available to you in your community. You will meet practitioners and providers who can educate you and help you. You will gather great strength from the people you meet.

Don't push your feelings away. Talk about them. You may feel both ambivalent and angry. Those are emotions to be expected. It's okay to feel conflicting emotions. Try to direct your anger towards the disorder and not towards your loved ones. When you find yourself arguing with your spouse over an autism related issue, try to remember that this topic is painful for both of you; and be careful not to get mad at each other when it really is the autism that has you so upset and angry.

Try to have some semblance of an adult life. Be careful to not let autism consume every waking hour of your life. Spend quality time with your typically developing children and your spouse, and refrain from constantly talking about autism. Everyone in your family needs support, and to be happy despite the circumstances.

Appreciate the small victories your child may achieve. Love your child and take great pride in each small accomplishment. Focus on what they can do instead of making comparisons with a typically developing child. Love them for who they are rather than what they should be.

Get involved with the autism community. Don't underestimate the power of community. You may be the captain of your team, but you can't do everything yourself. Make friends with other parents who have children with autism. By meeting other parents you will have the support of families who understand your day to day challenges. Getting involved with autism advocacy is empowering and productive. You will be doing something for yourself as well as your child by being proactive.

## *Five Tips for Brothers and Sisters*

Remember that you are not alone. Every family is confronted with life's challenges—and yes, autism is challenging—but, if you look closely, nearly everyone has something difficult to face in their families.

Be proud of your brother or sister. Learn to talk about autism and be open and comfortable describing the disorder to others. If you are comfortable with the topic, they will be comfortable too. If you are embarrassed by your brother or sister, your friends will sense this and it will make it awkward for them. If you talk openly to your friends about autism, they will become comfortable. But, like everyone else, sometimes you will love your brother or sister, and sometimes you will hate them. It's okay to feel your feelings. And, often it's easier when you have a professional counselor to help you understand them—someone special who is here just for you. Love your brother or sister the way they are.

While it is okay to be sad that you have a brother or sister affected by autism, it doesn't help to be upset and angry for extended periods of time. Your anger doesn't change the situation; it only makes you unhappier. Remember your mom and dad may have those feelings too.

Spend time with your mom and dad alone. Doing things together as a family with and without your brother or sister strengthens your family bond. It is okay for you to want alone time. Having a family member with autism can often be very time consuming, and attention grabbing. You need to feel important too. Remember, even if your brother or sister didn't have autism, you would still need alone time with Mom and Dad.

Find an activity you can do with your brother or sister. You will find it rewarding to connect with your brother or sister, even if it is just putting a simple puzzle together. No matter how impaired they may be, doing something together creates a closeness. They will look forward to these shared activities and greet you with a special smile.

### *Five Tips for Grandparents and Extended Family*

Family members have a lot to offer. Each family member is able to offer the things they have learned to do best over time. Ask how you can be helpful to your family.

Your efforts will be appreciated whether it means taking care of the child so that the parents can go out to dinner, or raising money for the special school that helps your family's child. Organize a lunch, a theatre benefit, a carnival, or a card game. It will warm your family's hearts to know that you are pitching in to create support and closeness.

Seek out your own support. If you find yourself having a difficult time accepting and dealing with the fact that your loved one has autism, seek out your own support. Your family may not be able to provide you with that kind of support so you must be considerate and look elsewhere. In this way you can be stronger for them, helping with the many challenges they face.

Be open and honest about the disorder. The more you talk about the matter, the better you will feel. Your friends and family can become your support system, but only if you share your thoughts with them. It may be hard to talk about it at first, but as time goes on it will be easier. In the end, your experience with autism will end up teaching you and your family profound life lessons.

Put judgment aside. Consider your family's feelings and be supportive. Respect the decisions they make for their child with autism. They are working very hard to explore and research all options, and are typically coming to well thought out conclusions. Try not to compare children (this goes for typically developing kids as well). Children with autism can be brought up to achieve their personal best.

Learn more about autism. It affects people of all social and economic standing. There is promising research with many possibilities for the future. Share that sense of hope with your family while educating yourself about the best ways to help manage this disorder.

Carve out special time for each child. You can enjoy special moments with both typically developing family members and the family member with autism. Yes, they may be different, but both children look forward to spending time with you. Children with autism thrive on routines, so find one thing that you can do together that is structured, even if it is simply going to a park for fifteen minutes. If you go to the same park every week, chances are over time that activity will become easier and easier, it just takes time and patience. If you are having a difficult time trying to determine what you can do, ask your family. They will sincerely appreciate that you are making an effort.

# Part Four

# Conditions That
# May Accompany Autism
# Spectrum Disorders

# Chapter 22

# *ASD and Communication Difficulties*

## *Chapter Contents*

## Section 22.1

# *Communication Problems Associated with Autism*

This section includes excerpts from "Autism and Communication," National Institute on Deafness and Other Communication Disorders (NIDCD), NIH Pub. No. 09–4315, June 29, 2010; and excerpts from "Statistics on Voice, Speech, and Language," NIDCD, June 7, 2010.

### *How does autism affect communication?*

The word autism has its origin in the Greek word *autos*, which means self. Children with autism often are self-absorbed and seem to exist in a private world where they are unable to successfully communicate and interact with others. Children with autism may have difficulty developing language skills and understanding what others say to them. They also may have difficulty communicating nonverbally, such as through hand gestures, eye contact, and facial expressions.

Not every child with an autism spectrum disorder will have a language problem. A child's ability to communicate will vary, depending upon his or her intellectual and social development. Some children with autism may be unable to speak. Others may have rich vocabularies and be able to talk about specific subjects in great detail. Most children with autism have little or no problem pronouncing words. The majority, however, have difficulty using language effectively, especially when they talk to other people. Many have problems with the meaning and rhythm of words and sentences. They also may be unable to understand body language and the nuances of vocal tones.

Following are some patterns of language use and behaviors that are often found in children with autism.

**Repetitive or rigid language:** Often, children with autism who can speak will say things that have no meaning or that seem out of context in conversations with others. For example, a child may count from one to five repeatedly. Or, a child may continuously repeat words he or she has heard, a condition called echolalia. Immediate echolalia occurs when the child repeats words someone has just said. For example, the child may respond to a question by asking the same question. In delayed echolalia, the child will repeat words heard at an earlier time. The child may say "Do you want something to drink?" whenever he or she asks for a drink.

Some children with autism speak in a high-pitched or singsong voice or use robot-like speech. Other children with autism may use stock phrases to start a conversation. For example, a child may say, "My name is Tom," even when he talks with friends or family. Still others may repeat what they hear on television programs or commercials.

**Narrow interests and exceptional abilities:** Some children may be able to deliver an in-depth monologue about a topic that holds their interest, even though they may not be able to carry on a two-way conversation about the same topic. Others have musical talents or an advanced ability to count and do math calculations. Approximately 10% of children with autism show savant skills, or extremely high abilities in specific areas, such as calendar calculation, music, or math.

**Uneven language development:** Many children with autism develop some speech and language skills, but not to a normal level of ability, and their progress is usually uneven. For example, they may develop a strong vocabulary in a particular area of interest very quickly. Many children have good memories for information just heard or seen. Some children may be able to read words before five years of age, but they may not comprehend what they have read. They often do not respond to the speech of others and may not respond to their own names. As a result, children with autism sometimes are mistakenly thought to have a hearing problem.

**Poor nonverbal conversation skills:** Children with autism often are unable to use gestures—such as pointing to an object—to give meaning to their speech. They often avoid eye contact which can make them seem rude, uninterested, or inattentive. Without meaningful gestures or the language to communicate, many children with autism become frustrated in their attempts to make their feelings and needs known. They may act out their frustrations through vocal outbursts or other inappropriate behaviors.

### *How are the speech and language problems of autism treated?*

If a doctor suspects a child has autism or another developmental disability, he or she usually will refer the child to a variety of specialists, including a speech-language pathologist. This is a health professional trained to treat individuals with voice, speech, and language disorders.

The speech-language pathologist will perform a comprehensive evaluation of the child's ability to communicate and design an appropriate treatment program. In addition, the pathologist might make a referral for audiological testing to make sure the child's hearing is normal.

Teaching children with autism how to communicate is essential in helping them reach their full potential. There are many different approaches to improve communication skills in a child with autism. The best treatment program begins early, during the preschool years, and is tailored to the child's age and interests. It also will address both the child's behavior and communication skills and offer regular reinforcement of positive actions. Most children with autism respond well to highly structured, specialized programs. Parents or primary caregivers as well as other family members should be involved in the treatment program so it will become part of the child's daily life.

For some younger children, improving verbal communication is a realistic goal of treatment. Parents and caregivers can increase a child's chance of reaching this goal by paying attention to his or her language development early on. Just as toddlers learn to crawl before they walk, children first develop pre-language skills before they begin to use words. These skills include using eye contact, gestures, body movements, and babbling and other vocalizations to help them communicate. Children who lack these skills may be evaluated and treated by a speech-language pathologist to prevent further developmental delays.

For slightly older children with autism, basic communication training often emphasizes the functional use of language, such as learning to hold a conversation with another person which includes staying on topic and taking turns speaking.

Experts estimate that as many as 25% of all children with autism may never develop verbal language skills. For some of these children, the goal may be to acquire gestured communication, such as the use of sign language. For others, the goal may be to communicate by means of a symbol system in which pictures are used to convey thoughts. Symbol systems can range from picture boards or cards to sophisticated electronic devices that generate speech through the use of buttons that represent common items or actions.

## Statistics on Voice, Speech, and Language

The functions, skills, and abilities of voice, speech, and language are related. Some dictionaries and textbooks use the terms almost interchangeably. But, for scientists and medical professionals, it is important to distinguish among them.

Voice (or vocalization) is the sound produced by humans and other vertebrates using the lungs and the vocal folds in the larynx, or voice box. Voice is not always produced as speech, however. Infants babble and coo, animals bark, moo, whinny, growl, and meow, and adult humans laugh, sing, and cry. Voice is generated by airflow from the lungs as the vocal folds are brought close together. When air is pushed past the vocal folds with sufficient pressure, the vocal folds vibrate. If the vocal folds in the larynx did not vibrate normally, speech could only be produced as a whisper. Your voice is as unique as your fingerprint. It helps define your personality, mood, and health.

### Speech Statistics

- The prevalence of speech sound disorder in young children is 8–9%. By the first grade, roughly 5% of children have noticeable speech disorders; the majority of these speech disorders have no known cause.

- Usually by six months of age an infant babbles or produces repetitive syllables such as "ba, ba, ba" or "da, da, da." Babbling soon turns into a type of nonsense speech called jargon that often has the tone and cadence of human speech but does not contain real words. By the end of their first year, most children have mastered the ability to say a few simple words. By 18 months of age most children can say 8–10 words and, by age two, are putting words together in crude sentences such as "more milk." At ages 3–5 a child's vocabulary rapidly increases, and he or she begins to master the rules of language.

- It is estimated that more than three million Americans stutter. Stuttering affects individuals of all ages but occurs most frequently in young children between the ages of 2–6 who are developing language. Boys are three times more likely to stutter than girls. Most children, however, outgrow their stuttering, and it is estimated that fewer than 1% of adults stutter.

- Autism is one of the most common developmental disabilities, affecting individuals of all races and ethnic and socioeconomic backgrounds. Current estimates suggest that approximately 400,000 individuals in the United States have autism. Autism is 3–4 times more likely to affect boys than girls and occurs in individuals of all levels of intelligence. Approximately 75% are of low intelligence while 10% may demonstrate high intelligence in specific areas such as math.

## *Language Statistics*

- Between 6–8 million people in the United States have some form of language impairment.

- Research suggests that the first six months are the most crucial to a child's development of language skills. For a person to become fully competent in any language, exposure must begin as early as possible, preferably before school age.

- More than 160 cases of Landau-Kleffner syndrome (LKS)—a childhood disorder involving loss of the ability to understand and use spoken language—have been reported from 1957 through 1990. Approximately 80% of children with LKS have one or more epileptic seizures that usually occur at night. Most children outgrow the seizures, and electrical brain activity on the electroencephalogram (EEG) usually returns to normal by age 15.

# Section 22.2

# *Auditory Processing Disorder in Children*

This section begins with excerpts from "Auditory Processing Disorder in Children," National Institute on Deafness and Other Communication Disorders (NIDCD), April 1, 2008; and continues with "Auditory Processing Problems in Autism," written by Stephen M. Edelson, PhD. © 2000 Autism Research Institute (http://legacy.autism.com). Reprinted with permission. Reviewed in October 2010 by David A. Cooke, MD, FACP.

Auditory processing is a term used to describe what happens when your brain recognizes and interprets the sounds around you. Humans hear when energy that we recognize as sound travels through the ear and is changed into electrical information that can be interpreted by the brain. The disorder part of auditory processing disorder means that something is adversely affecting the processing or interpretation of the information.

Children with auditory processing disorder (APD) often do not recognize subtle differences between sounds in words, even though the sounds themselves are loud and clear. For example, the request "Tell me how a chair and a couch are alike" may sound to a child with APD like "Tell me how a couch and a chair are alike." It can even be understood by the child as "Tell me how a cow and a hair are alike." These kinds of problems are more likely to occur when a person with APD is in a noisy environment or when he or she is listening to complex information.

APD goes by many other names. Sometimes it is referred to as central auditory processing disorder (CAPD). Other common names are auditory perception problem, auditory comprehension deficit, central auditory dysfunction, central deafness, and so-called word deafness.

### *What are the symptoms of possible auditory processing difficulty?*

Children with auditory processing difficulty typically have normal hearing and intelligence. However, they have also been observed to:

- have trouble paying attention to and remembering information presented orally,

- have problems carrying out multistep directions,

- have poor listening skills,

- need more time to process information,

- have low academic performance,

- have behavior problems,

- have language difficulty (for example, they confuse syllable sequences and have problems developing vocabulary and understanding language), and

- have difficulty with reading, comprehension, spelling, and vocabulary.

### How is suspected auditory processing difficulty diagnosed in children?

You, a teacher, or a day care provider may be the first person to notice symptoms of auditory processing difficulty in your child. So talking to your child's teacher about school or preschool performance is a good idea. Many health professionals can also diagnose APD in your child. There may need to be ongoing observation with the professionals involved.

Much of what will be done by these professionals will be to rule out other problems. A pediatrician or a family doctor can help rule out possible diseases that can cause some of these same symptoms. He or she will also measure growth and development. If there is a disease or disorder related to hearing, you may be referred to an otolaryngologist—a physician who specializes in diseases and disorders of the head and neck.

To determine whether your child has a hearing function problem, an audiologic evaluation is necessary. An audiologist will give tests that can determine the softest sounds and words a person can hear and other tests to see how well people can recognize sounds in words and sentences. For example, for one task, the audiologist might have your child listen to different numbers or words in the right and the left ear at the same time. Another common audiologic task involves giving the child two sentences, one louder than the other, at the same time. The audiologist is trying to identify the processing problem.

A speech-language pathologist can find out how well a person understands and uses language. A mental health professional can give you information about cognitive and behavioral challenges that may contribute to problems in some cases, or he or she may have suggestions that will be helpful. Because the audiologist can help with the functional problems of hearing and processing, and the speech-language pathologist is focused on language, they may work as a team with your child. All of these professionals seek to provide the best outcome for each child.

### What treatments are available for auditory processing difficulty?

Much research is still needed to understand APD problems, related disorders, and the best intervention for each child or adult. Several strategies are available to help children with auditory processing difficulties. Some of these are commercially available, but have not been fully studied. Any strategy selected should be used under the guidance of a team of professionals, and the effectiveness of the strategy needs to be evaluated. Researchers are currently studying a variety of approaches to treatment. Several strategies you may hear about include the following:

- Auditory trainers are electronic devices that allow a person to focus attention on a speaker and reduce the interference of background noise. They are often used in classrooms, where the teacher wears a microphone to transmit sound and the child wears a headset to receive the sound. Children who wear hearing aids can use them in addition to the auditory trainer.

- Environmental modifications such as classroom acoustics, placement, and seating may help. An audiologist may suggest ways to improve the listening environment, and he or she will be able to monitor any changes in hearing status.

- Exercises to improve language-building skills can increase the ability to learn new words and increase a child's language base.

- Auditory memory enhancement, a procedure that reduces detailed information to a more basic representation, may help. Also, informal auditory training techniques can be used by teachers and therapists to address specific difficulties.

- Auditory integration training may be promoted by practitioners as a way to retrain the auditory system and decrease hearing distortion. However, current research has not proven the benefits of this treatment.

253

## Auditory Processing Problems in Autism

Autistic individuals typically have problems processing auditory information. One auditory processing problem occurs when a person hears speech sounds but he/she does not perceive the meaning of the sounds. For example, if someone says the word shoe, the person may hear the speech sound, but he/she does not understand the meaning of the sound. Sometimes the lack of speech comprehension is interpreted by others as an unwillingness to comply. However, the person may not be able to retrieve the meaning of the sound at that particular time.

Eric Courchesne of the University of California at San Diego has found significant impairments in auditory processing in autistic individuals using P300 brain wave technology (see Courchesne, 1987 for a review). The P300 brain wave occurs 300 milliseconds after the presentation of a stimulus. (The P refers to the positive polarity of the brain wave.) The P300 is associated with cognitive processing, and this brain wave is considered an indication of long-term memory retrieval (Donchin, Ritter, and McCallum, 1978). Edelson et al. (1999) examined auditory P300 activity prior to and three months following auditory integration training (AIT). Three autistic individuals participated in the experimental AIT group and two autistic individuals participated in a placebo group. Prior to AIT, all five individuals had abnormal auditory P300 activity, indicating an auditory processing problem. Three months following AIT, the results showed dramatic improvement in P300 activity for those who received AIT (for example, a normalization of P300 activity) and found no change in those who received the placebo.

We do not know the underlying reason for auditory processing problems in autism; however, autopsy research by Drs. Bauman and Kemper have shown that an area in the limbic system, the hippocampus, is neurologically immature in autistic individuals (Bauman and Kemper, 1994). The hippocampus is responsible for sensory input as well as learning and memory. Basically, information is transferred from the senses to the hippocampus, where it is processed and then transferred to areas of the cerebral cortex for long-term storage. Since auditory information is processed in the hippocampus, the information may not be properly transferred to long-term memory in autistic individuals.

Auditory processing problems may also be linked to several autistic characteristics. Autism is sometimes described as a social-communication problem. Processing auditory information is a critical component of social-communication. Other characteristics that may be associated with auditory processing problems include: anxiety or confusion in social situations, inattentiveness, and poor speech comprehension.

Interestingly, those individuals who do not have auditory processing problems are often auditory learners. These children do very well using the Applied Behavior Analysis (ABA) approach, whereas those who are visual learners do not do as well with this approach (McEachin, Smith and Lovaas, 1993). Given this, one might suspect that many visual learners have auditory processing problems and that visual learners will do quite well with a visual communication/instruction approach. It is also possible to provide visual support with ABA programs that have an auditory component. In this way, the visual learner can process the auditory information more easily.

The better that autistic children understand auditory information, the better they can comprehend their environment, both socially and academically. The better we understand the autistic child, the better we can develop ways to intervene in an effective manner.

## References

Bauman, M.L., and Kemper, T.L. (1994). Neuroanatomic observations of the brain in autism. In M.L. Bauman and T.L. Kemper (Eds.), *The neurobiology of autism*. Baltimore: Johns Hopkins UP.

Courchesne, E. (1987). A neurophysiological view of autism. In E. Schopler & G.B. Mesibov (Eds.), *Neurological issues in autism*. New York: Plenum Press.

Donchin, E., Ritter, W., and McCallum, W.C. (1978). Cognitive psychophysiology: The endogenous components of the ERP. In E. Callaway, P. Tueting, and S. Koslow (Eds.), *Event-related brain potentials in man*. New York: Academic Press.

Edelson, S.M., Arin, D., Bauman, M., Lukas, S.E., Rudy, J.H., Sholar, M., and Rimland, B. (1999). Auditory integration training: A double-blind study of behavioral, electrophysiological, and audiometric effects in autistic subjects. *Focus on Autism and Other Developmental Disabilities, 14*, 73–81.

McEachin, J.J., Smith, T., and Lovaas, O.I. (1993). Long-term outcome for children with autism who received early intensive behavioral treatment. *American Journal of Mental Retardation, 97*, 359–372.

## Section 22.3

# *Autism Spectrum Disorders and Stuttering*

"Autism Spectrum Disorders and Stuttering," Kathleen Scaler
Scott, MS, CCC-SLP. © 2008 Stuttering Foundation of America
(www.stutteringhelp.org). Reprinted with permission.

### *What are autism spectrum disorders?*

Autism spectrum disorders (ASDs) include autism, pervasive developmental disorder not otherwise specified, and Asperger syndrome. All
three are characterized by impairments in 1) social interaction, 2) communication, and 3) restricted interests/repetitive behaviors. Specific
criteria distinguish one subgroup from another. ASDs are often first
diagnosed in childhood, and intelligence ranges from below to above
average. There is no definitive research regarding the cause of ASDs.

Although there are no specific statistics on the number of people
with ASDs who stutter, there have been numerous documented cases
of stuttering in ASDs. These range from typical forms of stuttering,
such as repetitions (c-c-cup), prolongations (cuuuup), or blocks (sound
gets stuck), to less typical stuttering, such as repetitions of the last
syllable of a word (sound-ound).

Speech may also sound disorganized due to a higher than average
number of normal disfluencies, interjections, repetitions of phrases,
and/or revisions of thoughts. Individuals may show different combinations and levels of awareness of these symptoms.

### *Diagnosis*

A professional specializing in pediatric development typically makes
the diagnosis of an ASD. Diagnosis often occurs between the age of
two and eight years. However, a speech-language pathologist (SLP)
typically diagnoses stuttering. Because children with ASDs have many
ongoing issues with social interaction and communication, stuttering is not always noticed and diagnosed until a child reaches school
age. Interactions between ASDs and stuttering present a complex
combination of disorders for which research is ongoing. An SLP who

has expertise in the area of fluency should evaluate stuttering in this population; those also familiar with ASDs are ideal evaluators. The evaluation should help distinguish typical disfluencies from stuttering and determine whether difficulties lie in speech production or other areas, such as organization of language. It is important to determine if the problem is motor- and/or language-based because treatment will be based upon this determination. After listening to the organization of a child's language during conversation and/or story retelling activities, an SLP may decide to test word finding or narrative language to determine whether accompanying language deficits are present. If both formal testing and observation of the child's speech in everyday settings reveal an underlying language deficit, the SLP should address the language issues along with the stuttering.

## *Treatment*

Treatment should always be based upon each client's needs, and this is particularly true with ASDs. Because stuttering interferes with effective conversation skills and therefore social interaction, treatment is crucial. Social interaction and self-monitoring can be more difficult for those with ASDs. So treatment will often focus upon use of fluency tools in social exchanges. Tools may include the following:

- **Traditional stuttering tools, such as easy onset or prolonged speech:** How the tools are taught will depend upon the child's level of comprehension. Those with a higher comprehension level will benefit from a description of techniques either written or in picture form coupled with practice. Carol Gray's model for Social Stories, www.thegraycenter.org and http://www.medical assistantschools.org/resources/autism.html, is often helpful for describing stuttering tools for those with ASDs. Children with a lower comprehension level will benefit from less description and more imitation of therapist models. Concrete visual models, such as stretching modeling clay for "stretchy," prolonged speech, are often helpful to demonstrate the skill. Self-monitoring in context can be difficult for those with ASDs, so consistent repeated practice is often necessary for mastery. To help ensure carryover to everyday environments, teachers, parents, and others who interact with the child should gently remind him about tool use.

- **Tools for organizing thoughts, such as visual organizers:** Story webs and visual mapping programs such as Inspiration or Kidspiration, www.inspiration.com, can be helpful in organizing thoughts. Once skills are demonstrated, they should be practiced in more to less structured settings.

- **Increase pausing to allow extra time:** To organize thoughts; breath in appropriate places; and apply fluency tools, such as easy onsets, easy starts, or prolonged speech. Pausing can be introduced by inserting visual markers to indicate where to pause when reading sentences or paragraphs. Model pausing if the child has difficulty with reading tasks.

## Tips for Parents

If your child is stuttering, treat him as you would any other child, with kindness and respect. Above all, convey total acceptance. Working on communication and fluency skills is a challenge that affects all areas of a child's day; therefore, the child needs as much support, encouragement, and acceptance as possible. When he is speaking, try to focus on the following:

- Listen to what your child has to say. Use facial expressions and other body language to convey that you are listening to the content of the message and not to how your child is talking. Maintain eye contact.

- Allow your child the time he needs to finish his thoughts.

- Help all members of the family learn to take turns talking and listening. Objects such a microphone or a salt shaker at the dinner table can be passed to indicate each person's turn. This provides a good model for the child with an ASD and helps her to feel like your family is in this together.

- Choose specific and brief times to work on strategies in the midst of everyday activities, such as 5–10 minutes during bath time. Short consistent practice is often most effective.

## Tips for Therapists in Structuring Sessions

Structure activities according to a consistent, organized schedule that the young person has helped to create. Post these routines in the therapy room so he is aware of the schedule and what comes next. The ASD population benefits most from direct engagement; this is contrary to the ADHD population who respond to rewards.

Therefore, you should teach and practice tools in the context of play or preferred activities to keep the young person engaged and to make activities meaningful. If activities are meaningful, she will re-member and use them outside therapy. Research indicates if children with ASDs are not first engaged, all the rewards in the world will not lead to generalization. Therefore, engagement is key. For example, if the child is engaged and motivated to have a snack, have her practice speech tools when asking for the snack. For more information, visit: http://icdl.com/staging and search for the Greenspan 2001 research document, The Affect Diathesis Hypothesis.

- Keep instructions simple, clear, and concise. Be sure that the child is engaged with you, and present directions multiple times if necessary. If there is no response, try simplifying the directions and/or adding visual/contextual cues. For example, simplify "Get your coat so we can go outside" to "Going outside. Get coat" while pointing to the child's coat.

- Provide visual cues, concrete examples, and drawings to increase comprehension. For example, try stretching Playdough while practicing easing in to a speech sound "e e e a s y."

- Increase the child's self-monitoring skills and awareness of how behaviors affect interactions with others. Focus on the accuracy of self-assessment of his speech in simple and complex speaking situations. Then, teach problem solving to allow him to change his speech accordingly.

- Keep in mind the child's level of functioning: some are quite lit-eral and need more concrete examples, such as rating their use of speech tools "thumbs up" or "thumbs down," while others can use more cognitively-based rating systems, such as using a scale from 1–5.

- Address overall communication skills. By introducing and modeling appropriate skills such as eye contact, volume, rate, and listening skills yourself, you will help to increase the child's confidence and self-esteem while reducing speech-related anxiety.

- Young people with ASDs benefit from working with socially stronger peers who can act as role models. To foster generaliza-tion of new skills, explore grouping the individual with others who have similar speech characteristics and who are good social models. This will provide an optimal setting to practice fluency tools, social skills, and overall self-monitoring.

# Chapter 23

# ASD, Seizures, and Epilepsy

Epilepsy is a brain disorder in which clusters of nerve cells, or neurons, in the brain sometimes signal abnormally. Neurons normally generate electrochemical impulses that act on other neurons, glands, and muscles to produce human thoughts, feelings, and actions. In epilepsy, the normal pattern of neuronal activity becomes disturbed, causing strange sensations, emotions, and behavior, or sometimes convulsions, muscle spasms, and loss of consciousness. During a seizure, neurons may fire as many as 500 times a second, much faster than normal. In some people, this happens only occasionally; for others, it may happen up to hundreds of times a day.

More than two million people in the United States—about one in 100—have experienced an unprovoked seizure or been diagnosed with epilepsy. For about 80% of those diagnosed with epilepsy, seizures can be controlled with modern medicines and surgical techniques. However, about 25% to 30% of people with epilepsy will continue to experience seizures even with the best available treatment. Doctors call this situation intractable epilepsy. Having a seizure does not necessarily mean that a person has epilepsy. Only when a person has had two or more seizures is he or she considered to have epilepsy.

Epilepsy is not contagious and is not caused by mental illness or mental retardation. Some people with mental retardation may experience seizures, but seizures do not necessarily mean the person has

This chapter includes text excerpted from "Seizures and Epilepsy: Hope through Research," National Institute of Neurological Disorders and Stroke (NINDS), NIH Publication No. 04–156, updated October 22, 2010.

or will develop mental impairment. Many people with epilepsy have normal or above-average intelligence. Seizures sometimes do cause brain damage, particularly if they are severe. However, most seizures do not seem to have a detrimental effect on the brain. Any changes that do occur are usually subtle, and it is often unclear whether these changes are caused by the seizures themselves or by the underlying problem that caused the seizures.

While epilepsy cannot currently be cured, for some people it does eventually go away. One study found that children with idiopathic epilepsy, or epilepsy with an unknown cause, had a 68% to 92% chance of becoming seizure-free by 20 years after their diagnosis. The odds of becoming seizure-free are not as good for adults or for children with severe epilepsy syndromes, but it is nonetheless possible that seizures may decrease or even stop over time. This is more likely if the epilepsy has been well-controlled by medication or if the person has had epilepsy surgery.

### What causes epilepsy?

Epilepsy is a disorder with many possible causes. Anything that disturbs the normal pattern of neuron activity—from illness to brain damage to abnormal brain development—can lead to seizures.

Epilepsy may develop because of an abnormality in brain wiring, an imbalance of nerve signaling chemicals called neurotransmitters, or some combination of these factors. Researchers believe that some people with epilepsy have an abnormally high level of excitatory neurotransmitters that increase neuronal activity, while others have an abnormally low level of inhibitory neurotransmitters that decrease neuronal activity in the brain. Either situation can result in too much neuronal activity and cause epilepsy. One of the most-studied neurotransmitters that plays a role in epilepsy is GABA, or gamma-aminobutyric acid, which is an inhibitory neurotransmitter. Research on GABA has led to drugs that alter the amount of this neurotransmitter in the brain or change how the brain responds to it. Researchers also are studying excitatory neurotransmitters such as glutamate.

In some cases, the brain's attempts to repair itself after a head injury, stroke, or other problem may inadvertently generate abnormal nerve connections that lead to epilepsy. Abnormalities in brain wiring that occur during brain development also may disturb neuronal activity and lead to epilepsy.

Research has shown that the cell membrane that surrounds each neuron plays an important role in epilepsy. Cell membranes are crucial for a neuron to generate electrical impulses. For this reason, researchers are studying details of the membrane structure, how molecules move in and out of membranes, and how the cell nourishes and repairs the membrane. A disruption in any of these processes may lead to epilepsy. Studies in animals have shown that, because the brain continually adapts to changes in stimuli, a small change in neuronal activity, if repeated, may eventually lead to full-blown epilepsy. Researchers are investigating whether this phenomenon, called kindling, may also occur in humans.

In some cases, epilepsy may result from changes in non-neuronal brain cells called glia. These cells regulate concentrations of chemicals in the brain that can affect neuronal signaling. About half of all seizures have no known cause. However, in other cases, the seizures are clearly linked to infection, trauma, or other identifiable problems.

**Genetic factors:** Research suggests that genetic abnormalities may be some of the most important factors contributing to epilepsy. Some types of epilepsy have been traced to an abnormality in a specific gene. Many other types of epilepsy tend to run in families, suggesting that genes influence epilepsy. Some researchers estimate that more than 500 genes could play a role in this disorder. However, it is increasingly clear that, for many forms of epilepsy, genetic abnormalities play only a partial role, perhaps by increasing a person's susceptibility to seizures that are triggered by an environmental factor.

Several types of epilepsy have now been linked to defective genes for ion channels, the "gates" that control the flow of ions in and out of cells and regulate neuron signaling. Another gene, which is missing in people with progressive myoclonus epilepsy, codes for a protein called cystatin B. This protein regulates enzymes that break down other proteins. Another gene, which is altered in a severe form of epilepsy called LaFora disease, has been linked to a gene that helps to break down carbohydrates.

While abnormal genes sometimes cause epilepsy, they also may influence the disorder in subtler ways. For example, one study showed that many people with epilepsy have an abnormally active version of a gene that increases resistance to drugs. This may help explain why anticonvulsant drugs do not work for some people. Genes also may control other aspects of the body's response to medications and each person's susceptibility to seizures, or seizure threshold. Abnormalities in the genes that control neuronal migration—a critical step in brain development—can lead to areas of misplaced or abnormally formed neurons, or dysplasia, in the brain that can cause epilepsy. In some cases, genes may contribute to development of epilepsy even in people with no family history of the disorder. These people may have a newly developed abnormality, or mutation, in an epilepsy-related gene.

**Other disorders:** In many cases, epilepsy develops as a result of brain damage from other disorders. For example, brain tumors, alcoholism, and Alzheimer disease frequently lead to epilepsy because they alter the normal workings of the brain. Epilepsy is associated with a variety of developmental and metabolic disorders, including cerebral palsy, neurofibromatosis, pyruvate dependency, tuberous sclerosis, Landau-Kleffner syndrome, and autism. Epilepsy is just one of a set of symptoms commonly found in people with these disorders.

# Chapter 24

# *Non-Verbal Learning Disability and Asperger Syndrome*

There is clearly a great deal of overlap between Asperger disorder (AD) and nonverbal learning disabilities (NVLD), so much so that it is possible that the symptoms of each describe the same group of children from different perspectives—AD from either a psychiatric/behavioral perspective, and NVLD from a neuropsychological perspective. The specific conventions of these diagnoses may lead to a somewhat different group of children meeting diagnostic criteria, but it is not clear that this reflects something true in nature. That is, it may only be convention that separates these two groups.

One is reminded of the story of the six blind men who were asked to describe an elephant. Each man grabbed a different part of the creature (the snake-like trunk versus the tree-like leg) and gave an accurate description from his own particular perspective—but each man thought the others were completely mistaken.

Studies conducted by the Yale Child-Study Group suggest that up to 80% of children who meet the criteria for AD also have NVLD. While there are no studies on overlap in the other direction, most likely children with the more severe forms of NVLD also have AD. Children from both groups are socially awkward and pay over-attention to detail and parts while missing main themes or underlying principles. However, by convention, the two groups differ in the range of severity. Professionals

"Asperger's Disorder and Non-Verbal Learning Disabilities: How Are These Two Disorders Related to Each Other," by Dr. David Dinklage. © 2008 Asperger's Association of New England (www.aane.org). Reprinted with permission.

reserve an AD diagnosis for children with more severe social impairment and behavioral rigidity; some symptoms may overlap with high functioning autism. There are degrees of severity within AD but not to the extent that is acceptable in diagnosing NVLD. These degrees can range from extreme autistic behavior to cases where the social difficulties are very subtle and the academic/cognitive difficulties are more prominent.

Here is a brief outline of the diagnostic criteria for AD and the pattern of neuropsychological findings in NVLD. While the overlap is apparent, the emphasis is different because criteria for NVLD focuses on academic issues as well as specific test findings and is not purely descriptive. This also results in different means of making the diagnosis (testing or observing).

## Asperger Disorder (AD) Characteristics

A. Qualitative impairment in social interaction.

1. Failure to use non-verbal social skills (such as eye contact, gestures, body posture, facial expressions).

2. Developmentally inappropriate peer relationships.

3. Lack of spontaneous sharing of enjoyment and interests with other people.

4. Lack of social and emotional reciprocity.

B. Restricted, repetitive and stereotyped patterns of behavior, interests, and activities.

1. Preoccupation that is overly intense and narrow.

2. Inflexible adherence to non-functional or peripheral routines.

3. Stereotyped or repetitive motor movements.

4. Persistent preoccupation with parts of objects.

C. These problems taken together (A plus B) result in significant challenges in the lives of people with AD as they attempt to live in a neuro-typical world and meet the expectations of others.

D. There is no general language delay.

E. There is no severe global cognitive impairment.

## Non-Verbal Learning Disability (NVLD)

A. NVLD can be conceptualized as an imbalance in thinking skills—intact linear, detail oriented, automatic processing with impaired appreciation of the big picture, gestalt, or underlying theme.

B. It is not nearly as common as language-based learning disabilities, but this may be a phenomenon created by environmental demands (for example, our societal demands for precision skills in reading assure that even the most subtle language-based learning disability [LD] cases are identified)

C. Typically social/psychiatric concerns are raised before academic problems are identified.

D. While the overlap is not complete, NVLD children may meet the criteria for pervasive developmental disorder not otherwise specified (PDDNOS), Asperger disorder, or schizotypal personality.

### *Neuropsychological Profile*

- Full range of intelligence quotient (IQ).

- Visual spatial deficits are most pronounced: poor appreciation of gestalt, poor appreciation of body in space, sometimes left side inattention/neglect, may have highly developed but ritualized drawing skills that are extremely detail oriented.

- Rote linguistic skills are normal (such as repetition, naming, fluency, syntactic comprehension), but pragmatic use of language is impaired: weak grasp of inference, little content, disorganized narrative despite good vocabulary and grammar. Rote recall of a story may be good, but the main point missed. Rhythm, volume, and prosody of speech are often disturbed.

- Motor and sensory findings are common: usually poor fine and gross motor coordination, left side worse than right.

- Attention is usually reported to be impaired and testing supports this, but the affect is desultory as opposed to distractingly impulsive, as in attention deficit/hyperactivity disorder (ADHD). It is as if people with NVLD do not know what to attend to, but once focused, can sustain attention to detail. The distinction between figure and ground is disturbed, resulting in attention errors.

## *Academics*

- Difficulties are often picked up late because decoding and spelling may be quite strong.

- Inferential reading comprehension is weak relative to decoding and spelling skills.

- Math is often the first academic subject to be viewed as problematic. Spatial and conceptual aspects of mathematics are a problem; math facts may be readily mastered. For example, a student may know the answer to a simple multiplication problem, but not understand what multiplication is.

- Due to spatial and fine motor problems, handwriting is usually poor.

- Organization skills are weak, particularly in written work.

## *Social/Emotional Issues*

- Peer relations are typically the greatest area of impairment; may play with much older or younger children than with same age peers where they must manage give and take.

- They often lack basic social skills; may stand too close, stare inappropriately or not make eye contact, have marked lack of concern over appearance, be oblivious to other's reactions, change topics idiosyncratically.

- Children with NVLD are seen as odd children who just don't get it socially. They may do better with adults, where they act dependent and immature, but may not be seen as odd.

- They may show poorly modulated affect, not matched to verbal content.

- Lack of empathy and social judgment may shield them from fully experiencing the hurt of peer rejection, while the same factors increase the likelihood of being rejected.

- History of unusual thinking can often be obtained: rituals, stereotypic behaviors, rigid routines, and magical/bizarre beliefs.

## Assessment of NVLD Compared with Assessment of AD

- NVLD should be diagnosed in the context of a comprehensive neuropsychological evaluation. It is not simply a matter of performance IQ being less than verbal IQ, since there may be many reasons for such a discrepancy besides NVLD. Furthermore, NVLD can be present even if no discrepancies between strong verbal ability and poor performance show up on the *Weschler Intelligence Scale for Children (WISC-III)*. One does not need to have every characteristic of NVLD in dramatic form for the diagnosis to be helpful in delineating the pattern of strength and weaknesses.

- NVLD can be complicated by an array of psychiatric and social/ familial problems, so it is important to assess the whole child-world system, not just the cognitive status.

- AD is best diagnosed from a detailed history, school reports, and observing the child. As parents vary in how they report symptoms, one good marker is whether or not the child had engaged in symbolic play as a toddler. Children with AD tend not to play with toys as the thing they represent. For example, they may collect fire trucks but not play fire. Parents may also report that their children use language instrumentally, rather than using it to trade ideas. The children do not seem to consider that the other may have different ideas.

- Because AD is diagnosed descriptively, one does not need neuropsychological testing to diagnose it. However, since there is so much overlap between AD and NVLD, neuropsychological testing is strongly recommended. Testing will identify any specific interference with academic functioning, and confirm imbalances in thinking skills that may have been observed.

In my practice I have seen a number of children with AD who would not meet the criteria for NVLD in any existing research studies. If these children had participated in the Yale study mentioned earlier in this article, they would probably have been in the 20% of the AD children who did not meet the NVLD criteria. It is possible that the AD children in that 20% may have had very high visual spatial scores, thus masking their over-attention to detail in problem solving. For example, they may have scored very high on the Block Design subtest of the IQ measure (using colored blocks to match a pattern given to them) with little or no appreciation of the gestalt. Their considerable skill and speed at analyzing detail would have allowed them to use this inefficient strategy effectively. With these very bright children, it may be that the tests are not sufficiently sensitive to discern a pattern of NVLD. On the other hand, some children with AD show diffuse difficulties in the language and attention domain, but may not exhibit the pronounced discrepancies associated with NVLD. Nonetheless, they may still struggle with the cognitive difficulties of NVLD. Conversely, a child meeting the criteria for NVLD, may not meet the criteria for AD, even though subtle characteristics of the disorder may be present.

A case example best illustrates how children who clearly have NVLD may not meet the criteria for AD as it is presently understood. I evaluated an eighth grade girl whose parents were concerned about her math performance. She had above average overall ability, but a 24-point discrepancy between her verbal and visual spatial skills on the IQ measure. On the neuropsychological measures, she clearly had the pattern of visual spatial deficits, left sided motor slowing, and poor math ability, while language skills were intact. She did not have any problems with inferential comprehension in reading. One would not even have considered Asperger disorder. She had had many good friends through elementary school and felt herself to be part of her peer group. Symbolic play development had been normal and she exhibited no repetitive behaviors. This is unusual in NVLD as well, but since much of the criteria for this neuropsychological diagnosis is cognitive and test-based, it was determined that she met enough of the criteria for a diagnosis of NVLD. I commented in the report that, unlike this girl, most children with NVLD have more social problems, tend to miss the point in social interactions, and have trouble in content areas in school because of inferential reading comprehension problems.

The parents came back to me when she was a senior. She was now isolated from her peers, who complained that she was too literal. Now she was struggling in literature and social studies; her papers tended to be more like lists and less integrated than those of her peers. I don't believe she was developing a new disorder. She had a classic NVLD, but it was relatively subtle, and it required more high-powered peer and academic demands to highlight her social perception and inferential reasoning weaknesses, much the same way that some mildly dyslexic individuals compensate reasonably well and go unnoticed until they flunk out of their first year of college. Given her history of good social adjustment, one would still never diagnose her with AD. One has to wonder whether her neurocognitive functioning indicated AD, but in a much milder form.

Asperger disorder was not originally thought of as having a continuum of severity that included these subtle forms, whereas NVLD did not start with the assumption of more extreme difficulties. As information about AD becomes more widely circulated more and more subtle cases are being identified and the culture is, in some manner, changing the original intention of the category. While that may dilute the meaning of the diagnosis, it will more accurately reflect the variety of developmental presentations in nature. As humans, we naturally want to categorize. The complex relationship between NVLD and AD may be an example of how categorizing too rigidly can confuse, rather than clarify, our thinking.

~Dr. David Dinklage is Director of Neuropsychology at Cambridge Hospital, and has a private practice in Belmont.

# Chapter 25

# *Co-Occurring Genetic Disorders in People with ASD*

## *Chapter Contents*

# Section 25.1

# *Angelman Syndrome*

Some of the associated clinical features of Angelman syndrome (AS) (for example: hand-flapping, stereotypic behaviors, deficits in expressive language), overlap with certain features of autism. Generally speaking, clinicians should exercise caution when examining symptoms of autism within AS, because some AS patients have been mistakenly identified as having autism in lieu of AS,[1] and some patients who exhibit features of autism when they are younger, may no longer exhibit these features as their cognition and their language skills improve.

There are, however, some studies that specifically examine the frequency and magnitude of autistic traits in individuals with AS. While some researchers demonstrate a lack of autistic traits or very low incidence of autism in individuals with AS,[2,3] several other studies have demonstrated that a percentage of individuals with AS do also meet criteria for autism.[4-6] Individuals with AS and co-morbid autism are more likely to show decreased eye gaze, fewer social overtures, use fewer nonverbal gestures, use another person's body as a "tool" to communicate "for" them, have decreased shared enjoyment in interactions, and fewer socially directed vocalizations.[4-6]

In considering the differences in findings and clinical opinions across these studies, it is important to note that differences in sample selection, including differences in autism symptom severity across molecular subtypes of AS play a major role. Specifically, recent studies demonstrate that it is primarily deletion positive individuals with AS that exhibit greater symptom severity associated with autism, and within the deletion positive group, primarily children with larger, Class I deletions.[7,8] Most recent findings indicate that these differences in symptoms of autism between the deletion subgroups are not related to differences in cognition (for example: children with greater symptom severity were not necessarily lower functioning).

To summarize, studies seem to indicate that severity of autism symptoms in AS only affects a small proportion of AS patients, is associated with deletion size, and with a more aloof/withdrawn behavioral phenotype. There are four genes (NIPA 1, NIPA 2, CYFIP1, and GCP5) missing in Class I and present in Class II deletions, one or more of which may have a role in the development of socialization skills and symptoms related to autism. For the small percentage of patients with AS who do exhibit more features of co-morbid autism, specific therapies such as applied behavioral analysis are quite helpful.

Repetitive behaviors (for example, using objects or toys inappropriately), sensory interests (licking/mouthing, sniffing objects), and stereotypic motor movements (rocking, hand-flapping) are common to all individuals with AS and do not differentiate between those individuals who also have co-morbid autism.[4,6,9] In fact, some individuals with AS do exhibit some compulsions, rituals (such as hoarding, hiding of food or objects, food fads), and repetitive interests/playing with unusual objects.[10] These behaviors are primarily noted in older, and/or higher functioning individuals with AS and do seem to overlap with behaviors associated with Prader-Willi syndrome; but the degree to which these associated behaviors are prevalent across the different molecular subclasses of individuals with AS has not yet been investigated. Additionally, the degree to which these behaviors may be responsive to pharmacological treatment has also not been investigated in formal clinical trials.

## References

1. Williams CA. Neurological aspects of the Angelman syndrome. *Brain Dev*, 2005. 27(2): p. 88–94.

2. Thompson RJ and Bolton PF. Case report: Angelman syndrome in an individual with a small SMC(15) and paternal uniparental disomy: a case report with reference to the assessment of cognitive functioning and autistic symptomatology. *J Autism Dev Disord*, 2003. 33(2): p. 171–6.

3. Veltman MW, Craig EE and Bolton PF. Autism spectrum disorders in Prader-Willi and Angelman syndromes: a systematic review. *Psychiatr Genet*, 2005. 15(4): p. 243–54.

4. Peters SU, Goddard-Finegold J, Beaudet AL, et al. Cognitive and adaptive behavior profiles of children with Angelman syndrome. *Am J Med Genet A*, 2004. 128(2): p. 110–3.

5. Trillingsgaard A and Ostergaard JR. Autism in Angelman syndrome: an exploration of comorbidity. *Autism*, 2004. 8(2): p. 163–74.

6. Bonati MT, Russo S, Finelli P, et al. Evaluation of autism traits in Angelman syndrome: a resource to unfold autism genes. *Neurogenetics,* 2007. 8(3): p. 169–78.

7. Sahoo T, Bacino CA, German JR, et al. Identification of novel deletions of 15q11q13 in Angelman syndrome by array-CGH: molecular characterization and genotype-phenotype correlations. *Eur J Hum Genet,* 2007. 15(9): p. 943–9.

8. Peters SU, Bird LM, Barbier-Welge R, et al. *The relationship between molecular subtype and autism symptom severity in Angelman Syndrome*. Presented at the International Meeting for Autism Research, 2008.

9. Walz NC, Beebe D and Byars K. Sleep in individuals with Angelman syndrome: parent perceptions of patterns and problems. *Am J Ment Retard,* 2005. 110(4): p. 243–52.

10. Barry RJ, Leitner RP, Clarke AR, et al. Behavioral aspects of Angelman syndrome: a case control study. *Am J Med Genet A,* 2005. 132(1): p. 8–12.

## Section 25.2

# *Fragile X Syndrome*

This section includes an excerpt from "Fragile X Syndrome Fact Sheet," Centers for Disease Control and Prevention (CDC), 2010; and "Brain Imaging Study of Infant Sibs at Risk for Autism Expands Scope." Reprinted with the permission of Autism Speaks, www.autismspeaks.org, © 2010.

Fragile X syndrome (FXS) is the most common known cause of intellectual disability (formerly referred to as mental retardation) that can be inherited, that is passed from parent to child. It is estimated that FXS affects about one in 4,000 boys and one in 6,000 to 8,000 girls. Both boys and girls can have FXS, but girls usually are more mildly affected.

The cause of FXS is genetic. FXS occurs when there is a change in a gene on the X chromosome called FMR1. The FMR1 gene makes a protein needed for normal brain development. In FXS, the FMR1 gene does not work properly. The protein is not made, and the brain does not develop as it should. The lack of this protein causes FXS.

Children with FXS might have learning disabilities, speech and language delays, and behavioral problems such as attention-deficit/ hyperactivity disorder (ADHD) and anxiety. Some older males can develop aggressive behavior. Depression can also occur. Boys with FXS usually have a mild to severe intellectual disability. Many girls with FXS have normal intelligence. Others have some degree of intellectual disability, with or without learning disabilities. Autism spectrum disorders (ASDs) occur more often among children with FXS.

### Brain Imaging Study of Infant Sibs at Risk for Autism Expands Scope

Researchers at the University of North Carolina, Children's Hospital of Philadelphia, University of Washington in Seattle, and Washington University in St. Louis, are currently conducting a multi-center study to examine brain development in infants who have an older sibling with autism spectrum disorder (ASD). Infants are being seen at six, 12, and 24 months. Infants who have an older sibling with

277

ASD are at higher risk of developing the disorder than the general population. The goal of the Infant Brain Imaging Study (IBIS), funded in part by Autism Speaks and an Autism Center of Excellence grant from the National Institutes of Health, is to better understand early brain development in very young infants at risk for ASD, which will eventually lead to ways of identifying ASD early in life and developing interventions. Recently, new funding from the Eunice Kennedy Shriver National Institute of Child Health and Development has expanded this project to include infants and toddlers with fragile X syndrome. The study is seeking participation from families with an infant who has an older sibling with ASD or with an infant diagnosed with fragile X. All infants will receive developmental screening for ASD as part of the study.

Fragile X is a neurodevelopmental disorder caused by a single gene mutation. Because approximately 1/3 of children with fragile X also receive a diagnosis of autism, studying the brain development of these individuals very early on in life will provide important clues about what happens during brain development, when, and why.

Research suggests that early overgrowth of the brain in children with autism may coincide with the onset of autistic symptoms at the end of the first year of life. By conducting both magnetic resonance imaging (MRI) brain scans and behavioral assessments at these three time points, researchers hope to be able to understand the relationship between brain development and the onset of autistic symptoms in children at higher risk for autism (infants with older brothers and sisters with autism). Findings from this study may provide important clues to early detection and intervention. Moreover, data from this study is forming part of an even larger collaboration, announced last year, which is focusing upon understanding the influence of gene X environment interactions on brain development. A total of 1500 children will be examined as part of this large collaboration.

# Section 25.3

# *Landau-Kleffner Syndrome*

Excerpted from "Landau-Kleffner Syndrome Information Page,"
National Institute of Neurological Disorders and Stroke (NINDS),
October 17, 2008.

Landau-Kleffner syndrome (LKS) is a rare, childhood neurological disorder characterized by the sudden or gradual development of aphasia (the inability to understand or express language) and an abnormal electroencephalogram (EEG). LKS affects the parts of the brain that control comprehension and speech. The disorder usually occurs in children between the ages of five and seven years. Typically, children with LKS develop normally but then lose their language skills for no apparent reason. While many of the affected individuals have seizures, some do not. The disorder is difficult to diagnose and may be misdiagnosed as autism, pervasive developmental disorder, hearing impairment, learning disability, auditory/verbal processing disorder, attention deficit disorder, mental retardation, childhood schizophrenia, or emotional/behavioral problems.

Treatment for LKS usually consists of medications, such as anticonvulsants and corticosteroids, and speech therapy, which should be started early. A controversial treatment option involves a surgical technique called multiple subpial transection in which the pathways of abnormal electrical brain activity are severed

The prognosis for children with LKS varies. Some affected children may have a permanent severe language disorder, while others may regain much of their language abilities (although it may take months or years). In some cases, remission and relapse may occur. The prognosis is improved when the onset of the disorder is after age six and when speech therapy is started early. Seizures generally disappear by adulthood.

## Section 25.4

# *Mitochondrial Disease*

Excerpted from "Mitochondrial Disease: Frequently Asked Questions,"
Centers for Disease Control and Prevention (CDC), March 31, 2010.

Mitochondria are tiny parts of almost every cell in your body. Mitochondria are like the power house of the cells. They turn sugar and oxygen into energy that the cells need to work. In mitochondrial diseases, the mitochondria cannot efficiently turn sugar and oxygen into energy, so the cells do not work correctly.

There are many types of mitochondrial disease, and they can affect different parts of the body: the brain, kidneys, muscles, heart, eyes, ears, and others. Mitochondrial diseases can affect one part of the body or can affect many parts. They can affect those part(s) mildly or very seriously.

Not everyone with a mitochondrial disease will show symptoms. However, when discussing the group of mitochondrial diseases that tend to affect children, symptoms usually appear in the toddler and preschool years.

A child with autism may or may not have a mitochondrial disease. When a child has both autism and a mitochondrial disease, they sometimes have other problems as well, including epilepsy, problems with muscle tone, and/or movement disorders.

### What is regressive encephalopathy and is there a relationship between autism and encephalopathy?

Encephalopathy is a medical term for a disease or disorder of the brain. It usually means a slowing down of brain function. Regression happens when a person loses skills that they used to have like walking or talking or even being social. Regressive encephalopathy means there is a disease or disorder in the brain that makes a person lose skills they once had.

We know that sometimes children with mitochondrial diseases seem to be developing as they should, but around toddler or preschool age, they regress. The disease was there all the time, but something happens that sets it off. This could be something like malnutrition, an illness such as flu, a high fever, dehydration, or it could be something else.

Most children with an autism spectrum disorder do not and have not had an encephalopathy. Some children with an autism spectrum disorder have had regression and some have had a regressive encephalopathy.

# Section 25.5

# *Moebius Syndrome*

Excerpted from "Moebius Syndrome Information Page," National Institute of Neurological Disorders and Stroke (NINDS), September 16, 2008.

Moebius syndrome is a rare birth defect caused by the absence or underdevelopment of the 6th and 7th cranial nerves, which control eye movements and facial expression. Many of the other cranial nerves may also be affected, including the 3rd, 5th, 8th, 9th, 11th, and 12th. The first symptom, present at birth, is an inability to suck. Other symptoms can include: feeding, swallowing, and choking problems; excessive drooling; crossed eyes; lack of facial expression; inability to smile; eye sensitivity; motor delays; high or cleft palate; hearing problems and speech difficulties. Children with Moebius syndrome are unable to move their eyes back and forth. Decreased numbers of muscle fibers have been reported. Deformities of the tongue, jaw, and limbs, such as clubfoot, and missing or webbed fingers may also occur. As children get older, lack of facial expression and inability to smile become the dominant visible symptoms. Approximately 30%–40% of children with Moebius syndrome have some degree of autism.

**Treatment:** There is no specific course of treatment for Moebius syndrome. Treatment is supportive and in accordance with symptoms. Infants may require feeding tubes or special bottles to maintain sufficient nutrition. Surgery may correct crossed eyes and improve limb and jaw deformities. Physical and speech therapy often improves motor skills and coordination, and leads to better control of speaking and eating abilities. Plastic reconstructive surgery may be beneficial in some individuals. Nerve and muscle transfers to the corners of the mouth have been performed to provide limited ability to smile.

**Prognosis:** There is no cure for Moebius syndrome. In spite of the impairments that characterize the disorder, proper care and treatment give many individuals a normal life expectancy.

## Section 25.6

# *Prader-Willi Syndrome*

Excerpted from "Prader-Willi Syndrome,"
Genetics Home Reference, July 2009.

Prader-Willi syndrome is a complex genetic condition that affects many parts of the body. In infancy, this condition is characterized by weak muscle tone (hypotonia), feeding difficulties, poor growth, and delayed development. Beginning in childhood, affected individuals develop an insatiable appetite, which leads to chronic overeating (hyperphagia) and obesity. Some people with Prader-Willi syndrome, particularly those with obesity, also develop type 2 diabetes mellitus (the most common form of diabetes).

People with Prader-Willi syndrome typically have mild to moderate intellectual impairment and learning disabilities. Behavioral problems are common, including temper tantrums, stubbornness, and compulsive behavior. Many affected individuals also have sleep abnormalities. Additional features of this condition include distinctive facial features, short stature, and small hands and feet. Some people with Prader-Willi syndrome have unusually fair skin and light-colored hair. Both affected males and affected females have underdeveloped genitals. Puberty is delayed or incomplete, and most affected individuals are unable to have children (infertile).

**Genetic changes:** Prader-Willi syndrome is caused by the loss of genes in a specific region of chromosome 15. People normally inherit one copy of this chromosome from each parent. Some genes are turned on (active) only on the copy that is inherited from a person's father (the paternal copy). This parent-specific gene activation is caused by a phenomenon called genomic imprinting. Prader-Willi syndrome occurs when the region of the paternal chromosome 15 containing these genes is missing.

Most cases of Prader-Willi syndrome are not inherited, particularly those caused by a deletion in the paternal chromosome 15 or by maternal uniparental disomy. These genetic changes occur as random events during the formation of reproductive cells (eggs and sperm) or in early embryonic development. Affected people typically have no history of the disorder in their family.

Rarely, a genetic change responsible for Prader-Willi syndrome can be inherited. For example, it is possible for a genetic defect that abnormally inactivates genes on the paternal chromosome 15 to be passed from one generation to the next.

## Section 25.7

# *Smith-Lemli-Opitz Syndrome*

Excerpted from "Smith-Lemli-Opitz Syndrome,"
Genetics Home Reference, July 2007.

Smith-Lemli-Opitz syndrome is a developmental disorder that affects many parts of the body. This condition is characterized by distinctive facial features, small head size (microcephaly), intellectual disability or learning problems, and behavioral problems. Many affected children have the characteristic features of autism, a developmental condition that affects communication and social interaction. Malformations of the heart, lungs, kidneys, gastrointestinal tract, and genitalia are also common. Infants with Smith-Lemli-Opitz syndrome have weak muscle tone (hypotonia), experience feeding difficulties, and tend to grow more slowly than other infants. Most affected individuals have fused second and third toes (syndactyly), and some have extra fingers or toes (polydactyly).

The signs and symptoms of Smith-Lemli-Opitz syndrome vary widely. Mildly affected individuals may have only minor physical abnormalities with learning and behavioral problems. Severe cases can be life-threatening and involve profound intellectual disability and major physical abnormalities.

**Prevalence:** Smith-Lemli-Opitz syndrome affects an estimated one in 20,000 to 60,000 newborns. This condition is most common in Caucasians (whites) of European ancestry, particularly people from Central European countries such as Slovakia and the Czech Republic. It is very rare among African and Asian populations.

**Genes:** Mutations in the DHCR7 gene cause Smith-Lemli-Opitz syndrome. The DHCR7 gene provides instructions for making an enzyme called 7-dehydrocholesterol reductase. Cholesterol plays a role in the production of certain hormones and digestive acids. Mutations in the DHCR7 gene reduce or eliminate the activity of 7-dehydrocholesterol reductase, preventing cells from producing enough cholesterol. A lack of this enzyme also allows potentially toxic byproducts of cholesterol production to build up in the blood, nervous system, and other tissues. The combination of low cholesterol levels and an accumulation of other substances likely disrupts the growth and development of many body systems. It is not known, however, how this disturbance in cholesterol production leads to the specific features of Smith-Lemli-Opitz syndrome.

## Section 25.8

# *Tourette Syndrome*

Excerpted from "Tourette Syndrome Fact Sheet," National Institute of
Neurological Disorders and Stroke (NINDS), July 16, 2010.

Tourette syndrome (TS) is a neurological disorder characterized by repetitive, stereotyped, involuntary movements and vocalizations called tics. The early symptoms of TS are almost always noticed first in childhood, with the average onset between the ages of 7–10 years. TS occurs in people from all ethnic groups; males are affected about three to four times more often than females. It is estimated that 200,000 Americans have the most severe form of TS, and as many as one in 100 exhibit milder and less complex symptoms such as chronic motor or vocal tics or transient tics of childhood. Although TS can be a chronic condition with symptoms lasting a lifetime, most people with the condition experience their worst symptoms in their early teens, with improvement occurring in the late teens and continuing into adulthood.

### Symptoms

Tics are classified as either simple or complex. Simple motor tics are sudden, brief, repetitive movements that involve a limited number of muscle groups. Some of the more common simple tics include eye blinking and other vision irregularities, facial grimacing, shoulder shrugging, and head or shoulder jerking. Simple vocalizations might include repetitive throat-clearing, sniffing, or grunting sounds. Complex tics are distinct, coordinated patterns of movements involving several muscle groups. Complex motor tics might include facial grimacing combined with a head twist and a shoulder shrug. Other complex motor tics may actually appear purposeful, including sniffing or touching objects, hopping, jumping, bending, or twisting. Simple vocal tics may include throat-clearing, sniffing/snorting, grunting, or barking. More complex vocal tics include words or phrases. Perhaps the most dramatic and disabling tics include motor movements that result in self-harm such as punching oneself in the face, or vocal tics including coprolalia (uttering swear words) or echolalia (repeating the words or phrases of others). Some tics are preceded by an urge or sensation in the affected muscle group, commonly called a premonitory urge. Some with TS will describe a need to complete a tic in a certain way or a certain number of times in order to relieve the urge or decrease the sensation.

Tics are often worse with excitement or anxiety and better during calm, focused activities. Certain physical experiences can trigger or worsen tics, for example tight collars may trigger neck tics, or hearing another person sniff or throat-clear may trigger similar sounds. Tics do not go away during sleep but are often significantly diminished.

### What is the course of TS?

Tics come and go over time, varying in type, frequency, location, and severity. Most patients experience peak tic severity before the mid-teen years with improvement for the majority of patients in the late teen years and early adulthood. Approximately 10% of those affected have a progressive or disabling course that lasts into adulthood.

### What disorders are associated with TS?

Many with TS experience additional neurobehavioral problems including inattention; hyperactivity and impulsivity (attention deficit hyperactivity disorder—ADHD), and related problems with reading, writing, and arithmetic; and obsessive-compulsive symptoms such as intrusive thoughts/worries and repetitive behaviors. For example, worries about dirt and germs may be associated with repetitive hand-washing, and concerns about bad things happening may be associated with ritualistic behaviors such as counting, repeating, or ordering and arranging. People with TS have also reported problems with depression or anxiety disorders, as well as other difficulties with living, that may or may not be directly related to TS. Given the range of potential complications, people with TS are best served by receiving medical care that provides a comprehensive treatment plan.

## Inheritance

Evidence from twin and family studies suggests that TS is an inherited disorder. The sex of the person also plays an important role in TS gene expression. At-risk males are more likely to have tics and at-risk females are more likely to have obsessive-compulsive symptoms. People with TS may have genetic risks for other neurobehavioral disorders such as depression or substance abuse. Genetic counseling of individuals with TS should include a full review of all potentially hereditary conditions in the family.

Section 25.9

# *Tuberous Sclerosis*

First described in 1943 as a syndrome impacting behavior, autism is typically diagnosed within the first three years of a child's life. The three areas evaluated to reach a diagnosis of autism are:

1. An impairment in the ability to interact socially with people; often demonstrating a lack of eye contact and disinterest in physical contact such as hugging or hand-holding;

2. An impairment in the ability to communicate using speech and/or gestures; and

3. A tendency to have narrow patterns of interests and activities coupled with repetitive and obsessive behaviors, and a lack of pretend or imaginative play; often children with autism find it necessary to have rigid and structured routines.

There are a wide range of variants and degree of demonstrated behavior such that autism is often defined as autistic spectrum disorder, or ASD. Some children have clear signs of ASD in two of the main areas required for diagnosis, but have less obvious features in the third. In these instances, individuals are said to have an atypical form of autism. When the intellectual abilities are normal, early language development is not significantly delayed and speech is well developed, then individuals may meet criteria for another variant called Asperger syndrome. A third variant, termed pervasive developmental disorder (not otherwise specified) or PDD, describes individuals who have difficulties in all three areas but fail to meet full criteria in any of the areas.

### *What is the link between autism spectrum disorder and tuberous sclerosis complex?*

Over the years, it has become recognized that between one-fourth and one-half of all children with tuberous sclerosis complex (TSC) develop ASD. The rate of ASD in the general population is substantially lower (around 0.5% or 0.6% of the total population), so there is clearly a very substantial increase in the rate of ASD in children with TSC. Likewise, the rate of TSC in children diagnosed with ASD is around 1%. Although this is a relatively low rate it is still clearly much higher than the rate of TSC in the general population, which is somewhere between one in 6,000 individuals. Either way, the overlap between ASD and TSC is clear.

ASD is usually diagnosed in young children between the ages of 2–4, but in individuals with TSC, the diagnosis of ASD may go unrecognized or be delayed due to other developmental disabilities. The importance of an accurate diagnosis of ASD for individuals with TSC is so that the individual can receive appropriate educational services and life-long support, as needed.

### *Why do individuals with TSC frequently develop ASD?*

Current research does not definitely answer the questions related to the increase of ASD in individuals with TSC. However, some important leads are beginning to form the basis of an explanation for the link. In general, it is believed the abnormalities in brain development that occur in TSC sometimes interfere with the proper development of brain areas that are important for the development of social communication skills (the ability to appropriately interact with other individuals).

Evidence is beginning to emerge that shows that if cortical tubers (which develop in earlier stages of brain development) in individuals with TSC involve the region of the brain called the temporal lobes, then there is an increased likelihood of an ASD developing. The temporal lobes are important for processing auditory information, especially speech sounds as well as information about faces and facial expressions. Interference with the development of these key skills may then lead to the social communication difficulties that characterize ASD.

It seems, however, that the presence of cortical tubers in the temporal lobes is not sufficient on its own to produce ASD. Instead, it appears that when temporal lobe tubers occur in conjunction with the onset of seizures at a young age, often presenting as infantile spasms, then this combination of factors leads to the much higher chance of ASD. Although the link with early-onset epilepsy and infantile spasms raises the possibility that the seizures may play a role in interfering with normal development of brain systems important in social communication, it is possible that the link with early seizures instead reflects the presence of cortical tubers and related structural abnormalities in key locations in the brain. These structural abnormalities may give rise to both the seizures as well as ASD. Further research to try to determine which of these two explanations is correct is required, especially as it has such important implications for treatment.

### Is it important to diagnose ASD in individuals with TSC?

Some people express the view that it is enough that an individual has TSC, so another diagnosis such as ASD is unnecessary. Although it makes sense to avoid adding diagnoses and labels, the diagnosis of an ASD is important for several reasons. A diagnosis can often help parents make sense of a range of rather unusual behaviors that otherwise seem extremely puzzling. Often, parents feel that somehow they have been doing something wrong in how they are parenting their child, and that the difficulties that the child is having in relating to others, communicating, or playing is somehow the parents' fault. It can be quite helpful for parents to discover that some of the unusual behaviors their child may be demonstrating are part of the developmental delays a child may be experiencing related to the autistic process.

In addition, the diagnosis is important because children with ASD often benefit from early intervention services that support improvement in speech, language, and behaviors. Early intervention services are available for very young children and their families. These services include physical therapy, speech therapy, and occupational therapy. Early intervention services work with not only the child with ASD, but also the parents and siblings. The goal of early services is to foster the development of children with ASD.

### How is the diagnosis made?

The diagnosis of an ASD is based on a report of the child's early development, detailing the way in which he or she acquired skills and the areas in which he or she has struggled, coupled with careful observations and assessments. These evaluations need to be performed by individuals who are experienced in evaluating individuals with complex developmental disabilities and ASD. The assessments are lengthy, and it may be necessary for the evaluator to see the child at home or in the playgroup or nursery setting, often referred to as a functional contextual assessment, before the diagnosis can be confirmed. The diagnosis of ASD is made through a team evaluation, including reports from therapists, pediatricians, teachers, parents, and psychologists.

There are several assessments that are used to reach a diagnosis of ASD; the most commonly used is called the Autism Diagnostic Observation Schedule (ADOS). This assessment should be performed by someone familiar with ASD who is trained to utilize the ADOS.

## When is diagnosis possible?

To some extent the answer to this depends on the individual's overall level of ability. In individuals who have the most severe cognitive disabilities, it can sometimes be extremely difficult to make a definitive diagnosis. In general it is hard to make a confident diagnosis before the individual's cognitive age level is at least equivalent to that of an 18-month to 2-year-old child. In less affected individuals, it might well be possible to make a diagnosis around the age of two, whereas in the individuals with very significant delays in development it may not be possible until they are much older. Research is continuing to identify the early markers of ASD so early treatments can be implemented.

## What treatment is suggested?

Treatment options vary based on the individual's age and ability. The focus of the treatment is often targeted at strengthening skills in individual areas of difficulty. Special education provisions and accommodations are incorporated in a child's individual education plan (IEP). This often includes the individual working with a multidisciplinary team of clinical professionals that provide several different services, including speech and language therapists, developmental and child psychologists and pediatricians.

According to the Autism Society of America, treatment approaches include these:

- Applied Behavioral Analysis (ABA) and Discrete Trial Training

- Treatment of Autistic and Related Communication Handicapped Children (TEACCH)

- Picture Exchange Communication System (PECS)

**ABA and Discrete Trial Training** are often used interchangeably. These methods include intense repetitive, structured tasks in which good behavior is rewarded and undesirable behavior is ignored. It is time intensive and focuses on changing current behaviors and does not prepare individuals to respond in new situations. Some individuals with TSC who have ASD have significantly benefited from ABA programs.

**TEACCH (Treatment of Autistic and Related Communication Handicapped Children)** was developed at the University of North Carolina. TEACCH focuses on adapting the environment to the individual with ASD instead of trying to make the individual adapt to the environment. This is achieved through high structure, organizational charts and schedules. While many favor this approach, some feel that it is too structured and makes the individual too dependent on charts and other organizational tools.

**PECS (Picture Exchange Communication System)** is used to encourage communication. By using pictures, an individual can point to or hand an object to someone to demonstrate what he or she wants.

Options vary and the treatment program needs to be tailored to the individual's age and ability. Treatment is targeted at fostering skills in the three main areas of difficulty— social and communication skills and the development of imaginative play. In addition, treatment aims to ensure that the repetitive or obsessive behaviors do not become too marked or prominent and do not interfere with family life. Lastly, the treatment aims to help parents foster their child's development and support them during the early, often very demanding, years.

There is growing evidence to suggest that early intervention programs may be one of the most effective current forms of treatment in individuals with ASD, but it is not yet known to what extent the intervention programs of this kind are helpful for children with TSC. Research is needed to evaluate effectiveness of these programs for individuals with TSC who have ASD.

### What will the future hold?

Detailed knowledge about the way individuals with TSC and ASD develop is currently being gained through studies in the United States and the United Kingdom, so for now we can only be guided by the development of individuals with ASD who do not have TSC. The range of outcomes here is very great. At one extreme, individuals can have persisting serious problems throughout childhood and into adult life. Some individuals with ASD are prone to self-injury, particularly if they get upset or frustrated when their routines or activities are interrupted, or if they get frustrated over their communication difficulties.

At the other extreme, individuals with Asperger syndrome or high-functioning ASD can largely outgrow their difficulties and lead an independent or semi-independent life in adulthood. The outcome is to some extent related to the severity of the associated cognitive impairments or a demonstrated level of cognitive disabilities. Individuals who have severe or profound forms of cognitive ability are likely to have persisting difficulties. In addition, the amount of useful speech that the individual acquires indicates how they will fare in the future. Lastly, the severity of the social and communication difficulties and behavior problems is also helpful in determining what the outcome will be. The more severe the problems, the more persistent they tend to be.

Chapter 26

# *Other Conditions That May Accompany ASD*

## *Chapter Contents*

Section 26.1

# *Thin Bones and ASD*

Excerpted from "Thin Bones Seen in Boys with Autism and Autism
Spectrum Disorder," *NIH News*, National Institutes of Health (NIH),
January 29, 2008.

Results of an early study suggest that dairy-free diets and uncon-
ventional food preferences could put boys with autism and autism
spectrum disorder (ASD) at higher than normal risk for thinner, less
dense bones when compared to a group of boys the same age who do not
have autism. The study, by researchers from the National Institutes of
Health and Cincinnati Children's Hospital Medical Center, was published online in *the Journal of Autism and Developmental Disorders*.

The researchers believe that boys with autism and ASD are at risk
for poor bone development for a number of reasons. These factors are
lack of exercise, a reluctance to eat a varied diet, lack of vitamin D,
digestive problems, and diets that exclude casein, a protein found in
milk and milk products. Dairy products provide a significant source of
calcium and vitamin D. Casein-free diets are a controversial treatment
thought by some to lessen the symptoms of autism. "Our results suggest
that children with autism and autism spectrum disorder may be at risk
for calcium and vitamin D deficiencies," Dr. Mary L. Hediger, said. "Parents of these children may wish to include a dietitian in their children's
health care team, to ensure that they receive a balanced diet."

Dr. Hediger stressed that the current study results need to be
confirmed by larger studies. Until definitive information is available,
however, it would be prudent for parents of children with autism and
ASD to include a dietitian in their care, particularly if the children's
diets do not include dairy products, or they are not otherwise eating
a balanced diet, she said. Because girls are much less likely to have
autism or ASD than are boys, the researchers were unable to enroll a
sufficient number of girls within the short time frame of the study to
allow them to draw firm conclusions. Dr. Hediger added that if a girl
with autism or ASD is not eating dairy products or eating a balanced
diet, it would be prudent for a dietitian to be included in her health
care team.

When the boys were enrolled in the study, the researchers asked the boys' parents if the boys were taking over-the-counter or prescription medications, were taking any vitamin or mineral supplements, or were on a restricted diet. During the study, researchers X-rayed the hands of 75 boys between the ages of four and eight years old who had been diagnosed with autism or ASD. The researchers then measured the thickness of the bone located between the knuckle of the index finger and the wrist and compared its development to a standardized reference based on a group of boys without autism. Dr. Hediger said that the research team measured cortical bone thickness. She added that this procedure was done as a substitute for a conventional bone scan, which measures bone density. Bone density is an indication of bones' mineral content. Less dense bones may indicate a risk of bone fracture.

The investigators found that the bones of the boys with autism were growing longer but were not thickening at a normal rate. During normal bone development, material from inside the bone is transferred to the outside of the bone, increasing thickness, while at the same time, the bones are also growing longer. At five or six years of age, the bones of the autistic boys were significantly thinner than the bones of boys without autism and the difference in bone thickness became even greater at ages seven and eight. The bone thinning was particularly notable because the boys with autism and ASD were heavier than average and would therefore be expected to have thicker bones.

The researchers do not know for certain why the boys had thinner than normal bones. A possible explanation is lack of calcium and vitamin D in their diets. Dr. Hediger explained that a deficiency of these important nutrients in the boys' diets could result from a variety of causes. Many children with autism, she said, have aversions to certain foods. Some will insist on eating the same foods nearly every day, to the exclusion of other foods. So while they may consume enough calories to meet their needs—or even more calories than they need—they may lack certain nutrients, like calcium and vitamin D.

Other children with autism may have digestive problems which interfere with the absorption of nutrients. Moreover, many children with autism remain indoors because they require supervision during outdoor activity. Lack of exercise hinders proper bone development, she said. Similarly, if children remain indoors and are not exposed to sunlight, they may not make enough vitamin D which is needed to process calcium into bones. The boys in the study who were on a casein-free diet had the thinnest bones. In fact, the nine boys who were on a casein-free diet had bones that were 20% thinner than normal for children their age. Boys who were not on a casein-free diet showed a

10% decrease in bone thickness when compared to boys with normal bone development.

The study authors wrote that bone development of children on casein-free diets should be monitored very carefully. They noted that studies of casein-free diets had not proven the diets to be effective in treating the symptoms of autism or ASD. Only nine boys on casein-free diets were available to participate in the study, Dr. Hediger said. When conducting a scientific study, it's easier to obtain statistically valid results by studying a larger number of individuals than with a smaller number of individuals. However, the dramatic difference in the boys' bone thickness when they were either on a casein-free diet or an unrestricted diet and when compared to normally developing bones strongly suggests that the bone thinning the researchers observed was statistically valid.

## Section 26.2

# *High Growth Hormones in Boys with ASD*

Excerpted from "Boys with Autism, Related Disorders, Have High Levels of Growth Hormones," *NIH News*, National Institutes of Health (NIH), June 27, 2007.

Boys with autism and autism spectrum disorder (ASD) had higher levels of hormones involved with growth in comparison to boys who do not have autism, reported researchers from the National Institutes of Health, the Centers for Disease Control and Prevention, the Cincinnati Children's Hospital, and the University of Cincinnati College of Medicine.

The researchers believe that the higher hormone levels might explain the greater head circumference seen in many children with autism. Earlier studies had reported that many children with autism have very rapid head growth in early life, leading to a proportionately larger head circumference than children who do not have autism. The researchers found that, in addition to a larger head circumference, the boys with autism and autism spectrum disorder who took part in the current study were heavier than boys without these conditions.

"The study authors have uncovered a promising new lead in the quest to understand autism," said Duane Alexander, MD, Director of the National Institute of Child Health and Human Development. "Future research will determine whether the higher hormone levels the researchers observed are related to abnormal head growth as well as to other features of autism." The study was published on line in *Clinical Endocrinology*.

The researchers compared the height, weight, head circumference, and levels of growth-related hormones to growth and maturation in 71 boys with autism and with ASD to a group of 59 boys who did not have these conditions. The investigators found that the boys with autism had higher levels of two hormones that directly regulate growth (insulin-like growth factors 1 and 2). These growth-related hormones stimulate cellular growth. The researchers did not measure the boys' levels of human growth hormone which for technical reasons is difficult to evaluate. The boys with autism also had higher levels of other hormones related to growth, such as insulin-like growth factor binding protein and growth hormone binding protein.

In addition to greater head circumference, the boys with autism and those with autism spectrum disorders weighed more and had a higher body mass index (BMI). BMI is a ratio of a person's weight and height. A higher BMI often indicates that a person is overweight or obese. The boys' higher BMI may be related to their higher hormone levels, said the study's principal investigator, NICHD's James L. Mills, MD, a senior investigator in the Division of Epidemiology, Statistics and Prevention Research's Epidemiology Branch. Dr. Mills and his coworkers also found that there was no difference in height between the two groups of boys.

The levels of growth-related hormones were significantly higher in the boys with autism even after the researchers compensated for the fact that higher levels of these hormones would be expected in children with a greater BMI. "The higher growth-related hormone levels are not a result of the boys with autism simply being heavier," said Dr. Mills. While it has long been noted that many children with autism have a larger head circumference than other children, few studies have investigated whether these children are also taller and heavier, Dr. Mills added.

Researchers analyzed medical records and blood samples from 71 boys diagnosed with autism and ASD who were patients at Cincinnati Children's Hospital Medical Center from March 2002 to February 2004. The researchers compared the information on the boys with autism and autism spectrum disorders to other boys treated for other conditions at the hospital and who do not have autism. Children with conditions that may have affected their growth—such as being born severely premature, long-term illness, or the genetic condition fragile X were not included in the study. Girls are much less likely to develop autism than are boys, and the researchers were unable to recruit a sufficient number of girls with autism to participate in the study.

Dr. Mills explained that the bone age of the boys with autism—the bone development assessed by taking X-rays and comparing the size and shape of the bones to similarly-aged children—were not more advanced in the group of boys with autism. For this reason, Dr. Mills and his coworkers ruled out the possibility that they were merely maturing more rapidly than were the other boys. Dr. Mills said that future studies could investigate whether the higher levels of growth hormones seen in children with autism could be directly related to the development of the condition itself.

# Part Five

# Interventions and Treatments for Autism Spectrum Disorder

# Chapter 27

# *Choosing Professionals and Coordinating Services*

Because autism and its related disabilities are difficult to diagnose, a child may be evaluated by a variety of professionals before a final diagnosis is determined.

Unless specifically trained in the area of developmental disabilities, physicians and psychologists may have little experience with autism spectrum disorders. Many have never seen a child with autism or a related disability such as PDDNOS (pervasive development disorder not otherwise specified), Rett syndrome, or Asperger syndrome when a parent brings their child in with the first signs of the disability emerging.

The following are brief descriptions of the specialists most commonly associated with diagnosis, intervention, and treatment of autism spectrum disorder and suggestions about how to select professionals to work with you and your child.

## *Specialists*

**Developmental pediatrician:** A physician specializing in diagnosing and treating children with developmental disabilities from birth to adolescence.

"Choosing Professionals and Coordinating Services," © 2005 Center for Autism and Related Disabilities (CARD)–University of Central Florida. Reprinted with permission. Reviewed in October 2010 by David A. Cooke, MD, FACP.

**Psychiatrist:** A physician who focuses on diagnosing and treating mental illnesses from a biological and psychological perspective and may prescribe various medications for treatment.

**Psychologist:** A licensed practitioner specializing in understanding a person's behavior, emotions, and cognitive skills. They may recommend strategies to aid growth and development or help with challenging behaviors.

**Neurologist/pediatric neurologist:** A physician specializing in diagnosing and treating disorders of the nervous system.

**Geneticist:** A physician specializing in the study of disorders associated with heredity.

## The Selection Process

Choosing a professional is not always easy. When choosing a professional to work with you and your child, it is important to look for someone who shows respect for the parents and regards parents as experts on their children. The professional should convey a sense of hope and have a philosophy similar to your own. Look for a professional who takes an individualized approach to treatment and intervention—one who does not say that all people with autism exhibit the same characteristics.

Based on your child's needs, it will take various professionals working together with you to develop a treatment and intervention plan. The most effective treatment of people with autism almost always involves a long-term team approach. Visits to the classroom, home, and community usually provide the most useful information about the child. Since frequent visits may not be possible, the professional may collect information through interviews and questionnaires.

Just as professionals ask many questions, so should you. Remember, no questions you have regarding your child are trivial or unimportant. You may want to ask some of the following questions of the physicians and therapists:

- What are my child's strengths? How can they be maximized?
- What specific activities or interventions should I do at home?
- What kind of testing and evaluations should my child have?
- Why should my child have these tests and evaluations?
- How is each test or evaluation performed?
- How will the results influence my child's intervention or treatment?

- Can you put me in touch with another family you are currently working with?

- Do you have any articles or resources on autism or autism spectrum disorders?

- Can I have a copy of your report? How soon will it be until I receive it?

Obtaining and reviewing all reports is very helpful in understanding your child's needs, progress, and how recommendations can maximize your child's potential.

## Service Coordination

Sometimes evaluations and recommendations may be different or conflicting. This can be confusing and exhausting. A case manager or service coordinator can help when questions, problems, or concerns arise. A case manager keeps current records and, when appropriate, shares information about a child with professionals involved in that child's care. It's one very effective way to make sure a child's needs are being met. Case managers may also help by making sure all appointments are scheduled, tests are performed, evaluations conducted, and that appropriate and effective follow-up care is being provided.

If an evaluation has been performed at a Child Development and Evaluation Center, or if the child is receiving services through a state funded program, chances are that one person has been designated as a service coordinator or case manager. If this is not the case, you can ask for help from your pediatrician or family physician, local Autism Society of America chapter, your local school district special education department, or Center for Autism and Related Disabilities (CARD). Some parents elect to perform this role themselves.

## Working Together

Parents and professionals communicating effectively and respectfully as partners is an important factor in achieving progress and success for any person with autism or a related disability. Working as a team by sharing information and responsibility can be the most effective approach when developing a treatment plan. Parents often have the best understanding of their children's behavior, communication, preferences, and motivations.

Professionals may suggest various ways to help a child but parents know what activities are practical for their family life. Parental perspective is integral when developing an intervention plan. Professionals, specializing in autism and related disabilities, have specific knowledge and training with regard to evaluation and development of education and treatment plans. By working together and respecting each other as equally important partners in a child's care, parents and professionals can optimize the potential for a child's development.

# Chapter 28

# *Evidence for ASD Interventions*

## *Chapter Contents*

# Section 28.1

# *Treatment Integrity*

"Improving Treatment Plan Implementation for Individuals with Special Needs," by Patrick F. Heick, PhD, BCBA. © 2010 May Institute (www.mayinstitute.org). Reprinted with permission.

Individuals with disabilities often rely on others to teach them the skills they need to enjoy meaningful and independent lives. The success of a young student with a learning disability in a school setting or an elderly adult with autism in a community-based residence, for example, often depends upon the quality of instruction provided by a teacher's aide or a direct care staff member. It is crucial, therefore, that these paraprofessionals have the training and support they need to become effective teachers and caregivers.

Children with disabilities in school settings have individualized education programs (IEPs). Similarly, adults with disabilities in day or residential settings have individualized support plans (ISPs). Both IEPs and ISPs are likely to have goals to help individuals gain skills. In some cases, they will also have objectives aimed at reducing challenging behavior. In both cases, teachers and caregivers develop and implement treatment plans—sometimes referred to as instructional strategies or behavior support plans—in an effort to teach functional skills. These plans are the keystones to effective treatment.

How well an instructional strategy or behavior support plan is implemented as it was designed refers to its treatment integrity. There are several factors that should be considered when developing, teaching, and monitoring a treatment plan to ensure its implementation integrity and the subsequent success of teachers and students.

The way a treatment plan is developed is likely to influence how well it is carried out. Research on the effectiveness of behavioral consultation in schools has shown the importance of change agents—those who implement or oversee plans—in the planning process. Actively involving these people in the initial problem-solving and brainstorming makes it more likely that plans will be viewed as acceptable and feasible and will be implemented accurately.

How paraprofessionals are trained to implement treatment plans also impacts their future effectiveness as teachers and caregivers. Research findings in the areas of school-based prevention and staff training strongly support the use of active teaching methods, such as role playing, modeling, and coaching. These methods provide opportunities for prompting and reinforcement of specific skills, ideally under conditions similar to those paraprofessionals will actually encounter. More traditional or passive teaching approaches, such as didactic (lecture) instruction, are not as effective.

After paraprofessionals have learned the skills they need to correctly implement treatment programs, they should be monitored to ensure they are using these skills consistently. Many research studies show that newly acquired skills can change or fade over time—a consequence referred to as drift. To protect against drift, educators and clinicians often use performance feedback—direct observation, corrective feedback, and reinforcing selected skills. It is important that new staff members receive very clear information on how well they implemented treatment strategies. For example, giving them feedback about which steps they completed both correctly and incorrectly has been shown to be very effective in maintaining and improving high levels of treatment integrity.

Professionals working in the fields of education and human services understand that changing the behavior of individuals with disabilities starts with changing the behavior of the teachers or care providers who work directly with them. We can improve the lives of children and adults with special needs by teaching skills that foster and support greater independence. How well we do that depends on the quality of the treatment plans and how successfully we carry them out.

A collaborative approach, paired with staff training that includes active teaching methods and ongoing performance feedback, appears to be the most effective way to develop, teach, and monitor treatment programs that will have the greatest likelihood of success for teachers and for those they serve.

Section 28.2

# *Review of ASD Interventions*

Excerpted from "Interventions for Autism Spectrum Disorders: State of the Evidence–Report of the Children's Services Evidence-Based Practice Advisory Committee, October 2009." Produced by the Maine Department of Health and Social Services, Maine Department of Health, and Cutler Institute for Health and Social Policy, University of Southern Maine. Reprinted with permission. The complete text of this report including references is available at http://muskie.usm.maine.edu/Publications/cutler/autism-spectrum-disorders-report2009.pdf.

The number of children in Maine with autism spectrum disorders (ASD) has increased significantly over the past decade. Since 2000, the number of children receiving special education services for ASD in Maine schools jumped from 594 to 2,231 in 2008—an increase of 276%. A recent study estimated that the total cost of caring for a person with autism over his or her lifetime can reach $3.2 million, with more than $35 billion spent collectively per year. To conserve already scarce resources and offer the best possible services to children with ASD, it is necessary to identify and understand the treatments and methods that produce positive outcomes as proven by research. Science helps to clarify some of the confusion about what works and enables evidence-informed treatment decisions, thus saving precious time and resources.

Autism spectrum disorders are a category of neurodevelopmental disorders characterized by distinct and pervasive impairment in multiple developmental areas, particularly social skills and communication. Children with ASD exhibit atypical patterns of social interaction and communication that are not consistent with their developmental age. These patterns become apparent in the first few years of life and are generally lifelong challenges. Early, intensive identification and intervention can greatly improve outcomes for children with ASD. Early and effective treatment also offers opportunity for significant cost/benefit improvement through regained productivity of individuals with ASD and their caregivers.

## Evidence-Based Practice

Evidence-based practice is a framework for integrating what is known from research into real-world settings in a manner that responds to the individual characteristics and values of the individual being served. There are three main components to evidence-based practice:

**Best research evidence:** In order to integrate research into practice, it is critical to be aware of the scope and quality of the literature. The quality and type of research is an important factor in the evaluation of evidence. Efficacy, the extent to which the treatment had the desired effect on the outcomes, is the critical determinant of empirical evidence.

**Clinical expertise and judgment:** Practitioners in an evidence-informed framework exercise their clinical judgment to select methods that address the client's needs by taking into account the client's environment, life circumstances, strengths, and challenges.

**Values:** Evidence-based practice is consistent with the child and family's values and perspectives. Engaging families in the process of evaluating, identifying, and implementing evidence-based interventions is critical. Family engagement promotes collaboration between families and practitioners and better informs individual treatment planning.

This project focused on the first factor in evidence-based practice—best research evidence. The purpose of this work was two-fold: Systematically review the research literature for treatment in ASD and subsequently determine the levels of empirical evidence for treatments commonly used for children with ASD. It is hoped that addressing this first element of evidence-based practice will enable providers, families, and systems to use the latest research to better inform treatment planning, decision making, policy making, and resource development.

## Process

In response to a growing need for information on evidence-based treatments for ASD, the Maine Department of Education and the Maine Department of Health and Human Services led a partnership of stakeholders in a systematic review of the latest research on treatment for ASD. This review was designed as an update to the Maine Administrators of Services for Children with Disabilities (MADSEC) Autism Task Force Report issued in 2000, one of the first efforts in

**Table 28.1.** Findings

| Level of Evidence | Intervention Category | Intervention(s) |
|---|---|---|
| **Established Evidence** | Applied Behavior Analysis | Applied Behavior Analysis for Challenging Behavior<br>Applied Behavior Analysis for Communication<br>Early Intensive Behavioral Intervention (EIBI) |
| | Augmentative and Alternative Communication | Picture Exchange Communication System (PECS) |
| | Pharmacological Approaches | Haloperidol (Haldol)–Effective for aggression<br>Methylphenidate (Ritalin)–Effective for hyperactivity<br>Risperidone (Risperdal)–Effective for irritability, social withdrawal, hyperactivity, and stereotypy |
| **Promising Evidence** | Applied Behavior Analysis<br>Augmentative and Alternative Communication<br>Psychotherapy | Applied Behavior Analysis for Adaptive Living Skills<br>Voice Output Communication Aid (VOCA)<br>Cognitive-Behavioral Therapy (CBT) for Anxiety |
| **Preliminary vidence** | Applied Behavior Analysis<br>Augmentative and Alternative Communication<br>Developmental, Social-Pragmatic Models<br>Diet and Nutritional Approaches<br>Pharmacological Approaches<br>Psychotherapy<br>Sensory Integration Therapy<br>Other | Applied Behavior Analysis for Academics–Numeral recognition, reading instruction, grammatical morphemes, spelling.<br>Applied Behavior Analysis for Vocational Skills<br>Sign Language<br>Developmental, Social-Pragmatic Models - Eclectic Models<br>Vitamin C–Modest effect on sensorimotor symptoms only<br>Atomoxetine (Strattera) –Effective for attention deficit and hyperactivity<br>Clomipramine (Anafranil) –Effective for stereotypy, ritualistic behavior, social behavior<br>Clonidine (Catapres) –Effective for hyperactivity, irritability, inappropriate speech, stereotypy, and oppositional behavior<br>CBT for Anger Management<br>Touch Therapy/Massage<br>Hyperbaric Oxygen Treatment |

**Table 28.1.** *continued*

| Level of Evidence | Intervention Category | Intervention(s) |
|---|---|---|
| **Studied and No Evidence of Effect** | Pharmacological Approaches | DMG<br>Secretin |
| **Insufficient Evidence** | Applied Behavior Analysis | Applied Behavior Analysis for Academics–Cooperative earning groups |
| | Augmentative and Alternative Communication | Facilitated Communication |
| | Diet and Nutritional Approaches | Gluten-Casein Free Diets<br>Omega-3 Fatty Acid Supplements<br>Vitamin B6/Magnesium Supplements |
| | Developmental, Social Pragmatic Models | DIR/Floortime<br>RDI<br>SCERTS<br>Solomon's PLAY model |
| | Pharmacological Approaches | Guanfacine (Tenex)<br>Intravenous Immunoglobin<br>Melatonin<br>Naltrexone (ReVia)<br>SSRIs: Citalopram (Celexa), Fluoxetine (Prozac)<br>Valproic Acid (Depakote) |
| | Sensory Integration Therapy | Auditory Integration Training<br>Sensory Integration Training |
| | Social Skills Training | Social Skills Training<br>Social Stories™ |
| | Other | TEACCH |
| **Evidence of Harm** | Pharmacological Approaches | Intravenous Chelation Using Edetate Disodium |

311

Maine to review the treatment literature for ASD. Over the course of a year, laypersons, state agency staff, providers, and researchers, reviewed more than 150 studies of 43 different treatments for children with ASD.

The Committee objectively reviewed the research using a validated rubric, the Evaluative Method for Determining Evidence-Based Practice in Autism, and assigned each intervention a level of evidence rating. The quality of each study was carefully evaluated using a set of primary and secondary quality indicators and factored into the determination of the level of evidence using a corresponding rating scale.

## Levels of Evidence

**Established evidence:** The treatment has been proven effective in multiple strong or adequately rated group experimental design studies, single-subject studies, or a combination. Results must be replicated in studies conducted by different research teams.

**Promising evidence:** The intervention has been shown effective in more than two strong or adequately rated group experimental design studies or at least three single-subject studies. Additional research is needed by separate teams to confirm that the intervention is effective in across settings and researchers.

**Preliminary evidence:** The intervention has been shown effective in at least one strong or adequately rated group or single-subject design study. More research is needed to confirm results.

**Studied and no evidence of effect:** Numerous (three or more) strong or adequately rated studies have determined that the intervention has no positive effect on the desired outcomes.

**Insufficient evidence:** Conclusions cannot be drawn on the efficacy of the intervention due to a lack of quality research and/or mixed outcomes across several studies.

**Evidence of harm:** Studies or published case reports indicate that the intervention involves significant harm or risk of harm, including injury and death.

## Conclusions

Based on its investigation of the research literature, the Committee concludes the following:

- The research clearly indicates that there are effective treatments for some core deficits and related challenges of ASD. For instance, comprehensive behavioral treatment has some of the most compelling evidence which emphasizes the importance of early and intensive intervention for children with ASD.

- Substantial investment in quality research is needed to further define effective treatment for ASD.

- Research specific to educational and behavioral interventions for children with ASD in the context of schools is seriously lacking. This is of deep concern since children receive a great deal of services through the education system.

- Comparative research on the efficacy of various treatment models would be very valuable.

- There is a dearth of research on treatment of older youth, adolescents, and adults with ASD. This is worrisome given that the number of adults with ASD is expected to significantly increase in the coming years as children with ASD mature.

- Families should be informed consumers of treatment and ask questions of providers about the nature and quality of the research behind the treatment their child is receiving.

- Providers need to make treatment decisions in active partnership with families while integrating relevant research into their practice and treatment planning process.

- Resources are needed to build capacity throughout Maine in order to efficiently and effectively deliver evidence-based treatments to children in their schools, homes, and communities. This requires resources for training, evaluation, and workforce development. For example, ABA has some of the best evidence for treatment in ASD yet Maine has only 26 certified ABA practitioners, with most located in the southern counties.

Evidence-based practice does not seek to dictate the interventions that should be used at the expense of others. Rather, it is a framework to integrate what is known from research into real-world practice in a manner that is accessible to families, responsive to what children need, and consistent with what providers can accomplish given available skills and resources. The first step toward evidence-based practice is creating awareness of what the best available research says. It is no longer enough to use what we believe works, we must consider what we know works in order to close the gap between science and practice, utilize limited resources wisely, and best serve Maine children with ASD.

## Section 28.3

# *Recommendations for Treatment Selection*

Excerpted from "Findings and Conclusions–The National Autism Center's National Standards Project." © 2009 National Autism Center (www.nationalautismcenter.org). Reprinted with permission.

Treatment selection is complicated and should be made by a team of individuals who can consider the unique needs and history of the individual with autism spectrum disorder (ASD) along with the environments in which he or she lives. We do not intend for this section to dictate which treatments can or cannot be used for individuals on the autism spectrum.

Having stated this, we have been asked by families, educators, and service providers to recommend how our results might be helpful to them in their decision-making. As an effort to meet this request, we provide suggestions regarding the interpretation of our outcomes. In all cases, we strongly encourage decision-makers to select an evidence-based practice approach.

Research findings are not the sole factor that should be considered when treatments are selected. The suggestions we make here refer only to the research findings component of evidence-based practice and should be only one factor considered when selecting treatments.

## *Recommendations Based on Research Findings*

**Established treatments** have sufficient evidence of effectiveness. We recommend the decision-making team give serious consideration to these treatments because (a) these treatments have produced beneficial effects for individuals involved in the research studies published in the scientific literature, (b) access to treatments that work can be expected to produce more positive long-term outcomes, and (c) there

314

is no evidence of harmful effects. However, it should not be assumed that these treatments will universally produce favorable outcomes for all individuals on the autism spectrum.

**Given the limited research support for emerging treatments**, we generally do not recommend beginning with these treatments. However, emerging treatments should be considered promising and warrant serious consideration if established treatments are deemed inappropriate by the decision-making team. There are several very legitimate reasons this might be the case.

**Unestablished treatments** either have no research support or the research that has been conducted does not allow us to draw firm conclusions about treatment effectiveness for individuals with ASD. When this is the case, decision-makers simply do not know if this treatment is effective, ineffective, or harmful because researchers have not conducted any or enough high quality research. Given how little is known about these treatments, we would recommend considering these treatments only after additional research has been conducted and this research shows them to produce favorable outcomes for individuals with ASD.

These recommendations should be considered along with other sources of critical information when selecting treatments.

One of the primary objectives of this report is to identify evidence-based treatments. We are not alone in this activity. The National Standards Project is a natural extension of the efforts of the National Research Council (2001), the New York State Department of Health, Early Intervention Division (1999), and other related documents produced at state and national levels.

Knowing which treatments have sufficient evidence of effectiveness is likely to, and should, influence treatment selection. Evidence-based practice, however, is more complicated than simply knowing which treatments are effective. Although we argue that knowing which treatments have evidence of effectiveness is essential, other critical factors must also be taken into consideration.

We have identified the following four factors of evidence-based practice:

**Research findings:** The strength of evidence ratings for all treatments being considered must be known. Serious consideration should be given to established treatments because there is sufficient evidence that (a) the treatment produced beneficial effects; and, (b) they are not associated with unfavorable outcomes (for example, there is no evidence that they are ineffective or harmful) for individuals on the autism spectrum. Ideally, treatment selection decisions should involve discussing the benefits of various established treatments. Despite the fact there is compelling evidence to suggest these treatments generally produce beneficial effects for individuals on the autism spectrum, there are reasons alternative treatments (for example, emerging treatments) might be considered. A number of these factors are listed.

**Professional judgment:** The judgment of the professionals with expertise in autism spectrum disorders (ASD) must be taken into consideration. Once treatments are selected, these professionals have the responsibility to collect data to determine if a treatment is effective. Professional judgment may play a particularly important role in decision-making when the following occurs:

- A treatment has been correctly implemented in the past and was not effective or had harmful side effects. Even established treatments are not expected to produce favorable outcomes for all individuals with ASD.

- The treatment is contraindicated based on other information (for example, the use of extra-stimulus prompts for a child with a prompt dependency history).

- A great deal of research support might be available beyond the ASD literature and should be considered when required. For example, if an adolescent with ASD presents with anxiety or depression, it might be necessary to identify what treatments are effective for anxiety or depression for the general population. The decision to incorporate outside literature into decision-making should only be made after practitioners are familiar with the ASD-specific treatments. Research that has not been specifically demonstrated to be effective with individuals with ASD should be given consideration along with the ASD-specific treatments only if compelling data support their use and the ASD-specific literature has not fully investigated the treatment.

- The professional may be aware of well-controlled studies that support the effectiveness of a treatment that were not available when the National Standards Project terminated its literature search.

**Values and preferences:** The values and preferences of parents, care providers, and the individual with ASD should be considered. Stakeholder values and preference may play a particularly important role in decision-making when:

- a treatment has been correctly implemented in the past and was not effective or had harmful side effects;

- a treatment is contrary to the values of family members;

- the individual with ASD indicates that he or she does not want a specific treatment.

**Capacity:** Treatment providers should be well positioned to correctly implement the intervention. Developing capacity and sustainability may take a great deal of time and effort, but all people involved in treatment should have proper training, adequate resources, and ongoing feedback about treatment fidelity. Capacity may play a particularly important role in decision making when the following occurs:

- A service delivery system has never implemented the intervention before. Many of these treatments are very complex and require precise use of techniques that can only be developed over time.

- A professional is considered the local expert for a given treatment but he or she actually has limited formal training in the technique.

- A service delivery system has implemented a system for years without a process in place to ensure the treatment is still being implemented correctly.

## Section 28.4

# *Fad Treatments Are Unproven*

"As Autism Diagnoses Grow, so Do Number of Fad Treatments, Researcher Say," August 20, 2007, Ohio State University Research Communications. © 2007 Ohio State University. Reprinted with permission.

Ineffective or even dangerous fad treatments for autism, always a problem, seem to be growing more pervasive, according to researchers who studied the problem. "Developmental disabilities like autism are a magnet for all kinds of unsupported or disproved therapies, and it has gotten worse as more children have been diagnosed with autism," said James Mulick, professor of pediatrics and psychology at Ohio State University. "There's no cure for autism, and many parents are willing to believe anything if they come to think it could help their child."

Mulick chaired a symposium on "Outrageous Developmental Disabilities Treatments" Aug. 20, 2007 in San Francisco at the annual meeting of the American Psychological Association. The symposium included presentations by several of Mulick's students at Ohio State who participated in a graduate seminar on fad treatments in autism.

Tracy Kettering, a doctoral student in special education at Ohio State, said a Google search for the phrase "autism treatment" yields more than 2.2 million matches. "You get hundreds of different types of therapies that come up, and many have quotes from parents that claim a particular therapy 'cured' their child," Kettering said. "It's no wonder that parents want to believe. But very few of these treatments have any evidence to support them."

The number and range of fad treatments has seemed to grow in recent years as more children have been diagnosed with autism, said Mulick, who is also editor of a book on fad treatments called *Controversial Therapies for Developmental Disabilities: Fad, Fashion, and Science in Professional Practice*. Mulick said when he began treating autism in the 1970s about three children in 10,000 were said to have autism. Now, reports are one in 166 children have the condition. The number of cases has mushroomed because of better diagnoses, and a changing definition of autism that includes a broader range of disorders.

318

Some of the newer, more popular fad treatments for autism involve special diets or nutritional supplements. Megadoses of vitamins C and B6 are popular, as well as supplements with fatty acids like omega-3s. A casein and/or gluten-free diet, which involves eliminating dairy and wheat products, has also gained favor with some parents.

While many of these treatments have never been adequately studied, that doesn't mean they aren't promoted. "One of the characteristics of fad treatments is that they are discussed in the media and on the internet, where many parents can be exposed to them," said Anne Snow, an Ohio State psychology graduate student.

And while some fads are simply ineffective, others can even be dangerous, Mulick said. Chelation therapy, which involves taking medicines to remove the heavy metal mercury from the body, has reportedly led to the death of at least one autistic boy receiving that treatment. Chelation therapy was also touted years ago as a new treatment against some forms of cancer but was eventually shown to have no helpful effect.

Many parents try multiple approaches, hoping at least one will help. Kettering said one survey she found suggests that the average parent of a child with autism has tried seven different therapies. "We're not saying that all of these treatments don't work or that they are all dangerous," Kettering said. "But the research hasn't been done to suggest that most of them are effective or even safe."

Many of the treatments may have just enough basis in scientific fact to attract attention, even if the treatment itself is unproven. For instance, most scientists believe that many cases of autism are caused by genetic mutations, and some mutations can be caused by various chemicals that we encounter in our everyday lives, Mulick said. But still, there is no evidence that any particular chemical causes mutations that lead to autism, as some have claimed. "There's a shred of truth in the rationale presented for some fad treatments, and that is enough for some people to go with," he said.

Another reason that fad treatments persist has to do with the natural course of autism, Mulick said. Autism, like many conditions, has cycles in which symptoms get worse and then get better. Parents tend to search for treatments when symptoms are getting worse, and when their children get better—as they do in the normal course of disease—parents credit the new therapy. "It's natural to have this bias that the therapy you're trying has had some positive effect," he said. "People want to believe."

While other treatments are still being investigated, right now the only therapy that has been shown to have a long-term positive affect on autism is called Early Intensive Behavioral Intervention, Mulick said. EIBI is a highly structured approach to learning, in which children with autism are taught first to imitate their teachers. But this treatment is very time-consuming and labor intensive. It involves one-on-one behavioral treatment with the child for up to 40 hours a week for several years. "It's expensive and difficult for many parents to use," Mulick said. "That's got to be one reason other treatments look attractive to them."

Mulick said other treatments and therapies are being studied. However, it takes years to test treatments for autism because of the nature of the disease and problems with proving effectiveness. "Autism studies are a long, time-consuming, and expensive process," Mulick said. "And some of the fad treatments being used today would never be approved for testing—they are just too dangerous."

Chapter 29

# Early Intervention for Children with Developmental Delays

## Chapter Contents

## Section 29.1

# *Overview of Early Intervention*

This section includes excerpts from "Overview of Early Intervention,"
National Dissemination Center for Children with Disabilities
(www.nichcy.org), accessed April 2, 2010.

Broadly speaking, early intervention services are specialized health, educational, and therapeutic services designed to meet the needs of infants and toddlers, from birth through age two, who have a developmental delay or disability, and their families. At the discretion of each state, services can also be provided to children who are considered to be at-risk of developing substantial delays if services are not provided.

Sometimes it is known from the moment a child is born that early intervention services will be essential in helping the child grow and develop. Often this is so for children who are diagnosed at birth with a specific condition or who experience significant prematurity, very low birth weight, illness, or surgery soon after being born. Even before heading home from the hospital, this child's parents may be given a referral to their local early intervention office.

Some children have a relatively routine entry into the world, but may develop more slowly than others, experience setbacks, or develop in ways that seem very different from other children. For these children, a visit with a developmental pediatrician and a thorough evaluation may lead to an early intervention referral, as well. However a child comes to be referred, assessed, and determined eligible—early intervention services provide vital support so that children with developmental needs can thrive and grow.

In a nutshell, early intervention is concerned with all the basic and brand new skills that babies typically develop during the first three years of life, such as:

- physical (reaching, rolling, crawling, and walking);
- cognitive (thinking, learning, solving problems);
- communication (talking, listening, understanding);
- social/emotional (playing, feeling secure and happy); or,
- self-help (eating, dressing).

### My child seems to be developing much slower than other children. Would he/she be eligible for early intervention services?

It is possible that your child may be eligible for early intervention, but more investigation is necessary to determine that. If you think that your child is not developing at the same pace or in the same way as most children his or her age, it is often a good idea to talk first to your child's pediatrician. Explain your concerns. Tell the doctor what you have observed with your child. Your child may have a disability or what is known as a developmental delay, or he or she may be at risk of having a disability or delay.

Developmental delay is a term that means an infant or child is developing slower than normal in one or more areas; for example, he or she may not be sitting up (or walking or talking) when most children of that age are. The term at risk means that a child s development may be delayed unless he or she receives early intervention services. So, if you are concerned about your child's development, you will need to have your child evaluated to find out if he or she is eligible for early intervention services. This evaluation is provided at no cost to you. There are many people who can help you with this.

### Where do I go for help?

Call National Dissemination Center for Children with Disabilities at 800-695-0285, or visit the website at http://www.nichcy.org/Pages/StateSpecificInfo.aspx. All state resource sheets are available there. Or, ask your child's pediatrician or the pediatrics branch in a local hospital to put you in touch with the early intervention system in your community or region. It is very important to write down the names and phone numbers of everyone you talk to. Having this information available will be helpful to you later on.

### What do I say to the early intervention contact person?

Explain that you are concerned about your child's development. Say that you think your child may need early intervention services. Explain that you would like to have your child evaluated under IDEA. Write down any information the contact person gives you.

The person may refer you to what is known as Child Find. One of Child Find's purposes is to identify children who need early intervention services. Child Find operates in every state and conducts screenings to identify children who may need early intervention services.

These screenings are provided free of charge. Each state has one agency that is in charge of the early intervention system for infants and toddlers with special needs.

## *What happens next?*

Once you are in contact with the early intervention system, the system will assign someone to work with you and your child through the evaluation and assessment process. This person will be your temporary service coordinator. He or she should have a background in early childhood development and ways to help young children who may have developmental delays. The service coordinator should also know the policies for early intervention programs and services in your state. The early intervention system will need to determine if your child is eligible for early intervention services. To do this, the staff will set up and carry out a multidisciplinary evaluation and assessment of your child.

Under the Individuals with Disabilities Education Act (IDEA), infants and toddlers with disabilities are defined as children from birth through age two who need early intervention services because they are experiencing developmental delays, as measured by appropriate diagnostic instruments and procedures, in one or more of the following areas:

- cognitive development;
- physical development, including vision and hearing;
- communication development;
- social or emotional development;
- adaptive development; or
- have a diagnosed physical or mental condition that has a high probability of resulting in developmental delay.

The term may also include, if a state chooses, children from birth through age two who are at risk of having substantial developmental delays if early intervention services are not provided. (34 Code of Federal Regulations §303.16)

If your child and family are found eligible, you and a team will meet to develop a written plan for providing early intervention services to your child and, as necessary, to your family. This plan is called the individualized family service plan, or IFSP. It is a very important document, and you, as parents, are important members of the team that develops it.

Under IDEA, early intervention services must include a multidisciplinary evaluation and assessment, a written IFSP, service coordination, and specific services designed to meet the unique developmental needs of the child and family. Early intervention services may be simple or complex depending on the child's needs. They can range from prescribing glasses for a two-year-old to developing a comprehensive approach with a variety of services and special instruction for a child, including home visits, counseling, and training for his or her family. Depending on your child's needs, his or her early intervention services may include:

- family training, counseling, and home visits;
- special instruction;
- speech-language pathology services (sometimes referred to as speech therapy);
- audiology services (hearing impairment services);
- occupational therapy;
- physical therapy;
- psychological services;
- medical services (only for diagnostic or evaluation purposes);
- health services needed to enable your child to benefit from the other services;
- social work services;
- assistive technology devices and services;
- transportation;
- nutrition services; and
- service coordination services.

Early intervention services may be delivered in a variety of ways and in different places. Sometimes services are provided in the child's home with the family receiving additional training. Services may also be provided in other settings, such as a clinic, a neighborhood daycare center, hospital, or the local health department. To the maximum extent appropriate, the services are to be provided in natural environments or settings. Natural environments, broadly speaking, are where the child lives, learns, and plays. Services are provided by qualified personnel and may be offered through a public or private agency.

# Section 29.2

## *Early Services for ASD*

Excerpted from "Treatment, Autism Spectrum Disorders–NCBDDD," National Center on Birth Defects and Developmental Disabilities (NCBD-DD), Centers for Disease Control and Prevention (CDC), August 20, 2009.

There is no single best treatment for all children with autism spectrum disorders (ASDs). However, well-planned, structured teaching of specific skills is very important. Some children respond well to one type of treatment while others have a negative response or no response at all to the same treatment. Before deciding on a treatment program, it is important to talk with the child's healthcare providers to understand all the risks and benefits.

It is also important to remember that children with ASDs can get sick or injured just like children without ASDs. Regular medical and dental exams should be part of a child's treatment plan. Often it is hard to tell if a child's behavior is related to the ASD or is caused by a separate health condition. For instance, head banging could be a symptom of the ASD, or it could be a sign that the child is having headaches. In those cases, a thorough physical exam is needed. Monitoring healthy development means, not only paying attention to symptoms related to ASDs, but also to the child's physical and mental health as well.

### *Early Intervention Services*

Research shows that early intervention treatment services can greatly improve a child's development. Early intervention services help children from birth to three years old (36 months) learn important skills. Services include therapy to help the child talk, walk, and interact with others. Therefore, it is important to talk to your child's doctor as soon as possible if you think your child has an ASD or other developmental problem.

Even if your child has not been diagnosed with an ASD, he or she may be eligible for early intervention treatment services. The Individuals with Disabilities Education Act (IDEA) says that children under the age of three years (36 months) who are at risk of having developmental delays may be eligible for services. These services are provided through an early intervention system in your state. Through this system, you can ask for an evaluation. In addition, treatment for particular symptoms, such as speech therapy for language delays, often does not need to wait for a formal ASD diagnosis. While early intervention is extremely important, intervention at any age can be helpful.

## Types of Treatments

The National Institute of Mental Health and the Autism Society of America suggest a list of questions parents can ask when planning treatments for their child. There are many different types of treatments available. For example, auditory training, discrete trial training, vitamin therapy, anti-yeast therapy, facilitated communication, music therapy, occupational therapy, physical therapy, and sensory integration. The different types of treatments can generally be broken down into the following categories: behavior and communication approaches, dietary approaches, medication, and complementary and alternative medicine.

**Behavior and communication approaches:** According to reports by the American Academy of Pediatrics and the National Research Council, behavior and communication approaches that help children with ASDs are those that provide structure, direction, and organization for the child in addition to family participation. A notable treatment approach for people with an ASD is called applied behavior analysis (ABA). ABA has become widely accepted among healthcare professionals and used in many schools and treatment clinics. ABA encourages positive behaviors and discourages negative behaviors in order to improve a variety of skills. The child's progress is tracked and measured.

Other therapies that can be part of a complete treatment program for a child with an ASD include:

- Developmental, Individual Differences, Relationship-Based Approach (DIR; also called Floortime)
- Treatment and Education of Autistic and related Communication-handicapped CHildren (TEACCH)
- Occupational Therapy
- Sensory Integration Therapy
- Speech Therapy
- The Picture Exchange Communication System (PECS)

## Section 29.3

# *Autism Intervention for Toddlers Improves Developmental Outcomes*

Excerpted from "Autism Intervention for Toddlers Improves
Developmental Outcomes," National Institute of Mental Health
(NIMH), December 8, 2009.

Current guidelines by the American Academy of Pediatrics recommend screening children for autism spectrum disorder (ASD) by age 18 months. However, no randomized clinical trials of intensive interventions for this age group had been conducted. To address this gap, Geraldine Dawson, PhD, who was at the University of Washington at the time of the study, and colleagues randomly assigned 48 children, ages 18–30 months, to one of two intervention groups:

- Early Start Denver Model (ESDM), a comprehensive, developmental behavioral intervention designed for toddlers with ASD as young as 12 months old. ESDM combines aspects of applied behavioral analysis (ABA) with developmental and relationship-based approaches.

- Assess and Monitor (A/M), the comparison group intervention in which parents received recommendations on ASD interventions for their children, as well as referrals to local community providers of the interventions. A/M represents typical community-based care.

Children in the ESDM group were provided 20 hours per week of therapy from study clinicians, while their parents received related training to use ESDM strategies for at least five additional hours per week during their daily activities. Parents of all study participants were also free to receive other community services they thought appropriate.

All children in the study had been diagnosed with autism or a milder form of ASD called pervasive developmental disorder not otherwise specified (PDDNOS). They were assessed yearly for two years or until the child turned four years old, whichever was longer.

## Results of the Study

By the first- year assessment, children in the ESDM group gained 15.4 intelligence quotient (IQ) points on average, while children in the A/M group gained an average of 4.4 points. Over the two-year study period, children in the ESDM group consistently improved on measures of communication skills. They also showed improvements in motor skills, daily living skills, and other adaptive behaviors.

While children in the ESDM group were significantly delayed in their adaptive behaviors compared to typically developing children, they showed similar rates of improvement. In contrast, children in the A/M group fell further and further behind over time.

By the end of the study, more children who had received ESDM received improved diagnoses than children in the A/M group—seven children initially diagnosed with autistic disorder had their diagnosis change to PDDNOS after receiving ESDM (30%), compared to only one child in the A/M group (5%).

## Significance

According to the researchers, this is the first randomized controlled trial to study a potentially useful intensive intervention for very young children with ASD. The study's findings suggest that ESDM can help children with ASD achieve better outcomes in terms of IQ, language, and behavioral skills, and in severity of their ASD diagnosis, than if they receive community-based care. Compared to research on other, similar interventions, this study showed greater differences between groups, suggesting that ESDM, delivered at a very young age, may be more effective than other approaches. The researchers noted that parents' use of ESDM strategies at home may have been key to this intervention's effectiveness.

# Chapter 30

# *Interventions for Individuals with Asperger Syndrome*

## *General Intervention Strategies*

Specific interventions, such as teaching practices and approaches, behavioral management techniques, strategies for emotional support, and activities intended to foster social and communication competence, should be conceived and implemented in a thoughtful, consistent (across setting, staff members, and situations), and individualized manner. More importantly, the benefit (or lack thereof) of specific recommendations should be assessed in an empirical fashion (for example, based on an evaluation of events observed, documented or charted), with useful strategies being maintained and unhelpful ones discarded so as to promote a constant adjustment of the program to the specific conditions of the individual child with Asperger syndrome (AS). The following items can be seen as tentative suggestions to be considered when discussing optimal approaches to be adopted. It should be noted, however; that there are degrees of concreteness and rigidity, paucity of insight, social awkwardness, communicative one-sidedness, and so forth, characterizing individuals with AS. Care providers should embrace the wide range of expression and complexity of the disorder, avoiding dogmatism in favor of practical, individualized, and common-sensual clinical judgment. The following suggestions should be seen in this context:

Excerpted from "Asperger Syndrome: Treatment and Intervention," by Ami Klin, PhD., and Fred R. Voikmar, MD, © 2006. Reprinted with permission from MAAP Services for Autism and Asperger Syndrome. The complete text of this article including references is available at http://aspergersyndrome.org.

1.  Skills, concepts, appropriate procedures should be taught in an explicit and rote fashion using a parts-to-whole verbal teaching approach, where the verbal steps are in the correct sequence for the behavior to be effective.

2.  Specific problem-solving strategies should be taught for handling the requirements of frequently occurring troublesome situations. Training should also be necessary for recognizing situations as troublesome and applying learned strategies in discrepant situations.

3.  Social awareness should be cultivated, focusing on the relevant aspects of given situations, and pointing out the irrelevancies contained therein. Discrepancies between the individual's perceptions regarding the situation in question and the perceptions of others should be made explicit.

4.  Generalization of learned strategies and social concepts should be instructed, from the therapeutic setting to everyday life (for example, to examine some aspects of a person's physical characteristics as well as to retain full names in order to enhance knowledge of that person and facilitate interaction in the future).

5.  To enhance the individual's ability to compensate for typical difficulties processing visual sequences, particularly when these involve social themes, by making use of equally typical verbal strengths.

6.  The ability to interpret visual information simultaneously with auditory information should be strengthened, since it is important not only to be able to interpret other people's nonverbal behavior correctly but also to interpret what is being said in conjunction with these nonverbal cues.

7.  Self-evaluation should be encouraged. Awareness should be gained into which situations are easily managed and which are potentially troublesome. This is especially important with respect to perceiving the need to use pre-learned strategies in appropriate situations. Self-evaluation should also be used to strengthen self-esteem and maximize situations in which success can be achieved. Individuals with AS often have many cognitive strengths and interests that can be used to the individual's advantage in specific situations as well as in planning for the future.

8.    Adaptive skills intended to increase the individual's self-sufficiency should be taught explicitly with no assumption that general explanations might suffice nor that he/she will be able to generalize from one concrete situation to similar ones. Frequently occurring problematic situations should be addressed by teaching the individual verbally the exact sequence of appropriate actions that will result in an effective behavior. Rule sequences for shopping, using transportation, and so forth, should be taught verbally and repeatedly rehearsed with the help of the interventionist and other individuals involved in the individual's care. There should be constant coordination and communication between all those involved so that these routines are reinforced in the same way and with little variation between the various people. Verbal instructions, rote planning and consistency are essential. A list of specific behaviors to be taught may be derived from results obtained with the *Vineland Adaptive Behavior Scales, Expanded Edition* (Sparrow, Balla and Cicchetti, 1984), which assess adaptive behavior skills in the areas of communication, daily living (self-help) skills, socialization, and motor skills.

9.    The individual with AS should be instructed on how to identify a novel situation and to resort to a pre-planned, well-rehearsed list of steps to be taken. This list should involve a description of the situation, retrieval of pertinent knowledge and step-by-step decision-making. When the situation permits (another item to be explicitly defined), one of these steps might be reliance on a friend's or adult's advice, including a telephone consultation.

10.   The link between specific frustrating or anxiety-provoking experiences and negative feelings should be taught to the individual with AS in a concrete, cause-effect fashion, so that he/she is able to gradually gain some measure of insight into his/her feelings. Also, the awareness of the impact of his/her actions on other people's feelings should be fostered in the same fashion.

11.   Additional teaching guidelines should be derived from the individual's neuropsychological profile of assets and deficits; specific intervention techniques should be similar to those usually employed for many subtypes of learning disabilities, with an effort to circumvent the identified difficulties by means of

compensatory strategies, usually of a verbal nature. For example, if significant motor, sensory-integration, or visual-motor deficits are corroborated during the evaluation, the individual with AS should receive physical and occupational therapies. These latter should not only focus on traditional techniques designed to remediate motor deficits, sensory integration, or visual-motor deficits, but should also reflect an effort to integrate these activities with learning of visual-spatial concepts, visual-spatial orientation and causation, time concepts, and body awareness, making use of narratives and verbal self-guidance.

## *General Strategies for Communication Intervention and Social Skills Training*

For most individuals with AS, the most important item of the educational curriculum and treatment strategy involves the need to enhance communication and social competence. This emphasis does not reflect a societal pressure for conformity or an attempt to stifle individuality and uniqueness. Rather, this emphasis reflects the clinical fact that most individuals with AS are not loners by choice, and that there is a tendency, as children develop towards adolescence, for despondency, negativism, and sometimes, clinical depression, as a result of the individual's increasing awareness of personal inadequacy in social situations, and repeated experiences of failure to make and/or maintain relationships. The typical limitations of insight and self-reflection vis-a`-vis others often preclude spontaneous self-adjustment to social and interpersonal demands. The practice of communication and social skills do not imply the eventual acquisition of communicative or social spontaneity and naturalness. It does, however, better prepare the individual with AS to cope with social and interpersonal expectations, thus enhancing their attractiveness as conversational partners or as potential friends or companions. The following are suggestions intended to foster relevant skills in this important area:

1.  Explicit verbal instructions on how to interpret other people's social behavior should be taught and exercised in a rote fashion. The meaning of eye contact, gaze, various inflections as well as tone of voice, facial and hand gestures, non-literal communications such as humor, figurative language, irony, sarcasm, and metaphor, should all be taught in a fashion not unlike the teaching of a foreign language, for example, all elements

should be made verbally explicit and appropriately and repeatedly drilled. The same principles should guide the training of the individual's expressive skills. Concrete situations should be exercised in the therapeutic setting and gradually tried out in naturally occurring situations. All those in close contact with the individuals with AS should be made aware of the program so that consistency, monitoring, and contingent reinforcement are maximized. Of particular importance, encounters with unfamiliar people (making acquaintances) should be rehearsed until the individual is made aware of the impact of his/her behavior on other people's reactions to him/her. Techniques such as practicing in front of a mirror, listening to the recorded speech, watching a video recorded behavior, and so forth, should all be incorporated in this program. Social situations contrived in the therapeutic setting that usually require reliance on visual-receptive and other nonverbal skills for interpretation should be used and strategies for deciphering the most salient nonverbal dimensions inherent in these situations should be offered.

2.  The individual with AS should be taught to monitor his/her own speech style in terms of volume, rhythm, naturalness, adjusting depending on proximity to the speaker, context and social situation, number of people, and background noise.

3.  The effort to develop the individual's skills with peers in terms of managing social situations should be a priority. This should include topic management, the ability to expand and elaborate on a range of different topics initiated by others, shifting topics, ending topics appropriately, and feeling comfortable with a range of topics that are typically discussed by same-age peers.

4.  The individual with AS should be helped to recognize and use a range of different means to interact, mediate, negotiate, persuade, discuss, and disagree through verbal means. In terms of formal properties of language, the individual may benefit from help in thinking about idiomatic language that can only be understood in its own right, and practice in identifying them in both text and conversation. It is important to help the individual to develop the ability to make inferences, to predict, to explain motivation, and to anticipate multiple outcomes so as to increase the flexibility with which the person both thinks about and uses language with other people.

## General Guidelines for Behavior Management

Individuals with AS often exhibit different forms of challenging behavior. It is crucial that these behaviors are not seen as willful or malicious; rather, they should be viewed as connected to the individual's disability and treated as such by means of thoughtful, therapeutic, and educational strategies, rather than by simplistic and inconsistent punishment or other disciplinary measures that imply the assumption of deliberate misconduct. Specific problem-solving strategies, usually following a verbal rule, may be taught for handling the requirements of frequently occurring, troublesome situations (for example, involving novelty, intense social demands, or frustration). Training is usually necessary for recognizing situations as troublesome and for selecting the best available learned strategy to use in such situations. The following are some suggestions on how to approach behavioral management in the case of individuals with AS:

1.  Setting limits: A list of frequent problematic behaviors such preservations, obsessions, interrupting, or any other disruptive behaviors should be made and specific guidelines devised to deal with them whenever the behaviors arise. It is often helpful that these guidelines are discussed with the individual with AS in an explicit, rule-governed fashion, so that clear expectations are set and consistency across adults, settings, and situations is maintained. These explicit rules should be not unlike curriculum guidelines. The explicit approach should be devised based on the staff's ongoing experiences, determined empirically, and discussed in team meetings. An effort should be made to establish as much as possible all possible (though few) contingencies and guidelines for limit setting so that each staff member does not need to improvise and thus possibly trigger the individual's oppositionality or a temper tantrum. When listing the problematic behaviors, it is important that these are specified in a hierarchy of priorities, so that staff and the individual himself/herself concentrate on a small number of truly disruptive behaviors (to others or to self).

2.  Helping the individual with AS make choices: There should not be an assumption that the individual with AS makes informed decisions based on his/her own set of elaborate likes and dislikes. Rather he/she should be helped to consider alternatives of action or choices, as well as their consequences (rewards and displeasure) and associated feelings. The need for such and

artificial set of guidelines is a result of the individual's typical poor intuition and knowledge of self.

## Academic Curriculum

The curriculum content should be decided based on long-term goals, so that the utility of each item is evaluated in terms of its long-term benefits for the individual's socialization skills, vocational potential, and quality of life. Emphasis should be placed on skills that correspond to relative strengths for the individual as well as skills that may be viewed as central for the person's future vocational life (such as writing skills, computer skills, science). If the individual has an area of special interest that is not as circumscribed and unusual so as to prevent utilization in prospective employment, such an interest or talent should be cultivated in a systematic fashion, helping the individual learn strategies of learning (library, computerized data bases, internet, and so forth). Specific projects can be set as part of the person's credit gathering, and specific mentorships (topic-related) can be established with staff members or individuals in the community. It is often useful to emphasize the utilization of computer resources, with a view to (a) compensate for typical difficulties in graphing-motor skills, (b) to foster motivation in self-taught strategies of learning, including the use of online resources, and (c) to establish contact via electronic mail with other people who share some interests, a more non-threatening form of social contact that may evolve into relationships, including personal contact.

## Vocational Training

Often, adults with AS may fail to meet entry requirements (such as having a college-degree) for jobs in their area of training, or fail to attain a job because of their poor interview skills, social disabilities, eccentricities, or anxiety attacks. Having failed to secure skilled employment (commensurate with their level of instruction and training), sometimes these individuals may be helped by well-meaning friends or relatives to find a manual job. As a result of their typically very poor visual-motor skills they may once again fail, leading to devastating emotional implications. It is important, therefore; that individuals with AS are trained for and placed in jobs for which they are not neuro-psychologically impaired, and in which they will enjoy a certain degree of support and shelter. It is also preferable that the job does not involve intensive social demands. As originally emphasized by Hans Asperger, there is a need to foster the development of existent talents and special interests in a way as to transform them into marketable skills. However, this is only part of the task to secure (and maintain) a work placement. Equal attention should be paid to the social demands defined by the nature of the jobs, including what to do during meal breaks, contact with the public or co-workers, or any other unstructured activity requiring social adjustment or improvisation.

## Self-Support

As individuals with AS are usually self-described loners despite an often intense wish to make friends and have a more active social life, there is a need to facilitate social contact within the context of an activity-oriented group (such as church communities, hobby clubs, and self-support groups). The little experience available with the latter suggests that individuals with AS enjoy the opportunity to meet others with similar problems and may develop relationships around an activity or subject of share interest.

## Pharmacotherapy

Although little information about pharmacological interventions with individuals with AS is available, a conservative approach based on the evidence from autism should probably be adopted (McDougle, Price and Volkmar, 1994). In general, pharmacological interventions with young children are probably best avoided. Specific medication might be indicated if AS is accompanied by debilitating depressive symptoms, severe obsessions and compulsions, or a thought disorder. It is important for parents to know that medications are prescribed for the treatment of specific symptoms, and not to treat the disorder as a whole.

## Psychotherapy

Although insight-oriented psychotherapy has not been shown to be very helpful, it does appear that fairly focused and structured counseling can be very useful for individuals with AS, particularly in the context of overwhelming experiences of sadness or negativism, anxiety, family functioning, frustration in regard to vocational goals and placement, and ongoing social adjustment.

# Chapter 31

# *Behavior Therapies Often Effective for ASD*

## Chapter Contents

## Section 31.1

# *Applied Behavior Analysis (ABA) Therapy*

"Applied Behavior Analysis (ABA)," Reprinted with permission of
Autism Speaks, www.autismspeaks.org, © 2010.

Behavior analysis was originally described by B.F. Skinner in the
1930s. You may have learned about Skinner and operant conditioning when you studied science in school. The principles and methods
of behavior analysis have been applied effectively in many circumstances to develop a wide range of skills in learners with and without
disabilities.

### What is applied behavior analysis (ABA)?

Behavior analysis is a scientific approach to understanding behavior
and how it is affected by the environment. Behavior refers to all kinds
of actions and skills (not just misbehavior) and environment includes
all sorts of physical and social events that might change or be changed
by one's behavior. The science of behavior analysis focuses on principles
(that is, general laws) about how behavior works, or how learning takes
place. For example, one principle of behavior analysis is positive reinforcement. When a behavior is followed by something that is valued
(a reward), that behavior is likely to be repeated. Through decades of
research, the field of behavior analysis has developed many techniques
for increasing useful behaviors and reducing those that may be harmful or that interfere with learning. Applied behavior analysis (ABA) is
the use of those techniques and principles to address socially important
problems, and to bring about meaningful behavior change.

### Who can benefit from ABA?

ABA methods have been used successfully with many kinds of learners of all ages, with and without disabilities, in many different settings.
In the early 1960s, behavior analysts began working with young children
with autism and related disorders. Those pioneers used techniques in
which adults directed most of the instruction, as well as some in which

children took the lead. Since that time, a wide variety of ABA techniques have been developed for building useful skills in learners with autism of all ages. Those techniques are used in both structured situations (such as formal instruction in classrooms) and in more natural everyday situations (such as during play or mealtime at home), and in one-to-one as well as group instruction. They are used to develop basic skills like looking, listening and imitating, as well as complex skills like reading, conversing, and taking the perspective of others.

The use of ABA principles and techniques to help persons with autism live happy and productive lives has expanded rapidly in recent years. Today, ABA is widely recognized as a safe and effective treatment for autism. It has been endorsed by a number of state and federal agencies, including the U.S. Surgeon General and the New York State Department of Health.

## *What is the research on ABA for autism?*

Hundreds of published studies have shown that specific ABA techniques can help individuals with autism learn specific skills, such as how to communicate, develop relationships, play, care for themselves, learn in school, succeed at work, and participate fully and productively in family and community activities, regardless of their age. A number of peer-reviewed studies have examined the effects of combining multiple ABA techniques into comprehensive, individualized, intensive early intervention programs for children with autism. Comprehensive refers to the fact that intervention addresses all kinds of skills: communication, social, self-care, play, motor, pre-academic, and so on. Early means that intervention began before the age of four for most children. Intensive means that ABA methods were used to arrange large numbers of learning opportunities for each child every day in both structured and unstructured situations, which amounted to 25–40 hours per week during which children actively learned and practiced skills. That was done so that young children with autism would have experiences like typical toddlers, who get thousands of chances every day to learn by interacting with their parents and others. These studies showed that many children with autism who received 1–3 years of this type of treatment had large improvements on tests of their cognitive, communication, and adaptive skills. Some who participated in early intensive ABA for at least two years acquired enough skills to participate in regular classrooms with little, or no, ongoing help. Other children in the studies learned many skills through intensive ABA, but not enough to function independently in regular classrooms full time. Across studies, a small percentage of children improved relatively little. At this time, it is very difficult to predict in advance how far any individual child might go with this treatment. More research is needed to determine why some children with autism respond more favorably to early intensive ABA than others.

In some studies, intensive ABA was compared with less intensive ABA, typical early intervention or special education, and eclectic, mixed-method interventions done both intensively and non-intensively. The children with autism who received intensive ABA treatment made larger improvements in most skill areas than children who participated in the other interventions. Parents whose children received intensive ABA reported less stress than parents whose children received other treatments.

## Does ABA work with older learners with autism?

Yes. Research documents that many ABA techniques are effective for building skills of all kinds in children, adolescents, and adults with autism and related disorders. Additionally, ABA methods are useful for helping individuals and families manage some of the difficult behaviors that may accompany autism, without the side effects of drugs or other treatments. A number of programs have been combining many ABA techniques into comprehensive treatment programs for youths and adults with autism for many years. Many of those individuals have learned to work and live successfully in their communities thanks to ABA treatment. However, so far, there have been no studies of intensive ABA with older individuals with autism comparable to those that have been done with young children.

## What does ABA intervention involve?

Done correctly, ABA intervention for autism is not a "one size fits all" approach consisting of a canned set of programs or drills. On the contrary, every aspect of intervention is customized to each learner's skills, needs, interests, preferences, and family situation. For those reasons, an ABA program for one learner might look somewhat different than a program for another learner. But genuine, comprehensive ABA programs for learners with autism have certain things in common:

- Intervention designed and overseen directly by qualified, well-trained professional behavior analysts

- Detailed assessment of each learner's skills as well as learner and family preferences to determine initial treatment goals

- Selection of goals that are meaningful for the learner and the family
- Ongoing objective measurement of learner progress
- Frequent review of progress data by the behavior analyst so that goals and procedures can be fine-tuned as needed
- Instruction on developmentally appropriate goals in skill areas (communication, social, self-care, play and leisure, motor, and academic skills)
- Skills broken down into small parts or steps that are manageable for the learner, and taught from simple (such as imitating single sounds) to complex (carrying on conversations)
- An emphasis on skills that will enable learners to be independent and successful in both the short and the long run
- Use of multiple behavior analytic procedures—both adult-directed and learner-initiated—to promote learning in a variety of ways
- Many opportunities—specifically planned and naturally occurring—for each learner to acquire and practice skills every day, in structured and unstructured situations
- Intervention provided consistently for many hours each week
- Abundant positive reinforcement for useful skills and socially appropriate behaviors
- An emphasis on positive social interactions, and on making learning fun
- No reinforcement for behaviors that are harmful or prevent learning
- Use of techniques to help trained skills carry over to various places, people, and times, and to enable learners to acquire new skills in a variety of settings
- Parent training so family members can teach and support skills during typical family activities
- Regular meetings between family members and program staff to plan, review progress, and make adjustments

## *What kind of improvements can be expected from ABA?*

Competently delivered ABA intervention can help learners with autism make meaningful changes in many areas. But most learners require a great deal of carefully planned instruction and practice on most skills, so changes do not occur quickly. As mentioned earlier, quality ABA programs address a wide range of skill areas, but the focus is always on the individual learner, so goals vary from learner to learner, depending on age, level of functioning, family needs and interests, and other factors. The rate of progress also varies from one learner to the next. Some acquire skills quickly, others more slowly. In fact, an individual learner may make rapid progress in one skill area—such as reading—and need much more instruction and practice to master another, such as interacting with peers.

## *Who can provide ABA intervention?*

Because of the huge demand for ABA intervention for autism, many individuals and programs now claim to do ABA. Some are private practitioners or agencies that offer to provide services by periodically coming into a family's home; others operate private schools, and still others provide consultation services to public schools. Not all of them have the education and practical experience that the field of behavior analysis considers minimum requirements for practicing ABA. Family members and concerned professional are urged to be cautious when enlisting anyone to do ABA with a child, youth, or adult with autism.

Whether assembling or choosing an ABA program, keep in mind the following:

- Just as a medical treatment program should be directed by a qualified medical professional, ABA programs for learners with autism should be designed and supervised by qualified behavior analysts, preferably individuals who are board certified behavior analysts with supervised experience providing ABA treatment for autism, or who can clearly document that they have equivalent training and experience. Always check credentials of those who claim to be qualified in behavior analysis.

- An ABA program should have the components and features listed previously.

- Monitor the program by observing sessions and participating in training sessions and consultations.

## Section 31.2

# *ABA Therapy at a Younger Age Leads to Faster Learning*

© 2009 Center for Autism and Related Disorders, Inc. (www.centerforautism.com). Reprinted with permission.

Researchers at the Center for Autism and Related Disorders, Inc. (CARD) found that increasing treatment hours within an early intensive behavioral intervention program resulted in greater efficiency in new skill acquisition. This effect was the strongest in younger children within their study.

In *Effects of age and treatment intensity on behavioral intervention outcomes for children with autism spectrum disorders*, published in the September 2009 edition of *Research in Autism Spectrum Disorders*, CARD researchers Doreen Granpeesheh, Dennis R. Dixon, Jonathan Tarbox, Andrew M. Kaplan, and Arthur E. Wilke found that an increase in treatment hours and a decrease in child age predicted an increase in the number of skills learned per hour of treatment. For example, a child between two to five years old, receiving 150 therapy hours per month would master an average of 54 skills per month. If this same child received only 40 therapy hours per month they would on average master 21 skills per month. This is contrasted to a child between five to seven years, who would master 57 skills per month if given 150 monthly therapy hours. And, an average of 15 skills per month if given 40 therapy hours per month.

The 245 participants were selected from a pool of clients receiving behavioral intervention services at a CARD, a nationwide provider of applied behavior analysis based treatment programs for children and young adults with autism spectrum disorders (ASDs). The participants were between 16 months and 12 years old, received an average of 20 or more hours of intervention per month, and had mastered at least one skill per month. Participants were from California, Arizona, Illinois, Texas, Virginia, and New York.

"While several studies have addressed the association between age and treatment intensity or hours of therapy received, this study is one of only two that used such a large sample of children," Tarbox said. "Plus, since CARD serves a large number of children across the United States, we were able to investigate questions at a scale that isn't normally possible. The size and geographic diversity of the study population decreases the likelihood that there are regional biases and increases the likelihood that these outcomes can be generalized across a larger region. Only one other autism treatment study, based in Canada, included a larger number of participants. It included over 300 children residing in Ontario, Canada.

The study outcomes showed that younger children learned faster than the older children, all other things being equal. It also showed that increases in therapy hours resulted in increases in new learned skills. "This is what we have suspected all along, but it wasn't until now that we had data across such a large group of children that really showed it clearly," Dixon said. "It's important to keep in mind, though, that this does not mean older kids on the spectrum can't learn—they certainly can and do—it just means you get a larger effect out of the same dose of behavioral treatment when the treatment is implemented early."

The study also showed no point of diminishing returns as hours were increased. Meaning that 20 hours per week was better than 10, 30 hours per week was better than 20, and 40 was better than 30. The degree of improvement did not decrease as treatment intensity approached 40 hours per week.

"It's common for therapy programs to max out at 40 hours per week, however, based on our findings the magic number of 40 hours per week may not really be the upper limit at all," Tarbox said. "We may actually be able to get even better outcomes with a larger intensity of treatment—but, of course, more research would be needed before we could make conclusions such as those."

# Section 31.3

# *Verbal Behavior Therapy*

Another behavioral (based on the principles of applied behavior analysis [ABA]) therapy method with a different approach to the acquisition and function of language is verbal behavior (VB) therapy.

In his 1957 book, "Verbal Behavior," B.F. Skinner detailed a functional analysis of language. He described all of the parts of language as a system. Verbal behavior uses Skinner's analysis as a basis for teaching language and shaping behavior. Skinner theorized that all language could be grouped into a set of units, which he called operants. Each operant identified by Skinner serves a different function. The most important of these operants, or units, he named echoics, mands, tacts, and intraverbals: The function of a mand is to request or obtain what is wanted. For example, the child learns to say the word cookie when he is interested in obtaining a cookie. When given the cookie, the word is reinforced and will be used again in the same context. In a VB program the child is taught to ask for the cookie anyway he can (vocally, sign language, and so forth). If the child can echo the work, he will be motivated to do so to obtain the desired object.

The operant for labeling an object is called a tact. For example, the child says the word cookie when seeing a picture and is thus labeling the item. In VB, more importance is placed on the mand than on the tact, theorizing that using language is different from knowing language.

An intraverbal describes conversational or social, language. Intraverbals allow children to discuss something that isn't present. For example, the child finishes the sentence, "I'm baking…" with the intraverbal fill-in cookies. Intraverbals also include responses to questions from another person, usually answers to wh- questions (Who? What? When? Where? Why?). Intraverbals are strengthened with social reinforcement.

VB and classic ABA use similar behavioral formats to work with children. VB is designed to motivate a child to learn language by developing a connection between a word and its value. VB may be used as an extension of the communication section of an ABA program.

### Who provides VB?

VB is provided by VB-trained psychologists, special education teachers, speech therapists, and other providers.

### What is the intensity of most VB programs?

VB programs usually involve 30 or more hours per week of scheduled therapy. Families are encouraged to use VB principles in their daily lives.

## Section 31.4

# *Pivotal Response Treatment*

"Pivotal Response Treatment." Reprinted with the permission of
Autism Speaks, www.autismspeaks.org, © 2010.

Pivotal response treatment, or PRT, was developed by Dr. Robert L. Koegel, Dr. Lynn Kern Koegel, and Dr. Laura Shreibman, at the University of California, Santa Barbara. Pivotal response treatment was previously called the natural language paradigm (NLP), which has been in development since the 1970s. It is a behavioral intervention model based on the principles of ABA.

### What is PRT?

PRT is used to teach language, decrease disruptive/self-stimulatory behaviors, and increase social, communication, and academic skills by focusing on critical, or pivotal, behaviors that affect a wide range of behaviors. The primary pivotal behaviors are motivation and child's initiations of communications with others.

The goal of PRT is to produce positive changes in the pivotal behaviors, leading to improvement in communication skills, play skills, social behaviors and the child's ability to monitor his own behavior. Unlike the discrete trial teaching (DTT) method of teaching, which targets individual behaviors, based on an established curriculum, PRT is child directed. Motivational strategies are used throughout intervention as often as possible. These include the variation of tasks, revisiting mastered tasks to ensure the child retains acquired skills, rewarding attempts, and the use of direct and natural reinforcement. The child plays a crucial role in determining the activities and objects that will be used in the PRT exchange. For example, a child's purposeful attempts at functional communication are rewarded with reinforcement related to their effort to communicate (for example, if a child attempts a request for a stuffed animal, the child receives the animal).

### *Who provides PRT?*

Psychologists, special education teachers, speech therapists and other providers specifically trained in PRT such as the Koeg Certification program.

### *What is a typical PRT therapy session like?*

Each program is tailored to meet the goals and needs of the child as well as family routines. A session typically involves six segments during which language, play and social skills are targeted in structured and unstructured formats. Sessions change to accommodate more advanced goals and the changing needs as the child develops.

### *What is the intensity of a PRT program?*

PRT programs usually involve 25 or more hours per week. Everyone involved in the child's life is encouraged to use PRT methods consistently in every part of the child's life. PRT has been described as a lifestyle adopted by the affected family.

## Section 31.5

## *Virtual Games Teach Skills to Students with ASD*

"Virtual games teach real-world skills to kids with autism,"
by Virginia Hughes, © 2010 Simons Foundation Autism Research
Initiative (SFARI). Reprinted with permission.

On May 13, 2008, Matthew Belmonte received a curious e-mail from Google. For more than a year, Belmonte, an assistant professor at Cornell University, and a team of student computer scientists had been designing a dynamic video game to test the social, sensory, and attentional abilities of children with autism. Belmonte had set up a website explaining the project and the game, called Astropolis, in which children act as pilots of their own spaceships. The site attracted a lot of online traffic. "We figured it would only be a matter of time before we heard from Google," he says, joking.

Chris Cronin, the business strategist who contacted Belmonte, had a vested interest in autism: He was part of a team working on SketchUp, Google's three-dimensional drafting software intended for architects and professional designers. Soon after SketchUp's release, Cronin and fellow Colorado-based business developer Tom Wyman began hearing from users that children with autism love using the software. "You hear it once, and it's a heartwarming story. Hear it twice, and it's a coincidence. Hear it three times, and you think, 'Gosh, there must be something going on here'," Wyman says. That led Cronin and Wyman, in late 2007, to launch Project Spectrum. The project initially sought to teach children with autism in the Boulder school system how to use SketchUp—giving them a creative outlet that they typically don't have through writing, speech, or social play. Word spread quickly about the software, and now many people with autism, from all over the world, have downloaded it and built floor plans, buildings, and landscapes of their own design. Project Spectrum's ultimate goal is to help children with autism communicate more effectively, as well as build self-esteem and skills for a rewarding career.

Cronin's e-mail to Belmonte launched a collaboration in which members of Project Spectrum build parts of the Astropolis virtual world. In

350

addition to teaching adolescents how to work cooperatively (they tend to get irritated and obstinate when programmers make even small modifications to their designs), Astropolis allows for the unprecedented testing of children with autism on a variety of cognitive skills, all at once, without the artificial, boring, and anxiety-ridden setup of a typical psychology lab. Gaming technology is more sophisticated, and more accessible, than ever before, and Belmonte is part of a burgeoning wave of researchers using it to test or train people with autism.

The first video and virtual reality games made for children with autism, developed about a decade ago, looked too simple and unrealistic, says Sarah Parsons, one of the leaders of these initial efforts and a senior research fellow in the School of Education at the University of Birmingham, United Kingdom (UK). "Now they have the potential to be very realistic in the way that they look, and you control everything that's seen and heard within them." In several studies over the years, Parsons has shown that children with autism usually recognize that virtual environments are meant to simulate reality.[1] Parsons is part of a new £1.65 million project in Europe, called COSPATIAL, which will place multi-player virtual reality programs into public schools, aiming to help high-functioning children with autism interact socially with their teachers and normal peers.

Using this technology is a particularly attractive method for studying autism because people with the disorder tend to have a knack for visual learning; some studies have even reported that they have superior visual acuity. "They're not so keen on interpersonal, face-to-face interaction, so there's something comfortable about using the computer," Parsons says. "And of course the visual stimuli appeal to a visual way of processing the world, which tends to favor people with autism."

For one piece of the COSPATIAL project, which launched in February, Parsons is developing virtual games that can be projected on to a piece of hardware that's already available in most UK classrooms: interactive whiteboards. To win the game, the children will need to work together with another player. "Their natural inclination is not to do that, but we hope that the games will be suitably motivating in order to help them learn social skills," Parsons says.

The project is still in the development phase, which has included significant input from autism teachers. The team plans to start testing this and similar technologies in early 2010 in mainstream and specialty schools in the UK and Israel. "We know that there are a lot of schools that are struggling to meet all the needs of young people on the spectrum," Parsons says. "The impact will be quite substantial if we design this in a way that allows it to be used quite easily in typical school contexts."

## Out of This World

Typical psychological experiments present two big problems for testing children with autism. First, they're long and tedious. Children with autism tend to have an increased ability to focus, and can repeat certain tasks over and over without a fuss. Healthy controls, in contrast, get "bored out of their skulls," Belmonte says. "What you end up measuring is the difference between boredom and nonboredom, instead of the difference between autistic and non-autistic," he says.

Second, psychological testing isn't done in a realistic environment. Children come to an unfamiliar space, surrounded by strangers, and perform tasks that may have no relevance to their daily life. This is particularly challenging for children with autism, who don't like novelty and are prone to social anxiety.

Belmonte envisioned Astropolis as a solution to both confounds. For instance, one of the program's mini-games, called Maritime Defender, puts a new twist on the classic "go/no-go" test meant to measure inhibition and executive function. In the classic lab paradigm, children are taught to press a button, as quickly as possible, when they see certain cues, but to refrain from pressing the button in response to other cues. In Astropolis, children see a series of spacecraft coming out of a wormhole. Some are enemy ships, which they must shoot as soon as possible; others are ships full of valuable resources.

In a different game, children must steer their ship through a starry black sky. The pattern of stars they see through the windshield shows them when their ship is starting to steer off course—and how well they steer gives Belmonte a measure of their motion perception. Astropolis even includes a Sally-Ann-type test of Theory of Mind, in which the player has to figure out where a space pirate believes that a precious resource is located. "The games are really fun—even my lab has fun playing it," Belmonte says.

So far, Belmonte has successfully piloted the games on healthy children and on some children with Project Spectrum. He's recruiting more children with autism for the first set of experiments and plans to loan participants a laptop, so they can practice the game at home—with the machine recording their behavioral data all the while. Once participants become comfortable with the game, Belmonte plans to bring them back into the lab, and have them play while they're hooked up to electroencephalography electrodes, which can measure their brain activity. "When we get these observations, a really interesting further question is, are social and non-social tasks being perturbed by some of the same sorts of neural properties? And if so, then could training in a non-social domain facilitate the development of social skills?" he asks.

One drawback of Astropolis is that it only works for individuals with high-functioning autism spectrum disorders, who can deftly use a mouse and sit in front of a computer for extended periods. "It's something that I honestly feel guilty about. None of the experiments I've done have addressed people like my brother," Belmonte says, referring to his older brother with autism, who does not speak and cannot sit still in front of a computer for extended periods. Down the line, Belmonte hopes to design similar games in which people with autism can experience full-body virtual worlds.

## Social Simulations

Though virtual reality may be useful in measuring the perceptual and cognitive skills of people with autism, it has shown mixed results when used as a method of therapy. Starting in the mid-1990s, computer scientist Dorothy Strickland began creating virtual environments that could help young children with autism learn safety measures, such as how to cross the street, or avoid a fire in their homes. Even with the cruder technology, these efforts worked fairly well.[2]

"Safety skills are pretty easy to teach actions on, because they give a good practice scenario situation," notes Strickland, a principal researcher at Do2Learn, which develops social learning games for children with disabilities, many of which are free to download on their website. She says the site gets about ten million views per month.

Attempts to do social-skills training in virtual reality, on the other hand, have proven more difficult because they require subtle actions and vary a lot from one situation to the next. For example, Strickland has completed a project in which people with autism learn how to enter a restaurant on Second Life, a popular online social world. Although the participants can learn a set of steps in one restaurant setting, they have trouble generalizing those lessons to a slightly different restaurant setting. "We introduce different parameters. So if someone comes up to them and are rude, then the individual with autism may lose all connection to the right steps because they personally feel threatened," she says. Strickland's team has found that it's more effective to combine virtual reality scenarios with explicit instructional videos that explain why various skills should be applied to different situations.

Peter Mundy has run up against similar hurdles in his work on children with autism. "The hardest thing is figuring out how to help them generalize what they learn in one context and apply it in a different context in the real world," says Mundy, director of educational research at the M.I.N.D. Institute at the University of California, Davis. Mundy has a two-year National Institutes of Health stimulus grant to set up virtual reality situations that teach children with autism to improve key social abilities. Data collection began in December, and Mundy plans to run these experiments on at least 40 high-functioning children with autism.

In one game, for example, kids strap on a headset and are asked to talk about themselves with a group of virtual peers. If they don't maintain eye contact, their friends will fade away. "We think we can build virtual social interactive situations that will help kids have a lot of opportunities to practice," he says. Virtual training might even supplement more traditional behavioral interventions, he adds. "If we use it in conjunction with social-skills training, or some sort of person-to-person intervention," he says, "we think the virtual practice will help the kids learn to apply what they are getting out of the intervention to a lot of different social contexts."

## References

1.  Parsons S. et al. *J. Autism Dev. Disord. 34*, 449–466 (2004) PubMed.

2.  Strickland D. et al. *J. Autism Dev. Disord. 26*, 651–659 (1996) PubMed.

Chapter 32

# Communication Therapies for ASD

## Chapter Contents

## Section 32.1

# *What a Speech Pathologist Does*

"Roles and Responsibilities of Speech-Language Pathologists in Diagnosis, Assessment, and Treatment of Autism Spectrum Disorders Across the Life Span [Position Statement]." © 2006 American Speech-Language-Hearing Association. All rights reserved. Available from www.asha.org/policy. This position statement is an official policy of the American Speech-Language-Hearing Association (ASHA). It was developed by ASHA's Ad Hoc Committee on Autism Spectrum Disorders. Members of the committee were Amy Wetherby (chair), Sylvia Diehl, Emily Rubin, Adriana Schuler, Linda Watson, Jane Wegner, and Ann-Mari Pierotti (ex officio). Celia Hooper, vice president for professional practices in speech-language pathology, 2003–2005, served as the monitoring officer. The ASHA (2001) *Scope of Practice in Speech-Language Pathology* states that the practice of speech-language pathology includes providing services for individuals with disorders of pragmatics and social aspects of communication, which would include individuals with autism spectrum disorders. This also includes individuals with severe disabilities and language disabilities in general. The ASHA (2004) Preferred Practice Patterns for the Profession of Speech-Language Pathology are statements that define universally applicable characteristics of practice. It is required that individuals who practice independently in this area hold the Certificate of Clinical Competence in Speech-Language Pathology and abide by the ASHA (2003) Code of Ethics, including Principle of Ethics II, Rule B, which states that "individuals shall engage in only those aspects of the professions that are within the scope of their competence, considering their level of education, training, and experience." This statement (LC_SLP/SLS_1-2006) was approved by ASHA's Speech-Language Pathology/Speech or Language Science Assembly of the Legislative Council on February 3, 2006.

## *Position Statement*

It is the position of the American Speech-Language-Hearing Association (ASHA) that speech-language pathologists play a critical role in screening, diagnosing, and enhancing the social communication development and quality of life of children, adolescents, and adults with autism spectrum disorders (ASD). The core features of ASD include impairments in reciprocal social interaction, impairments in verbal and nonverbal communication, and restricted range of interests and activities, which are due to neurobiological factors. There is great

356

heterogeneity in this population, evident in a broad range of cognitive, social, communication, motor, and adaptive abilities. Integral to the diagnostic criteria, all individuals with ASD are challenged in the area of social communication. Thus, many individuals with ASD have difficulty acquiring the form and content of language and/or augmentative and alternative communication systems, and all have needs in acquiring appropriate social use of communication. Therefore, problems in use of language and communication are overarching because ASD is primarily a social communication disability. These challenges result in far-reaching problems, including difficulties with joint attention, shared enjoyment, social reciprocity in nonverbal as well as verbal interactions, mutually satisfying play and peer interaction, comprehension of others' intentions, and emotional regulation. Due to the nature of ASD, family members, peers, and other communication partners may encounter barriers in their efforts to communicate and interact with individuals with ASD. Therefore, the speech-language pathologist's role is critical in supporting the individual, the environment, and the communication partner to maximize opportunities for interaction in order to overcome barriers that would lead to ever-decreasing opportunities and social isolation if left unmitigated.

Individuals with ASD should be eligible for speech-language pathology services due to the pervasive nature of the social communication impairment, regardless of age, cognitive abilities, or performance on standardized testing of formal language skills. As mandated by the Individuals with Disabilities Education Improvement Act of 2004 (Pub. L. 108-446), speech-language pathologists should avoid applying a priori criteria (for example: discrepancies between cognitive abilities and communication functioning, chronological age, or diagnosis) and make individualized decisions on eligibility for services. Because formal assessment tools may not accurately detect problems in the social use of language and communication, eligibility may need to be based on clinical judgment and more informal, observational measures.

Appropriate roles for speech-language pathologists include, but are not limited to, the following:

1.  Screening: Speech-language pathologists play a critical role in screening and early detection of individuals at risk for ASD and makes referrals to experienced professionals for diagnosis and intervention services.

2.  Diagnosis: Speech-language pathologists who acquire and maintain the necessary knowledge and skills can diagnose ASD, typically as part of a diagnostic team or in other

multidisciplinary collaborations, and the process of diagnosis should include appropriate referrals to rule out other conditions and facilitate access to comprehensive services.

3. Assessment and intervention: Speech-language pathologists should prioritize assessment and intervention in those aspects of development that are critical to the achievement of social communication competence and that honor and adapt to differences in families, cultures, languages, and resources. Speech-language pathologists should recognize the guidelines and active components of effective, evidence-based practice for individuals with ASD. They should draw on empirically supported approaches to meet specific needs of children with ASD and their families, thereby incorporating family preferences, cultural differences, and learning styles. Speech-language pathologists should assist communication partners in recognizing the potential communicative functions of challenging behavior and designing environments to support positive behavior. Embracing a broad view of communication, speech-language pathologists should assess and enhance the following:

- the initiation of spontaneous communication in functional activities across social partners and settings;
- the comprehension of verbal and nonverbal communication in social, academic, and community settings;
- communication for a range of social functions that are reciprocal and promote the development of friendships and social networks;
- verbal and nonverbal means of communication, including natural gestures, speech, signs, pictures, written words, functional alternatives to challenging behaviors, and other augmentative and alternative communication systems;
- access to literacy and academic instruction and curricular, extracurricular, and vocational activities.

4. Working with families: Speech-language pathologists should form partnerships with families in assessment and intervention with individuals with ASD because effective programs have active family involvement. Speech-language pathologists should provide counseling, education, and training, coordination of services, and advocacy for families.

358

5.  Collaboration: Speech-language pathologists should collaborate with families, individuals with ASD, other professionals, support personnel, peers, and other invested parties to identify priorities and build consensus on a service plan and functional outcomes.

6.  Professional development: Speech-language pathologists should participate as trainers and trainees in pre-service and continuing education designed to prepare and enhance the knowledge and skills of professionals who provide services for individuals with ASD.

7.  Research: Speech-language pathologists should be informed of current research and/or participate in and advance the knowledge base of the nature of the disability, screening, diagnosis, prognostic indicators, assessment, treatment, and service delivery of individuals with ASD.

8.  Advocacy: Speech-language pathologists also play an important role as advocates for individuals with ASD in promoting social communication skills that lead to greater independence in home, school, work, and community environments, and greater participation in social networks.

The broad impact of the social communication challenges and problems with generalization for individuals with ASD necessitates service delivery models and individualized programs that lead to increased active engagement and build independence in natural learning environments. Speech-language pathologists should recognize the importance of family involvement and collaboration with a variety of professionals and communication partners, the facilitation of peer-mediated learning, the continuity of services across environments, and the importance of matching service delivery to meaningful outcomes. Speech-language pathologists should provide services that are connected with functional and meaningful outcomes. Therefore, they should provide pull-out services only when repeated opportunities do not occur in natural learning environments or to work on functional skills in more focused environments. Because of the limited impact of pull-out services focused on discrete skills, speech-language pathologists should ensure that any pull-out services are tied to meaningful, functional outcomes and incorporate activities that relate to natural learning environments.

## References

American Speech-Language-Hearing Association. (2001). *Scope of practice in speech-language pathology*. Rockville, MD: Author.

American Speech-Language-Hearing Association. (2003). Code of ethics (Revised). *ASHA Supplement, 23*, 13–15.

American Speech-Language-Hearing Association. (2004*). Preferred practice patterns for the profession of speech-language pathology*. Available from http://www.asha.org/policy.

**Reference this material as:** American Speech-Language-Hearing Association. (2006). Roles and Responsibilities of Speech-Language Pathologists in Diagnosis, Assessment, and Treatment of Autism Spectrum Disorders Across the Life Span [Position Statement]. Available from www.asha.org/policy.

## Section 32.2

# *Speech and Language Therapy: A Key Intervention for Persons with ASD*

"IAN Research Findings: Speech and Language Therapy." Reprinted with permission from the Interactive Autism Network (IAN) Community (www.iancommunity.org), © 2008 Kennedy Krieger Institute.

Speech and language therapy, considered an essential intervention for any child with speech and language deficits, is mandated by the Individuals with Disabilities Education Act.[1] It is generally provided by a speech-language pathologist (SLP)—a professional expert in communication and social development. This person does much more than help a child learn to form words. The field of speech-language pathology is concerned with the study of communication, disorders of communication, and assessment and treatment of these disorders.

The following are areas targeted by an SLP:

- Articulation/phonology (movement of muscles used to produce speech; production of speech sounds)

- Morphology (grammatical rules)

- Syntax (sentence structure)

- Semantics (language content/meaning)

- Pragmatics (social use of language)
- Fluency (flowing, effortless speech)
- Prosody (variations in pitch, volume, and rate of speech)

A large percentage of people with autism do not use language functionally, that is, to communicate basic needs and wants. Even those who can speak will likely have difficulties with the pragmatic, or social, use of language, which includes understanding social cues, using appropriate conversational rules, and understanding age-appropriate humor. Whether a child is nonverbal or has a large vocabulary, has cognitive delays or has above-average intelligence, speech and language therapy can be a valuable piece of the therapeutic puzzle.

The setting for speech and language therapy will likely change as a child ages. Clinical services, school-based services, social skills groups with peers, and community training all may be part of the spectrum of therapy over time.

In the section that follows, we share the experience of families participating in IAN with regard to this crucial intervention.

## IAN Families and Speech and Language Therapy

Families participating in IAN Research have the opportunity to list all autism treatments they use, and to rate these. The IAN Research team then ranks all the treatments in two different ways. The first time, each individual treatment is ranked, so that every separate medication, vitamin, diet, or other intervention stands on its own. (see Table 32.1) When ranking treatments used by IAN families this way, speech and language therapy holds first place.

Next, treatments of a similar type or class are grouped together before being ranked. For example, Risperdal and Ritalin no longer appear separately, but are included with all other drugs under "prescription medications." In this grouped ranking of treatments used by IAN families, speech and language therapy is only second from the top. (see Table 32.2)

Who recommends speech and language therapy to families? This varies quite a bit. Most commonly, this recommendation is made by a team of professionals (30%), a pediatrician (19%), or a speech-language pathologist (15%).

## Obtaining the Therapy

One of the positive aspects of speech and language therapy is that most parents find it relatively easy to obtain. Gaining access to some

**Table 32.1.** Top Treatments Used by IAN Families: Individual Ranking

| Rank | Treatment |
|------|-----------|
| 1 | Speech and language therapy |
| 2 | Occupational therapy (OT) |
| 3 | Applied Behavior Analysis (ABA) |
| 4 | Social skills groups |
| 5 | Picture Exchange Communication Systems (PECS) |
| 6 | Sensory integration therapy |
| 7 | Visual schedules |
| 8 | Physical therapy (PT) |
| 9 | Social stories |
| 10 | Casein-free diet |
| 11 | Gluten-free diet |
| 12 | Weighted blanket or vest |
| 13 | Risperdal |
| 14 | Melatonin |
| 15 | Probiotics |

therapies requires a Herculean effort, but this did not seem to be the case for speech and language therapy, probably because it is an intervention mandated by the Individuals with Disabilities Education Act (IDEA) (see Table 32.3).

The action taken most often to make speech therapy possible was "quitting job (or significantly reducing hours) to take child to therapy or arrange treatment at home." Still, only 18% of families say they have taken such action. This compares with 31% of families who are using, for example, an intensive therapy like applied behavior analysis (ABA).

## Funding the Therapy

***What financial burden does providing speech and language therapy for their children with ASD place on families?***

Of those who answered questions about the cost of this therapy, 74% report obtaining it at no cost, while the remaining 26% report paying some portion of the expense. Of those who do pay something, more than half pay between $100 and $500 a month; overall, some pay as little as $1 and others pay in excess of $2,000.

**Table 32.2.** Top Treatments Used by IAN Families: Group Ranking

| Rank | Treatment |
|------|-----------|
| 1 | Prescription medications |
| 2 | Speech and language therapy |
| 3 | Occupational therapy (OT) |
| 4 | Applied Behavior Analysis (ABA) and related therapies |
| 5 | Treatments for sensory integration dysfunction |
| 6 | Casein/dairy-free and/or gluten-free diet |
| 7 | Social skills groups |
| 8 | Picture Exchange Communication System (PECS) |
| 9 | Visual schedules |
| 10 | Essential fatty acids |
| 11 | Physical therapy (PT) |
| 12 | Social stories |
| 13 | Greenspan—Floortime/developmental individual differences relationship-based approach (DIR) |
| 14 | Melatonin |
| 15 | Probiotics |

**Table 32.3.** Action Taken to Obtain Speech and Language Therapy

| Extra Action Taken to Obtain Therapy | Number of Families Who Took this Action |
|---|---|
| Move to another state | 5% |
| Move within a state to another county | 5% |
| Enroll in a research study | 5% |
| Travel more than 100 miles to see a professional or therapist | 6% |
| Pursue legal action | 7% |
| Go to a new doctor or specialist | 12% |
| Put child in a different school | 16% |
| Quit job or reduce hours to take child to therapy or do treatment at home | 18% |

### *How do so many families obtain this therapy at no cost?*

Many receive the therapy via an early childhood program or a public school. As might be expected, 91% of those who report receiving this therapy at no cost receive it via a publicly funded program. In addition, 53% of families who pay something for speech and language therapy also receive it through a publicly funded program. It may be that some parents, considering language a crucial part of their child's ability to progress, seek out additional speech therapy beyond that offered by schools or early intervention programs.

### *Does health insurance help parents pay for speech therapy for their child?*

Not often. Such costs are covered to some extent by private insurance or Medicaid in only 37% of families (19% have private insurance; 11% have Medicaid; and 7% have both). The remaining 63% of families report no insurance coverage for speech therapy costs.

## Hopes and Results

### *As a child begins this therapy, how optimistic do parents feel? As treatment progresses, are their expectations for their child's progress met?*

Parents are hopeful at the outset, with 90% expecting at least a moderate level of improvement in their child's communication and social interaction. Similarly, 90% report definite improvement in their child's skills. Of all parents rating their child's progress due to speech and language therapy, 42% reported a high or very high level of improvement. This compares to only 30% of parents reporting a high or very high level of improvement for all other current treatments being used by IAN families.

**Please note:** the information reported here reflects only parents' evaluation of current treatments. Because any treatment a child is currently receiving must be considered worthwhile by parents, we expect ratings to be fairly high at this point. As data is collected over time, and families can report on treatments they have dropped, there will likely be more negative reports.

The data make it clear that there are several reasons that speech and language therapy is in use by more than 2,000 of the families participating in IAN:

- It addresses key concerns in autism, including the ability to communicate and to interact socially.

- Fully 99% of parents feel that the therapy involves no, or very little, risk.

- Nearly 73% of parents feel that carrying out the therapy involves no, or very little, burden or difficulty.

- 81% of families receive at least some public funding for the therapy.

- 90% of families expected it to have a positive effect at the outset.

- 90% feel that it has alleviated their child's symptoms or improved his or her skills.

**Please note: These findings are preliminary.** The analyses presented here by the Interactive Autism Network are preliminary. They are based on information submitted via the internet by parents of children with autism spectrum disorders (ASDs) from the United States who choose to participate. They may not generalize to the larger population of parents of children with ASDs. The data have not been peer-reviewed—that is, undergone evaluation by researchers expert in a particular field—or been submitted for publication. IAN views participating families as research partners, and shares such preliminary information to thank them and demonstrate the importance of their ongoing involvement.

## *Reference*

1. National Research Council. (2001). *Educating children with autism.* Committee on Educational Interventions for Children with Autism, Division of Behavioral and Social Sciences and Education. Washington, D.C.: National Academy Press, pp. 138–139.

Section 32.3

# Language Instruction for Children with Autism: Learning Words

"Learning Word Meanings," by Karla McGregor, PhD, Allison Bean, MA, Elizabeth Walker, MA, and Derek Stiles, MA. Reprinted with permission from the Interactive Autism Network (IAN) Community (www.iancommunity.org), © 2008 Kennedy Krieger Institute. The complete document with references is available at http://www.iancommunity.org/cs/articles/wordmeanings.

Late emergence of spoken words is an early sign of autism spectrum disorders, but most children with autism spectrum disorders (ASD) acquire at least some spoken language, with approximately 80% producing more than five words. Expression of words may be stronger than understanding.

Words are the essential building blocks of spoken communication; therefore, it is important to understand how verbal children with ASD best learn words. In this section, we describe the components and processes of word learning and summarize relevant evidence from studies of children with ASD.

## What is involved in learning a word?

To know a word is to know its sound structure, its grammatical role, its meaning, and its appropriate usage. In our laboratory, we are particularly interested in what children know about the meanings of words and the processes involved in acquiring this knowledge.

The initial process of word learning is termed fast mapping because, indeed, both children and adults typically are quick to attach meaning to a new word. However, this new knowledge is fragile, in that it is easily forgotten, and incomplete, in that it does not encompass a full appreciation of the word's meaning. The subsequent process of word learning is referred to as slow mapping. Given additional experiences with the word in meaningful environments, the learner establishes a stronger memory and a deeper knowledge of the word meaning.

A third process of word learning is extension. With the exception of proper names, words extend to members of a category, not just to a single item. For example, dog refers to all dogs, not just the family pet. Typical children as young as 12 months have a basic understanding that words can refer to categories, and they can extend a new word to multiple items based on that understanding. Even with this general appreciation, some additional experience with a given word in multiple contexts may be required before knowledge of the conventional category boundary is acquired. The learning of a word extension, then, may involve both fast mapping and slow mapping. The learner may assume from his first meeting with the word that it refers to a category of things, not just to a single thing (for example, dog refers to all dogs), but he may need additional experience to establish the limits of that category (Siberian husky but not wolf) and the extent to which that category overlaps with or is encompassed within other categories (animal).

How do children accomplish fast mapping, slow mapping, and extension? We view these processes as the outcome of dynamic interactions between the child and his linguistic, social, and physical environments. Both the child and his communication partner—be it a parent, teacher, therapist, sibling, or peer—play a role in the creation and manipulation of those environments.

## Fast Mapping

Let us consider one simple, but not uncommon, environment. Imagine a child who is playing with two toys. One, a truck, is familiar; the other, a puzzle, is new. The child hears her father use a word she has never heard before, puzzle. How will the child know that the new word refers to the new toy? From a very young age, a typical child will figure this out by excluding the familiar toy as a potential reference—she already knows that toy is called a truck so she infers that the other toy must be the puzzle. Can children with ASD apply such principles? In 2005, Preissler and Carey demonstrated that they can. Five- to nine-year-olds with ASD were as able as their younger vocabulary-matched peers to make such inferences. This is an example of how the child with ASD and that child's environment interact during the process of word learning. It was the father (or the examiner) who provided the word at a time when the correct physical reference was present, but it was the child who applied her previous knowledge to finish the solution to the problem.

Let us imagine a slightly different environment. A child is again playing with two toys, but this time both are unfamiliar. When he hears his mother produce a new word, how will he know which toy

367

the mother is naming? A typical child will look toward his mother and read her eye gaze or other body gestures. If she is gazing toward one of the toys and not the other, the child will infer that the word she spoke names the toy to which she is attending. Do children with ASD use eye-gaze cues as a basis for inferring word meaning? Two studies, one by Baron-Cohen, Baldwin, and Crowson in 1997 and the other by Preissler and Carey in 2005, suggest that this is difficult for them. These two teams observed children, with ASD, developmental delay, or no impairment, in the type of word-learning environment described previously. When the new word was uttered, most of the children in the developmental-delay or no-impairment groups monitored the eye gaze of the speaker, shifted focus to the object, and mapped the word. Most of the children in the ASD group failed to monitor the eye-gaze cue, and so, they failed to map the word.

This environment could be restructured to facilitate fast mapping. In 2006, McDuffie, Yoder, and Stone presented one possibility. They heavily supported attention to a novel object as it was named by presenting only one object at a time, placing the object close to the child and gesturing to and moving the object. Under these conditions, children with ASD did look at the object, and they did so more often in conjunction with naming than in conjunction with other sorts of comments. Simpler and more redundant environments may help to focus attention and reduce demands on executive memory, processes known to relate to language learning and known to be challenging for children with ASD.

By gesturing toward and moving the object, McDuffie and her colleagues also enhanced the prominence of the attention-directing cue. In 2007, Parish-Morris, Hennon, Hirsh-Pasek, Golinkoff, and Tager-Flusberg also tried this strategy, this time in the context of two unfamiliar objects. They found that when the examiner pointed to or touched, as well as gazed at, one of the two objects, the children with ASD successfully oriented to the object and fast mapped its name. But, this happened only if the object was interesting to the child. If it was boring, then, even with the support of the point and touch gestures, the children with ASD were not successful.

Why do children with ASD fail to use eye gaze in service of fast mapping if it is not supported by extra gestures and simple or prominent object presentations? Eye gaze and other directional gestures such as pointing serve both to attract attention and to indicate intent. When the child sees his mother gaze toward an object while saying a word, he may follow the physical direction of her gaze and attend to that object; he also may infer that she intends to name that object. Therefore, we might ask whether the failure of children with ASD to use these cues is a failure to exploit their attentional or intentional meanings. Increasing evidence supports the latter explanation. Parish-Morris and her colleagues attempted to isolate social-intent cues from social-attention cues. Three- to seven-year-olds with ASD and two groups of typical children matched on the basis of either nonverbal intelligence or vocabulary level participated in a word-learning task that depended upon reading a social intent. An examiner pretended to unsuccessfully hunt for a *parlu* in a sack. She then asked the child to hunt through the sack and find it. The child had to infer that the unfamiliar object in the sack must be the object she intended, even though he had never seen the object while simultaneously hearing its name. Unlike the two comparison groups, the ASD group did not perform better than chance on this task. This finding demonstrates that children with ASD have difficulty using sophisticated combinations of cues, such as the language and facial expressions that might indicate frustration about not finding an object, to infer intent.

## Slow Mapping and Extension

Whereas we are beginning to understand the environments that promote or impede fast mapping by the child with ASD, we know little about his slow mapping and extension of words. Two studies from the 1980s suggest that children with ASD, like other children, appreciate that words extend to all members of a category. In those studies, children affected by ASD performed just as well as language- and intelligence quotient (IQ)-matched peers when asked to sort items into categories or to name categories and category members. A more recent study confirmed good performance by adults and adolescents with ASD on a task requiring generation of members of the category of animals.

In our own laboratory, we are collecting evidence on the outcomes of the slow-mapping process, if not the process itself. Specifically, we are finding that some children with ASD, aged 9–13 years, have a rather shallow understanding of word meanings. It isn't that they do not know the words; rather, they do not know them completely. That said, we find that other children with ASD have rich, age- and IQ-appropriate knowledge of word meanings. In 2005, Norbury drew similar conclusions. Rather than investigating depth of word knowledge, she focused on flexibility of word knowledge. Specifically, she asked whether these children aged 9–17 years with ASD knew not only dominant word meanings (bank as a place to keep money) but also secondary meanings

369

(bank as the edge of a river). Like us, she found that some children with ASD were limited in their knowledge of secondary meanings but that others had age-appropriate knowledge.

These are hopeful findings in that they suggest that the social deficits characteristic of autism do not necessarily limit successful slow mapping and extension of word meanings. But what of the child who does have these limitations? Can the environment be structured to support learning? Research on typically developing toddlers suggests that increasing the prominence of cues can enhance slow mapping and extension. Horst and Samuelson conducted four experiments in which typical two-year-olds were presented with names for unfamiliar objects, tested immediately, and tested again after a five-minute delay. In all four experiments, participants had no difficulty fast mapping word-object pairings. On the other hand, they were able to retain or extend novel names at better than chance levels only in the experiments that involved manipulation of the novel objects and direct naming. In other words, if the examiner was very direct in showing, pointing to, and labeling the object, the child was able to extend that name to other category members and to retain its name following a five-minute interval. Booth and her colleagues presented typical two-year-olds with two unfamiliar objects and named one of them. For some children, the examiner gazed toward the target object as she named it, for others, she gazed and pointed, and for others still she gazed and touched or manipulated the object. As the prominence of the gesture increased, from gaze, to point, to touch and manipulate, the toddlers' extension and retention of the new words during a period of 3–5 days increased, with the biggest difference being the benefit of gaze and point versus gaze alone. In 2005, Capone and McGregor found that toddlers recalled new words more readily and had a deeper knowledge of the word meanings if the words had been taught in the context of a gesture that emphasized the meaning (for example, shape or function) of the object than when the same words and objects were taught without gestural support. Although it is a leap to assume that these same strategies would support extension and slow mapping for children with ASD, these strategies do exploit the visual modality, a relative strength for many children with ASD.

## Conclusion

In summary, to the extent that word learning depends on the ability to read the social cues of others, children with ASD will face challenges in word learning. We know that these children have difficulties with fast mapping in situations where subtle social-attention cues like eye gaze or more sophisticated social cues to intention hold the key to success. We have little evidence to suggest that the inability to read social cues limits their slow mapping and extension of words; but, then again, we have little evidence about these processes period. We have found that some children with ASD can and do develop age-appropriate knowledge of word meaning, and fortunately, other investigators have found the same. We do not know for certain the best ways to help the children who do lag in the processes of word learning, but the literature demonstrates that children with ASD, like young typically developing children, learn better in environments where the complexity of competing information is reduced and the prominence of important attentional cues is enhanced.

## Section 32.4

# *Augmentative and Alternative Communication (AAC)*

This section includes text from "What is AAC?" and "Technology," undated, © International Society for Augmentative and Alternative Communication (ISAAC) (www.isaac-online.org). Reprinted with permission.

### *What is augmentative and alternative communication (AAC)?*

Augmentative and alternative communication (AAC) are the words used to describe extra ways of helping people who find it hard to communicate by speech or writing. AAC helps them to communicate more easily.

AAC includes many different methods. Signing and gesture do not need any extra bits and pieces and are called unaided systems. Others use picture charts, books, and special computers. These are called aided systems. AAC can help people understand what is said to them as well as being able to say and write what they want.

### *AAC Technologies*

Augmentative and alternative communication (AAC) equipment can be simple and cheap home-made aids that have no electronics. AAC equipment can also be very clever electronic aids.

Devices with no electronics include alphabet, symbol or picture boards where the user points to the letters, words, symbols or pictures which help to show what he wants to say. People can point with their finger, or a stick, or look specifically at a word or picture with their eyes.

Electronic aids are usually computers with extra bits that will speak for the user. These aids have several fancy names—speech generating devices (SGD), voice output communication aids (VOCAs), or voice output devices. There are many different types of electronic aids. Some take letters and words typed in by the user and speak them out loud like normal speech. Others show pictures, symbols, or words on the display and the user chooses one, or some, of these to be spoken out. Others have pages where all the words for a specific activity are displayed together. These pages can be for many different activities like ordering drinks or food in a pub, or for a geography lesson in school.

Most electronic aids can be worked in more than one way—touch screen, joystick, switches—to allow people with physical disabilities to use them.

All electronic aids can breakdown; batteries die, cables become disconnected, and sometimes they just will not work. It is a good idea for all users of electronic aids to carry some non-electronic system as a back-up.

# Chapter 33

# *ASD Medications*

## *Chapter Contents*

Section 33.1

# *Parent Training Complements Medication for Treating Behavioral Problems in Children with Pervasive Developmental Disorders*

Excerpted from "Parent Training Complements Medication for Treating Behavioral Problems in Children with Pervasive Developmental Disorders," National Institute of Mental Health (NIMH), November 20, 2009.

Treatment that includes medication plus a structured training program for parents reduces serious behavioral problems in children with autism and related conditions, according to a study funded by the National Institute of Mental Health (NIMH). The study, which was part of the NIMH Research Units on Pediatric Psychopharmacology (RUPP) Autism Network, was published in the December 2009 issue of the *Journal of the American Academy of Child and Adolescent Psychiatry*.

Results from a previous RUPP study reported in 2002 showed that the antipsychotic medication risperidone (Risperdal) reduced such behavior problems as tantrums, aggression, and self-injury in children with autism. However, most children's symptoms returned when the medication was discontinued.

"Medication alone has been shown to help with some symptoms of autism, but its potential is limited," said NIMH Director Thomas R. Insel. "This study shows promise of a more effective treatment protocol that could improve life for children with autism and their families."

In the study, the RUPP group tested the benefits of medication alone compared to medication plus a parent training program that actively involves parents in managing their children's severely disruptive and noncompliant behavior. Parents were taught to modify their children's behavior and learned to enhance their children's daily living skills.

The 24-week, three-site trial included 124 children ages 4–13 with pervasive developmental disorders (PDD) such as autism, Asperger syndrome, or related disorders accompanied by tantrums, aggression, and self-injury. The children were randomized to a combination of risperidone and parent training, or to risperidone only. Parents in

374

combination therapy received an average of 11 sessions of training over the course of the study.

Although both groups improved over the six-month trial, the group receiving combination therapy showed greater reduction in behavioral problems like irritability, tantrums, and impulsiveness compared to the group receiving medication only. The combination therapy group also ended the trial taking an average dose of 1.98 milligrams (mg) per day of risperidone, compared to 2.26 mg/day in the medication-only group—a 14% lower dose. However, children in both groups gained weight, indicating "a need to learn more about the metabolic consequences of medications like risperidone," said the authors.

## Section 33.2

# *Citalopram No Better Than Placebo Treatment for Children with ASD*

Excerpted from "Citalopram No Better Than Placebo Treatment
for Children with Autism Spectrum Disorders," National Institute
of Mental Health (NIMH), June 1, 2009.

Citalopram, a medication commonly prescribed to children with autism spectrum disorders (ASD), was no more effective than a placebo at reducing repetitive behaviors, according to researchers funded by the National Institute of Mental Health (NIMH) and other NIH institutes. The study was published in the June 2009 issue of *Archives of General Psychiatry*.

"Parents of children with autism spectrum disorders face an enormous number of treatment options, not all of which are research-based," said NIMH Director Thomas R. Insel, MD. "Studies like this help us to better understand which treatments are likely to be beneficial and safe."

The researchers say their findings do not support using citalopram to treat repetitive behaviors in children with ASD. Also, the greater frequency of side effects from this particular medication compared to placebo illustrates the importance of placebo-controlled trials in evaluating medications currently prescribed to this population.

Citalopram is in a class of antidepressant medications called selective serotonin reuptake inhibitors (SSRIs) that is sometimes prescribed for children with ASD to reduce repetitive behaviors. These behaviors, a hallmark of ASD, include stereotypical hand flapping, repetitive complex whole body movements (such as spinning, swaying, or rocking over and over, with no clear purpose), repetitive play, and inflexible daily routines.

Past research suggested that some children with ASD have abnormalities in the brain system that makes serotonin, a brain chemical that, among many other functions, plays an important role in early brain development. Children with obsessive compulsive disorder (OCD) may also have serotonin abnormalities and have repetitive or inflexible behaviors. OCD is effectively treated with SSRIs, leading some researchers to wonder whether similar treatment may reduce repetitive behaviors in children with ASD. So far, studies have produced mixed results, but SSRIs remain among the most frequently prescribed medications for children with ASD.

Researchers in the Studies to Advance Autism Research and Treatment (STAART) network, conducted a six-site, randomized controlled trial comparing the effectiveness and safety of using the SSRI citalopram (Celexa) versus placebo to treat repetitive behaviors in children with ASD. The study included 149 participants, ages 5–17, who had autism, Asperger disorder, or pervasive developmental disorder not otherwise specified (PDDNOS).

After 12 weeks of treatment, roughly one out of three children in both groups—32.9% of those treated with citalopram and 34.2% of those treated with placebo—showed fewer or less severe repetitive symptoms. According to the researchers, the study results may challenge the underlying premise that repetitive behaviors in children with ASD are similar to repetitive and inflexible behaviors in OCD.

# Section 33.3

# *Bonding Hormone Might Help Some with Autism*

People with high-functioning autism or Asperger syndrome were better able to catch social cues after inhaling the hormone oxytocin, new research shows. Oxytocin, which is produced in abundance when a mother is breast-feeding her baby, is known as the bonding hormone. Although there are many kinks to be worked out, experts feel the strategy holds promise to treat one of the core symptoms of autism spectrum disorder.

"When you start thinking of a hormone that can actually encourage pro-social behavior, you're talking about potentially significant changes in quality of life," said Clara Lajonchere, a vice president of clinical programs at the advocacy group Autism Speaks and a clinical assistant professor at the Keck School of Medicine, University of Southern California. "In the absence of intellectual deficits, the areas where they have the greatest struggle is around social communication and social connectedness," she continued. "These people can't interpret other people's perceptions, they can't read social cues, they don't make eye contact." While there are drugs for the secondary symptoms of autism, such as irritability and aggression, doctors have nothing yet for the core symptoms in the areas of language, social interaction and intellectual deficits.

Prior studies have shown a strong effect of oxytocin on people with autism, as well as on people who are not on the autism disorders spectrum. One study found that autistic people seem to have a lower sensitivity to oxytocin than people without the disorder. "There's no doubt that oxytocin has a big effect on social interactions in anyone. It's almost like a designer drug, a drug which has a selective effect on a behavior in the normal range," said Keith Young, vice chairman of research in psychiatry and behavioral science at the Texas A&M Health Science Center College of Medicine in Temple, and the neuroimaging and genetics core leader at the VA Center of Excellence for Research on Returning War Veterans at the Central Texas Veterans Health Care System.

The new study, led by Angela Sirigu at the Center for Cognitive Neuroscience in Lyon, France, was published in the February 2010 issue of *Proceedings of the National Academy of Sciences*. It involved 13 adults, most of them men, aged 17 to 39. All had high-functioning autism or Asperger syndrome. Participants performed different tasks—either after inhaling oxytocin or without using the hormone. When observed playing a virtual ball game, individuals who had inhaled oxytocin were able to interact better with their virtual partners compared to untreated participants. Also, after inhaling oxytocin, participants showed more alertness to socially important visual cues in pictures of human faces.

There were, however, wide variations in individual responses, the team noted. "It's not clear whether this would be effective at all in children or in young adults who had intellectual problems," warned Young.

The long-term effects of the hormone are also uncertain. "I really want to encourage clinical trials in this area because of its potential significance, but we have to be very careful in terms of safety data," Lajonchere said. "Safety data is really critical."

Also, scientists would need to come up with a different method of delivery, Young said. "The nasal [inhaled] drugs only work for a few minutes. Potentially it would be very difficult to be using this drug once an hour or something. It doesn't make a whole lot of sense," he pointed out. "But it does point the way to the possibility of raising oxytocin levels with other kinds of compounds to increase oxytocin levels more generally over a longer period of time. I don't know whether this is a realistic therapy as we have it now but, potentially, in the future it could really help these people whose primary autistic symptoms are having to do with reduction in social activity."

# Chapter 34

# *Treatments for Biological and Medical Conditions Associated with ASD*

These services are therapies that address symptoms commonly associated with autism, but not specific to the disorder. These are called related services.

**Speech-language therapy (SLT)** encompasses a variety of techniques and addresses a range of challenges for children with autism. For instance, some individuals are unable to speak. Others seem to love to talk. They may have difficulty understanding information or they may struggle to express themselves.

SLT is designed to coordinate the mechanics of speech and the meaning and social value of language. An SLT program begins with an individual evaluation by a speech-language pathologist. The therapy may then be conducted one-on-one, in a small group or in a classroom setting. The therapy may have different goals for different children. Depending on the verbal aptitude of the individual, the goal might be to master spoken language, or it might be to learn signs or gestures to communicate. In each case, the aim is to help the individual learn useful and functional communication. Speech-language therapy is provided by speech-language pathologists who specialize in children with autism. Most intensive therapy programs address speech-language therapy as well.

This chapter begins with "Treating Autism: Treatment for Biological and Medical Conditions Associated with Autism." Reprinted with the permission of Autism Speaks, www.autismspeaks.org, © 2010. The chapter concludes with "Center for Autism and Related Disorders Research Study Finds Chewing Gum an Effective Treatment for Children with Autism," © 2009 Center for Autism and Related Disorders, Inc. (www.centerforautism.com). Reprinted with permission.

**Occupational therapy (OT)** brings together cognitive, physical, and motor skills. The aim of OT is to enable the individual to gain independence and participate more fully in life. For a child with autism, the focus may be on appropriate play, learning, and basic life skills.

An occupational therapist will evaluate the child's development as well as the psychological, social, and environmental factors that may be involved. The therapist will then prepare strategies and tactics for learning key tasks to practice at home, in school, and other settings. Occupational therapy is usually delivered in a half hour to one hour session with the frequency determined by the needs of the child. Goals of an OT program might include independent dressing, feeding, grooming, and use of the toilet, and improved social, fine motor, and visual perceptual skills. OT is provided by certified occupational therapists.

**Sensory integration (SI) therapy** is designed to identify disruptions in the way the individual's brain processes movement, touch, smell, sight, and sound and help them process these senses in a more productive way. It is sometimes used alone, but is often part of an occupational therapy program. It is believed that SI does not teach higher-level skills, but enhances sensory processing abilities, allowing the child to be more available to acquire higher-level skills. Sensory integration therapy might be used to help calm your child, reinforce a desired behavior, or to help with transitions between activities.

Therapists begin with an individual evaluation to determine what your child's sensitivities are. The therapist then plans an individualized program for the child matching sensory stimulation with physical movement to improve how the brain processes and organizes sensory information. The therapy often includes equipment such as swings, trampolines, and slides. Certified occupational and physical therapists provide sensory integration therapy.

**Physical therapy (PT)** focuses on any problems with movement that cause functional limitations. Children with autism frequently have challenges with motor skills such as sitting, walking, running, and jumping. PT can also address poor muscle tone, balance, and coordination. A physical therapist will start by evaluating the abilities and developmental level of the child. Once they identify where the individual's challenges are, they design activities that target those areas. PT might include assisted movement, various forms of exercise, and orthopedic equipment. Physical therapy is usually delivered in a half hour to one-hour session by a certified physical therapist, with the frequency determined by the needs of the child.

**Picture exchange communication system (PECS)** is a learning system that allows children with little or no verbal ability to communicate using pictures. PECS can be used at home, in the classroom, or a variety of settings. A therapist, teacher, or parent helps the child build a vocabulary and articulate desires, observations, or feelings by using pictures consistently.

The PECS program starts by teaching the child how to exchange a picture for an object. Eventually, the individual is shown how to distinguish between pictures and symbols and use them to form sentences. Although PECS is based on visual tools, verbal reinforcement is a major component and verbal communication is encouraged. Standard PECS pictures can be purchased as a part of a manual or pictures can be gathered from photos, newspapers, magazines, or other books.

**Auditory integration therapy (AIT),** sometimes called sound therapy, is sometimes used to treat children with difficulties in auditory processing or sound sensitivity. Treatment with AIT involves the patient listening to electronically modified music through headphones during multiple sessions. There are different methods of AIT, including Tomatis and Berard. While some individuals have reported improvements in auditory processing resulting from AIT, there are no credible studies that demonstrate its effectiveness or support its use.

**Gluten free, casein free diet (GFCF):** Many families of children with autism are interested in dietary and nutritional interventions that might help some of their children's symptoms. Removal of gluten (a protein found in barley, rye, and wheat, and in oats through cross contamination) and casein (a protein found in dairy products) is a popular dietary treatment for symptoms of autism.

The theory behind this diet is that proteins are absorbed differently in some children. Rather than having an allergic reaction, children who benefit from the GFCF diet experience physical and behavioral symptoms. While there have not yet been sufficient scientific studies to support this theory, many families report that dietary elimination of gluten and casein has helped regulate bowel habits, sleep activity, habitual behaviors, and contributed to the overall progress in their individual child. Because no specific laboratory tests can predict which children will benefit from dietary intervention, many families choose to try the diet with careful observation by the family and intervention team.

Families choosing a trial of dietary restriction should make sure their child is receiving adequate nutrition. Dairy products are the most common source of calcium and vitamin D in young children in the United States. Many young children depend on dairy products for a balanced protein intake. Alternative sources of these nutrients require the substitution of other food and beverage products with attention to the nutritional content.

Substitution of gluten-free products requires attention to the overall fiber and vitamin content of a child's diet. Vitamin supplement use may have both positive effects and side effects. Consultation with a dietician or physician should be considered and can be helpful to families in the determination of healthy application of a GFCF diet. This may be especially true for children who are picky eaters.

## *What about other medical interventions?*

Many families are eager to try new treatments, even those that have not yet been scientifically proven to be effective. A family's hopes for a cure for their child may make them more vulnerable to the lure of untested treatments.

It's important to remember that just as each child with autism presents differently, so is their response to treatments. It may be helpful to collect information about a therapy that you are interested in trying and speak with a pediatrician as well as other team members, so that a discussion of the potential risks/benefits and measurable outcomes are addressed.

Parents of older children with autism can provide a history of therapies and biomedical interventions that have been promised as a cure for autism over the years. Some of them may have been meaningful for a small number of children. Upon further study, none of them, so far, has turned out to be a cure for many.

We do know that many children get better with intensive behavioral therapy. There is a large body of scientific evidence to support it. For this reason, it makes sense to engage a child in an intensive behavioral program before looking at other interventions.

## *Is there a cure? Is recovery possible?*

You may have heard about children who have recovered from autism. Experts disagree about whether or not this is possible.

Growing evidence suggests that a small minority of children with autism have progressed to the point where they no longer meet the criteria for a diagnosis. The theories behind the recovery of some children range from the assertion that the child was misdiagnosed to the belief that the child had a form of autism that may resolve as he matures to the opinion that the child benefited from successful treatment. You may also hear about children who reach best outcome status, which means they score normally on tests for intelligence quotient (IQ), language, adaptive functioning, school placement, and personality, but have mild symptoms on some personality and diagnostic tests. Some children who no longer meet the criteria for an autism diagnosis are later diagnosed as having ADHD, anxiety, or even Asperger syndrome.

We don't yet know what percentage of children with autism will recover, or what genetic, physiological, or developmental factors can predict which ones will. Recovery from autism is usually reported in connection with intensive early intervention, but we do not know how much or which type of intervention works best, or whether the recovery can be fully credited to the intervention. Presently, there is no way of predicting which children will have the best outcomes.

In the absence of a cure or even an accurate prognosis of a child's future, do not be afraid to believe in a child's potential. Most children with autism will benefit from intervention. Many, if not most, will make very significant, meaningful progress.

## Center for Autism and Related Disorders Research Study Finds Chewing Gum an Effective Treatment for Children with Autism

According to new research conducted by the Center for Autism and Related Disorders, Inc. (CARD), the "Chewing Gum as a Treatment for Rumination in a Child with Autism" study reveals the challenging behavior of rumination can be treated effectively by using chewing gum as a replacement behavior. The study was published in the September 2009 issue of the *Journal of Applied Behavior Analysis*.

Rumination involves regurgitation of previously ingested food, re-chewing the food, and re-swallowing it. The study examined a child with autism who displayed chronic rumination for approximately one year, resulting in the decay and subsequent removal of several teeth. After several treatments failed, including thickened liquids and starch satiation, the child was taught to chew gum. His rumination decreased significantly when gum was made available.

"The key findings of this research study are significant for both parents and practitioners," says researcher Denise Rhine, MS ED, BCBA. "The findings suggest that access to chewing gum may be an effective and practical treatment for rumination in some individuals with autism."

The complete "Chewing Gum as a Treatment for Rumination in a Child with Autism" study was published in the summer 2009 Edition of the *Journal of Applied Behavior Analysis*, pages 381–385. The study is also located online at http://seab.envmed.rochester.edu/jaba/toc/cur/jabacurrent.php.

# Chapter 35

# *Research Studies and ASD*

## *Chapter Contents*

## Section 35.1

# *Participating in ASD Research Studies*

## *Participating in Research Studies*

Autism research studies, especially in the area of applied research, are dependent on participation by individuals with an autism spectrum disorders (ASD) diagnosis. Parents of children with autism often seek to include their child in ongoing research studies in part to increase our understanding of autism and for the potential benefit to the child from receiving the intervention being used in the research study.

Researchers also actively recruit children with autism and family members to be participants in research studies. Participation in a research study is a decision that is both voluntary and personal. If you decide that you would like to have your child, family members, or yourself participate in a research study, please consider the following points and questions.

## *Ethical Considerations in Research with Human Participants*

The American Medical Association and the American Psychological Association have strict codes of ethics that all researchers must follow when conducting research with human participants. As a participant, you should be informed about all aspects of the research, including information about the following:

- Potential risks of participation: You should be informed of any potential risks to you or your child as a consequence of participating in a study.

- Potential benefits of participation: You should be informed of the benefits of participation.

- Assurance of confidentiality: You should be informed of how researchers are going to ensure the confidentiality of you and your child's identity.

- The right to withdraw from the research at any time: Your participation is voluntary and you have the right to withdraw from the study at any time with no penalty.

- Informed consent: Researchers must obtain your written informed consent for participation and this consent must be provided freely and without coercion (for example, "If you don't agree, we can no longer work with your child").

If you are not informed of any of these aspects of the research, do not participate in the study.

## Questions to Answer before Participating in Research Studies

Assuming that you have been fully informed and that the human subjects' protection requirements have been approved by an institutional review board (IRB), please ask yourselves the following questions and consider Organization for Autism Research (OAR)'s accompanying advice before enrolling your child, other family member, or yourself in any study.

### *Will I learn more about my child from participating in a study?*

Be sure you understand the purpose of a study. Generally, research studies are conducted to answer a very specific question, so you will probably not receive any information specific to your child as an individual.

### *How can I be sure that it is safe for my child to participate in a study?*

Inquire about the review process that the study had to undergo. Be sure that the research is being conducted in a controlled environment that is committed to the protection of participant rights. Studies conducted at universities and medical institutions must receive approval from institutional review boards (IRBs) whose job it is to make sure that the research is ethical and safe. Private facilities are not always as closely regulated, so be sure to inquire about their systems of review and safeguards.

### *How can I be sure that the study will not demand too much of my time?*

Be sure you understand the requirements of participation. Find out how long the study is expected to last, how much time you will have to commit, if you will have to participate on a daily or weekly basis, how many hours per day are required, and so forth.

### *If the study is using a randomized control design, how will I know if my child is in the control or the treatment group?*

Random assignment means that participants in a study are as-signed to be in either an experimental group or a control group using a method similar to flipping a coin, so that they have an equal chance of being in either group. Your child has a 50/50 chance of being assigned to either a treatment or a placebo group, and you will not be told of your child's group assignment until the conclusion of the study. For this reason, it is very important to be sure you understand whether or not you will be offered an opportunity to receive the treatment at the conclusion of the study if he or she is assigned to the placebo group. Sometimes, researchers use a cross-over design, in which groups switch conditions after a period of time. If this is the case, your child will be assured to receive the intervention. However, to keep you and your child "blind" to your group assignment, you will not always know that the research is using a cross-over design in advance of the study.

# Section 35.2

# *Why Some Research Studies Are Flawed*

This section provides reasons why individual research studies into autism interventions may not be fully valid or reliable.

## *Purpose of the Research*

- The study may not address a clearly defined issue.

- The study may not answer the key questions raised.

## *Objectivity of the Researchers*

The researchers who carried out the study may not be completely independent. For example,

- they may have a biased hypothesis (they are setting out to prove something they already know is right), or

- they may stand to gain financially if they claim that an intervention is successful.

## *Methodology Used in the Research*

- The study may not have lasted long enough for the results to be valid. For example, the study may only have lasted for a few weeks, while the effect of the intervention may not be apparent until months later.

- The study may have used techniques that are more likely to produce a biased result. For example, an observational study is more likely to be biased than an experimental study, and a non-randomized control study is more likely to be biased than a randomized control trial.

- The researchers may not have reported any confounders—things which may have influenced the results.

## Participants Included in the Research

- The study may not include enough participants for the results to be statistically significant. For example, a study which looks at one or two people is much less likely to be statistically significant than a study which looks at more than twenty people.

- The study may not record vital information about the participants in the study group, such as the type of autistic spectrum disorder they had, or whether they had any other conditions which might have affected the result.

- The study may not record whether the intervention is specifically relevant to people with autistic spectrum disorders. This sometimes happens when people with autism are included in a research study alongside other groups of people.

## Interventions Being Researched

- The study may not record detailed information about the intervention and how it was delivered. This makes it more difficult for other researchers to replicate the study and check the accuracy of the findings.

- The study may not record detailed information about the intervention received by the control group. This makes it more difficult to compare the effects of the intervention on the study group compared to the intervention received by the control group.

- The study may not record information about other things which may have affected the result. For example, family circumstances or other treatments being received at the same time as the intervention could affect the results of the study into the intervention.

## Outcomes and Measures

- The study may not use standardized outcome measures—ways of measuring improvements in the participants. This makes it difficult to compare the results with other studies

- The study may use different measures before and after the intervention. This makes it difficult to compare the effect of the intervention.

- The study may only use subjective measures such parental observations of children's behavior. This makes the results less reliable.

- The assessors—the people evaluating the study—may know which participants received which intervention. This makes it more likely they could influence the results, however subconsciously.

# Part Six

# Education and Autism Spectrum Disorder

# Chapter 36

# *A Child's Rights to Public Education*

Your special needs child has the right to a free and appropriate education. The *Individuals with Disabilities Education Act* (IDEA), which was first enacted in 1975 and most recently revised in 2004, mandates that each state provide all eligible children with a public education that meets their individual needs.

The *Individuals with Disabilities Act* (IDEA) was most recently revised in 2004 (and, in fact, renamed the *Individuals with Disabilities Education Improvement Act*, but most people still refer to it as IDEA). The law mandates that the state provide all eligible children with a free and appropriate public education that meets their unique individual needs.

IDEA specifies that children with various disabilities, including autism, are entitled to early intervention services and special education. If your child has been diagnosed with a form of autism, the diagnosis is generally sufficient to gain access to the rights afforded by IDEA.

The IDEA legislation has established an important role for parents in their children's education. You, as a parent, are entitled to be treated as an equal partner with the school district in deciding on an education plan for your child and his or her individual needs. This enables you to be a powerful advocate for your child. It also means that you must be an informed, active participant in planning and monitoring your child's unique program and legal rights.

"Your Child's Rights." Reprinted with the permission of Autism Speaks, www.autismspeaks.org, © 2010.

# What is a free and appropriate public education (FAPE)?

As described, IDEA provides for a free and appropriate education for all children with disabilities. Each word in this phrase is important, but appropriate is the one that relates specifically to your special needs child. Your child is entitled to an education that is tailored to his or her special needs and a placement that will allow him or her to make educational progress.

Although you and your child's teachers or therapists may want to provide your child with the best or optimal program and services, the school district is not required to provide the best or optimal but rather an appropriate education. One of the challenges here is working with the school district to determine what is appropriate, and therefore, what will be provided for your child. This is a collaborative process that may involve considerable negotiation to secure the services from the school.

# What is least restrictive environment (LRE)?

As specified in the IDEA, your child is also entitled to experience the least restrictive environment. This means that your child should be placed in the environment in which he or she has the greatest possible opportunity to interact with children who do not have a disability and to participate in the general education curriculum. This is commonly referred to as mainstreaming or inclusion. In the general education setting, providing the least restrictive environment can sometimes be accomplished with accommodations, such as using a one-on-one aide who is trained to work with children with autism. While it may be true that seeking the least restrictive environment is beneficial for children with autism, it's important to consider whether or not an option such as inclusion is right for your child. It may or may not be more appropriate for your child to be placed in a special education program, in a school for children with special needs, or in a home instruction program.

**Early intervention services (EI):** The IDEA provides states with federal grants to institute early intervention programs. Any child younger than age three who has a developmental delay or a physical or mental condition likely to result in a developmental delay is eligible to receive early intervention services through these programs. If a child is determined to be eligible, these early intervention services must be provided to the child at no cost.

EI services can vary widely from state to state and region to region. However, the services should address a child's unique needs rather than being limited to what is currently available or customary in your area. The document that spells out a child's needs and the services that will be provided is the individual family service plan (IFSP). The IFSP should be based on a comprehensive evaluation of a child. It should describe the child's current levels of functioning and the anticipated goals. It should also list the specific services that will be provided to a child and your family.

EI services are aimed at minimizing the impact of disabilities on the development of a child. Services for a child may include, but are not limited to, speech and language instruction, occupational therapy, physical therapy, Applied Behavior Analysis (ABA), and psychological evaluation. Services for families may include training to help reinforce the affected child's new skills and counseling to help the family adapt.

**Special education services** pick up where early intervention services leave off, at age three. Your local school district provides these services through their special education department. The focus of special education is different from that of early intervention. While early intervention addresses your child's overall development, special education focuses on providing your child with an education, regardless of disabilities or special needs. The document that spells out your child's needs and how these needs will be met is the individualized education program (IEP).

Like the IFSP, the IEP describes your child's strengths and weaknesses, sets goals and objectives, and details how these can be met. Unlike the IFSP, the IEP is almost entirely related to how the needs of your child will be met within the context of the school district and within school walls.

**Extended school year (ESY) services:** If there is evidence that a child experiences a substantial regression in skills during school vacations, he or she may be entitled to ESY services. These services would be provided over long breaks from school (summer vacation) to prevent substantial regression, but not to acquire new skills. It is important for the family to remain involved in determining appropriate goals, communicating with the educational team about progress, and working to provide consistency between home and school.

## How to Get Services Started for a Child

**For early intervention services,** if a child is under the age of three, call the local early intervention agency.

**For special education services,** if a child is three or older, contact the local school district.

**Before services can be provided,** it may be necessary to complete further assessments and evaluations. These may include: an unstructured diagnostic play session, a developmental evaluation, a speech-language assessment, a parent interview, an evaluation of current behavior, or an evaluation of adaptive or real life skills.

Having to wait for the completion of these additional evaluations, which may be required by the school district or Early Intervention, may be frustrating for parents. Often, the evaluations provide much more in-depth information about a child's symptoms, strengths, and needs, and will be helpful for accessing and planning therapy services in the long run.

If parents find they are spinning their wheels, waiting for them, there are things you can be doing to in the meantime. Talk to other parents about what services have been helpful for their children, investigate therapies, and start reading about autism.

Chapter 37

# *Understanding the Special Education Process*

## *Chapter Contents*

## Section 37.1

# *Special Education Overview for Parents*

From "Understanding the Special Education Process: An Overview for Parents," by the Families and Advocates Partnership for Education (FAPE). © PACER Center Inc. Used with permission from PACER Center Inc., Minneapolis, MN, (952) 838-9000. www.pacer.org. All rights reserved.

This section offers an overview of the special education process. It is not designed to show all steps or the specific details. It shows what happens from the time a child is referred for evaluation and is identified as having a disability, through the development of an individualized education program (IEP). The process begins when someone (school staff, parents, and so forth) makes a referral for an initial evaluation.

## *How the Process Works*

1.  Parents, school personnel, students, or others may make a request for evaluation. If you request an evaluation to determine whether your child has a disability and needs special education, the school district must complete a full and individual evaluation. If it refuses to conduct the evaluation, it must give you appropriate notice and let you know your rights. You must give permission in writing for an initial (first-time) evaluation and for any tests that are completed as part of a reevaluation.

2.  A team of qualified professionals and you will review the results of the evaluation and determine if your child is eligible for special education services.

3.  If your child is not eligible, you will be appropriately notified and the process stops. However, you have a right to disagree with the results of the evaluation or the eligibility decision. If you disagree with the results of an evaluation, you have a right to an independent educational evaluation (IEE). Someone who does not work for the school district completes the IEE. The school district must pay for the IEE or show at an impartial due process hearing that its evaluation is appropriate.

4. If you and the school district agree that your child is eligible for services, you and the school staff will plan your child's individualized education program (IEP) at an IEP team meeting. You are an equal member of this team. Some states may have a different name for the IEP team meeting.

5. The IEP lists any special services your child needs, including goals your child is expected to achieve in one year and objectives or benchmarks to note progress. The team determines what services are in the IEP, as well as the location where those services and modifications will occur. At times, the IEP and placement decisions will take place at one meeting. At other times, placement may be made at a separate meeting (usually called a placement meeting). Placement for your child must be in the least restrictive environment (LRE) appropriate to your child's needs. He or she will be placed in the regular classroom to receive services unless the IEP team determines that, even with special additional aids and services, the child cannot be successful there. You are part of any group that decides what services your child will receive and where they will be provided.

6. If you disagree with the IEP and/or the proposed placement, you should first try to work out an agreement with your child's IEP team. If you still disagree, you can use your due process rights.

7. If you agree with the IEP and placement, your child will receive the services that are written into the IEP. You will receive reports on your child's progress at least as often as parents are given reports on their children who do not have disabilities. You can request that the IEP team meet if reports show that changes need to be made in the IEP.

8. The IEP team meets at least once per year to discuss progress and write any new goals or services into the IEP. As a parent, you can agree or disagree with the proposed changes. If you disagree, you should do so in writing.

9. If you disagree with any changes in the IEP, your child will continue to receive the services listed in the previous IEP until you and the school staff can reach agreement. You should discuss your concerns with the other members of the IEP team. If you continue to disagree with the IEP, you have several options, including asking for additional testing or an independent educational evaluation (IEE), or resolving the disagreement using due process.

10. Your child will continue to receive special education services if the team agrees that the services are needed. A reevaluation is completed at least once every three years to see if your child continues to be eligible for special education services and to decide what services he or she needs.

If you would like more information about special education or about your rights, call your state Parent Training and Information Center. If you do not know the number, call PACER Center at the national toll-free number: 888-248-0822.

## Important Terms

**Due process:** Protects the right of parents to have input into their child's educational program and to take steps to resolve disagreements. When parents and school districts disagree with one another, they may ask for an impartial hearing to resolve issues. Mediation must also be available.

**Mediation**: A meeting between parents and the school district with an impartial person, called a mediator, who helps both sides come to an agreement that each finds acceptable.

**Impartial due process hearing:** A meeting between parents and the school district. Each side presents its position, and a hearing officer decides what the appropriate educational program is, based on requirements in law.

School districts must give parents a written copy of special education procedural safeguards. This document outlines the steps for due process hearings and mediation. Parents must be given a copy when their child is first referred for an evaluation and each time they are notified of an IEP meeting for their child.

# Section 37.2

# *Individualized Education Plan (IEP)*

## *What's an IEP?*

Kids with delayed skills or other disabilities might be eligible for special services that provide individualized education programs in public schools, free of charge to families. Understanding how to access these services can help parents be effective advocates for their kids.

The passage of the updated version of the Individuals with Disabilities Education Act (IDEA 2004) made parents of kids with special needs even more crucial members of their child's education team. Parents can now work with educators to develop a plan—the individualized education plan (IEP)—to help kids succeed in school. The IEP describes the goals the team sets for a child during the school year, as well as any special support needed to help achieve them.

## *Who needs an IEP?*

A child who has difficulty learning and functioning and has been identified as a special needs student is the perfect candidate for an IEP. Kids struggling in school may qualify for support services, allowing them to be taught in a special way, for reasons such as:

- learning disabilities,
- attention deficit hyperactivity disorder (ADHD),
- emotional disorders,
- mental retardation,
- autism,
- hearing impairment,

403

- visual impairment,
- speech or language impairment,
- developmental delay.

### *How are services delivered?*

In most cases, the services and goals outlined in an IEP can be provided in a standard school environment. This can be done in the regular classroom (for example, a reading teacher helping a small group of children who need extra assistance while the other kids in the class work on reading with the regular teacher) or in a special resource room in the regular school. The resource room can serve a group of kids with similar needs who are brought together for help.

However, kids who need intense intervention may be taught in a special school environment. These classes have fewer students per teacher, allowing for more individualized attention. In addition, the teacher usually has specific training in helping kids with special educational needs. The children spend most of their day in a special classroom and join the regular classes for nonacademic activities (like music and gym) or in academic activities in which they don't need extra help.

Because the goal of IDEA is to ensure that each child is educated in the least restrictive environment possible, effort is made to help kids stay in a regular classroom. However, when needs are best met in a special class, then kids might be placed in one.

## The Referral and Evaluation Process

The referral process generally begins when a teacher, parent, or doctor is concerned that a child may be having trouble in the classroom, and the teacher notifies the school counselor or psychologist. The first step is to gather specific data regarding the student's progress or academic problems.

This may be done through:

- a conference with parents,
- a conference with the student,
- observation of the student,
- analysis of the student's performance (attention, behavior, work completion, tests, classwork, homework, and so forth).

This information helps school personnel determine the next step. At this point, strategies specific to the student could be used to help the child become more successful in school. If this doesn't work, the child would be tested for a specific learning disability or other impairment to help determine qualification for special services. It's important to note, though, that the presence of a disability doesn't automatically guarantee a child will receive services. To be eligible, the disability must affect functioning at school.

To determine eligibility, a multidisciplinary team of professionals will evaluate the child based on their observations; the child's performance on standardized tests; and daily work such as tests, quizzes, classwork, and homework.

### Who's on the team?

The professionals on the evaluation team can include: a psychologist, a physical therapist, an occupational therapist, a speech therapist, a special educator, a vision or hearing specialist, and others, depending on the child's specific needs.

As a parent, you can decide whether to have your child assessed. If you choose to do so, you'll be asked to sign a permission form that will detail who is involved in the process and the types of tests they use. These tests might include measures of specific school skills, such as reading or math, as well as more general developmental skills such as speech and language. Testing does not necessarily mean that a child will receive services.

Once the team members complete their individual assessments, they develop a comprehensive evaluation report (CER) that compiles their findings, offers an educational classification, and outlines the skills and support the child will need. The parents then have a chance to review the report before the IEP is developed. Some parents will disagree with the report, but they will have the opportunity to work together with the school to come up with a plan that best meets the child's needs.

### Developing an IEP

The next step is an IEP meeting at which the team and parents decide what will go into the plan. In addition to the evaluation team, a regular teacher should be present to offer suggestions about how the plan can help the child's progress in the standard education curriculum.

At the meeting, the team will discuss your child's educational needs—as described in the CER—and come up with specific, measurable short-term and annual goals for each of those needs. If you attend this meeting, you can take an active role in developing the goals and determining which skills or areas will receive the most attention.

The cover page of the IEP outlines the support services your child will receive and how often they will be provided (for example, occupational therapy twice a week). Support services might include special education, speech therapy, occupational or physical therapy, counseling, audiology, medical services, nursing, vision or hearing therapy, and many others.

If the team recommends several services, the amount of time they take in the child's school schedule can seem overwhelming. To ease that load, some services may be provided on a consultative basis. In these cases, the professional consults with the teacher to come up with strategies to help the child but doesn't offer any hands-on instruction. For instance, an occupational therapist may suggest accommodations for a child with fine-motor problems that affect handwriting, and the classroom teacher would incorporate these suggestions into the handwriting lessons taught to the entire class.

Other services can be delivered right in the classroom, so the child's day isn't interrupted by therapy. The child who has difficulty with handwriting might work one on one with an occupational therapist while everyone else practices their handwriting skills. When deciding how and where services are offered, the child's comfort and dignity should be a top priority.

The IEP will be reviewed annually to update the goals and make sure the levels of service meet your child's needs. However, IEPs can be changed at any time on an as-needed basis. If you think your child needs more, fewer, or different services, you can request a meeting and bring the team together to discuss your concerns.

### *Your Legal Rights*

Specific timelines ensure that the development of an IEP moves from referral to providing services as quickly as possible. Be sure to ask about this timeframe and get a copy of your parents' rights when your child is referred. These guidelines (sometimes called procedural safeguards) outline your rights as a parent to control what happens to your child during each step of the process.

The parents' rights also describe how you can proceed if you disagree with any part of the CER or the IEP—mediation and hearings both are options. You can get information about low-cost or free legal representation from the school district or, if your child is in Early Intervention (for kids ages 3–5), through that program. Attorneys and paid advocates familiar with the IEP process will provide representation if you need it. You also may invite anyone who knows or works with your child whose input you feel would be helpful to join the IEP team.

## *A Final Word*

Parents have the right to choose where their kids will be educated. This choice includes public or private elementary schools and secondary schools, including religious schools. It also includes charter schools and home schools.

It is important to understand that the rights of children with disabilities who are placed by their parents in private elementary schools and secondary schools are not the same as those of kids with disabilities who are enrolled in public schools or placed by public agencies in private schools when the public school is unable to provide a free appropriate public education (FAPE).

Two major differences that parents, teachers, other school staff, private school representatives, and the kids need to know about are:

1.  Children with disabilities who are placed by their parents in private schools may not get the same services they would receive in a public school.

2.  Not all kids with disabilities placed by their parents in private schools will receive services.

The IEP process is complex, but it's also an effective way to address how your child learns and functions. If you have concerns, don't hesitate to ask questions about the evaluation findings or the goals recommended by the team. You know your child best and should play a central role in creating a learning plan tailored to your child's specific needs.

For more information, the government has a website to educate anyone about IDEA: http://idea.ed.gov.

Section 37.3

# *Including Children with ASD in Regular Classrooms*

Your classroom is already a diverse place. With the increasing inclusion of students with autism, the challenges associated with managing a classroom will grow. This section outlines a simple and highly flexible six-step plan you and your team can use to prepare for the inclusion of a child with autism in your classroom.

## *Step 1: Educate Yourself*

You must have a working understanding of autism and what that means for your particular student(s). Different behaviors are very much a part of autism. Sometimes children with autism may behave in inappropriate or disruptive ways but their behaviors are more related to their autism than they are deliberate, negative acts. Learning about autism and about how it affects your student specifically is the first step to success.

Your education about autism will evolve as your relationship with the family and the student develops and your knowledge about the disorder and skills in dealing with its impact on the classroom grows. Maintaining an open attitude to learning and working closely with the parents and school team will help you succeed in the long term.

## *Step 2: Reach Out to the Parents*

Parents are your first and best source of information about their child. Step 2 is establishing a working partnership with your student's parents. Ideally, it will begin with meetings before the school year. After that, establishing mutually agreed modes and patterns of communication with the family throughout the school year is critical.

Building trust with the parents is essential. Communication with families about the progress of the student should be ongoing. While the information you exchange may often focus on current classroom challenges, strategies employed, and ideas for alternative solutions, do not forget to include positive feedback on accomplishments and milestones reached.

## Step 3. Prepare the Classroom

There are ways you can accommodate some of the needs of children with autism in your classroom that will enhance their opportunity to learn without sacrificing your plans for the class in general. Of course, there are practical limitations on how much you can modify the physical characteristics of your classroom, but even a few accommodations to support a child with autism may have remarkable results. *The Educator's Guide to Autism* provides a schematic that offers a visual representation of the ideal classroom for a child with autism.

## Step 4: Educate Peers and Promote Social Goals

You must make every effort to promote acceptance of the child with autism as a full member and integral part of the class, even if that student only attends class for a few hours a week. As the teacher of a child with autism, you must create a social environment that encourages positive interactions between the child with autism and his or her typically developing peers throughout the day. Children with autism, by definition, have difficulties in socialization and in understanding language and social cues. But with appropriate assistance, children with autism can engage with peers and establish mutually enjoyable and lasting interpersonal relationships.

Research shows that typically developing peers have more positive attitudes, increased understanding, and greater acceptance of children with autism when provided with clear, accurate, and straightforward information about the disorder. Assuming there are no restrictions on disclosing that your student has autism, educating your class about autism and its effect on their fellow student can be an effective way to increase positive, social interactions between the child with autism and his classroom peers.

Remember that many social interactions occur in settings outside the classroom. Without prior planning and extra help, students with autism may end up isolated during these unstructured times. You may want to create a "circle of friends," a rotating group of responsible, peer buddies for the student with autism, who will not abandon him, serve as a model of appropriate social behavior, and protect against teasing or bullying. This tactic can also be encouraged outside of school.

## Step 5. Collaborate on the Implementation of an Educational Plan

Since your student with autism has special needs beyond academics, his or her educational plan is defined by an individualized education program (IEP). The IEP is a blueprint for everything that will happen to a child in the next school year. As the principal observer and teacher of the child, you play a key role in the development, implementation, and evaluation of the child's IEP. You will be responsible for reporting back to the IEP team on the student's progress toward meeting specific academic, social, and behavioral goals and objectives in the IEP. You will also be asked for input about developing new goals for the student in subsequent IEP meetings.

IEPs are created by a multidisciplinary team of education professionals, along with the child's parents, and are tailored to the needs of the individual student. Special and general education teachers, speech and language therapists, occupational therapists, school psychologists, and families form the IEP team and meet regularly to discuss student progress on IEP goals.

Before the IEP team meets, an assessment team gathers information about the student to make an evaluation and recommendation. Then, one person on the evaluation team coordinates all the information, and the team meets to make recommendations. The IEP team then meets to write the IEP based on the evaluation and team member suggestions.

IEPs always include annual goals, short-term objectives, special education services required by the student, and a yearly evaluation to see if the goals were met. Annual goals must explain measurable behaviors so that it is clear what progress should have been made by the end of the year. The short-term objectives should contain incremental and sequential steps toward meeting each annual goal.

## Step 6. Manage Behavioral Challenges

For students with autism, problem behaviors may be triggered for a variety of reasons. Such behaviors may include temper tantrums, running about the room, loud vocalizations, self-injurious activities, or other disruptive or distracting behaviors. Because children with autism often have difficulties communicating in socially acceptable ways, they may act out when they are confused or fearful about something.

Your first challenge is to decipher the cause, or function, of the particular behavior. Look for patterns in these behaviors such as when they do, or do not, consistently occur. Communicating with families and other team members and observing the behavior in the context in which it occurs is essential to learning the function of the behavior.

It's important to use consistent, positive behavioral reinforcement techniques to promote positive and pro-social behaviors for children with autism. The student's IEP should contain concrete and explicit positive behavioral goals, as well as a wide range of methods for promoting these goals. The student's parents and IEP team may be able to suggest visual recognition techniques and incentive systems that you can use to reinforce positive behaviors.

Teachers may choose to ignore other negative behaviors or give predetermined consequences. The key is to be consistent with how you react to the behaviors over time and to use as many positive strategies to promote pro-social behaviors as possible.

As you follow these steps and learn more about children with differences, you will become a mentor to other educators when they face similar challenges for the first time. Your curiosity will fuel your education about autism; your communication skills will help you create a meaningful alliance with parents. Most of all, your collaboration skills will help you work as a key part of the team that will support the child with autism throughout the course of the school year, and your patience, kindness, and professionalism will make a difference in the lives of all your students.

Section 37.4

# *Individuals with Disabilities Education Act (IDEA) Summary*

From "IDEA 2004 Summary," by the Families and Advocates Partnership for Education (FAPE). © PACER Center Inc. Used with permission from PACER Center Inc., Minneapolis, MN, (952) 838-9000. www.pacer.org. All rights reserved.

This is a summary of some of the most critical changes affecting children with disabilities and their families in the Individuals with Disabilities Education Act (IDEA) 2004, concentrating on the individual education program (IEP) process, due process, and the discipline provisions. How these changes affect our children will depend, at least in part, on how the U.S. Department of Education interprets them through policies and regulations and how they are implemented at the state, district, and school level. Most of these changes were effective as of July 1, 2005.

A new provision in the Act authorizes the Secretary to issue only regulations necessary to secure compliance with the statute. This provision may limit the Secretary's authority to issue regulations that could be useful in clarifying ambiguities. A new section of the Act also suggests that states minimize the number of rules, regulations, and policies to which the school districts are subject.

This law, as amended by the 2004 changes, will not provide mandatory full funding. Although the annual amounts now authorized (permitted) to be spent on IDEA would achieve full funding in six years, that assumes these amounts will actually be appropriated (spent), and explains why mandatory funding of IDEA is so important. In fact, two days after Congress passed the *IDEA Conference Report* with its "glide path to full funding" it appropriated significantly less funding for special education than it had just promised.

## *IEP Process*

1. **Short-term objectives:** The long established obligation for IEP teams to spell out short-term objectives for meeting each child's measurable annual IEP goals no longer exists for

most children. Such short-term objectives are only required for the very small percentage of children (generally less than 1% of students with disabilities) who are taking alternate assessments aligned to alternate achievement standards. The *No Child Left Behind Act* (NCLB) limits participation on these assessments to students with the most significant cognitive disabilities. NCLB also provides that both grade-level and alternate achievement standards should be aligned with state content standards. Parents should ensure that their child's academic IEP goals are also aligned with these standards. Short-term objectives are essential stepping stones toward these goals for all students with disabilities, not just a very small percentage. In states that offer alternate assessments aligned to alternate achievement standards, it is the IEP team that determines whether a child fits the criteria for students with the most significant cognitive disabilities. Parents, as members of the IEP team, may feel pressure to agree that their child fits these criteria in order to retain short-term objectives. Such pressure directly undermines the accountability provisions of NCLB. Even if these short-term objectives are not mandated by law, all parents can still request their child's IEP team to identify them. IDEA 2004 still requires a description of how progress toward meeting goals will be measured and parents can contend that short-term objectives are the answer. Without short-term objectives, parents will have virtually no way of measuring whether their children are making progress in achieving their annual goals and will not be informed participants in their child's education. In addition, teachers will not have a guide as to the intervening steps that should be taken towards achieving these goals and when they should be taken. Teachers will also have great difficulty developing meaningful progress reports to the parents.

2. **IEP progress reports:** The progress the child is making toward meeting the annual goals must be reported, but there is no longer a reference to "the extent to which the progress is sufficient to attain the goal by the end of the year." This information seems especially important to parents and teachers if there is a shared commitment to help all children learn to high standards set for all. Parents may see progress all year only to realize in June that the progress was not sufficient to meet the goal.

3. **Transition information in IEP:** The amendments clarify that the transition process for a student with a disability now begins at age 16 and is not merely a plan for transition. Parents should request that the student's IEP, when appropriate, include a statement of inter-agency responsibilities and any needed linkages since this language is no longer in the statute.

4. **IEP attendance and participation:** A new section allows IEP team members to be excused from attendance if their area is not being discussed. When this section is read with new provisions allowing alternate means of meeting participation (such as conference calls), consolidation of reevaluation meetings and other IEP meetings, and a pilot program authorizing up to 15 states to use multi-year IEPs, the combined effect is a revolution in the traditional IEP meeting. Some say these are positive changes. Others are concerned that these provisions will limit cross fertilization of ideas and undermine the interdisciplinary nature of IEP meetings (team members each bring areas or disciplines of expertise to the table). While written parental consent is required before these actions can occur, parents may find that they are under considerable pressure to provide their consent. At least once a year, the parents should be able to get all the members of their child's team in one room, all sharing ideas for the benefit of the child. The potential richness of these conversations cannot be anticipated in written reports submitted by excused members and conference calls do not allow for the same flow of ideas. You never know which IEP team member will turn the tide of a meeting.

5. **Pilot program for multi-year IEPs:** The Secretary of Education is authorized to approve proposals from up to 15 states to allow local school districts to offer, with parental consent, a multi-year IEP, not to exceed three years. This option will limit parent participation in their child's education by not having a comprehensive annual IEP review, except in certain situations. Also, three-year IEPs will contain multi-year goals which can be expected to be less specific and harder to measure than annual goals—especially when benchmarks and short-term objectives are no longer required for all but those students with the most significant cognitive disabilities. Another serious problem is that the required elements under IDEA for these multi-year IEPs are not as inclusive as for annual IEPs. This is true with respect to statements on progress reports, accommodations,

supplementary aids and services, and more. While, the states may include these as required elements in the multi-year IEPs, IDEA does not mandate that they do so. Parents in these states will have to consent to the three-year IEPs that must be reviewed at natural transition points by the IEP team. Therefore, it will be critical that parents are informed, knowledgeable, and well prepared to deal with any pressure that may be put on them.

6. **Pilot program for paperwork reduction:** The Secretary of Education is authorized to grant waivers of statutory and regulatory requirements, for a period not to exceed four years, to 15 states proposing to reduce excessive paperwork and non-instructional time burdens. The Secretary is prohibited from waiving requirements related to civil rights or the right of a child to a free appropriate public education (FAPE). How this process is implemented is a matter of special concern to parents, who worry that many requirements in the IEP process which parents consider to be related to civil rights and FAPE may be seen as contributors to the paperwork burden. Another significant concern is that "pilot" implies that this is the first step toward expanding these programs beyond the 15 states.

7. **IEP team transition:** Parents of a child transitioning from part C services (early childhood) to part B services (school-age) can request an invitation to the initial IEP meeting be sent to representatives of the part C system to assist with a smooth transition of services. This provision doesn't require a part C representative to attend, but it does encourage collaboration.

8. **Transfers between school districts:** Services comparable to those described in the IEP in effect before a child's transfer must be provided by the new school district. These services must continue until the previous IEP is adopted, or a new IEP is developed, adopted, and implemented in the case of a transfer in the same state, or until a new IEP is developed in the case of a transfer outside the state. This new provision will help parents of transferring students know what they can expect from their new schools.

## Due Process

1. **Procedural safeguards notice:** The procedural safeguards notice will be distributed only once a year except that a copy will be distributed upon initial referral, when a parent makes

a request for an evaluation, when a due process complaint has been filed, or if a parent requests a copy. The notice will no longer be automatically distributed with the IEP team notice or upon reevaluation. This is only a problem if parents are unaware of their rights including the right to request this notice if they need one.

2. **Statute of limitations:** Parents now have two years in which to exercise their due process rights after they knew or should have known that an IDEA violation has occurred. The interpretation of the language "should have known" will be critical.

3. **Due process complaint notice:** Parents who feel their child's educational rights are being compromised must file a complaint with the school district (with a copy to the state) identifying the name and contact information of the child, describing the nature of the problem with supporting facts, and a proposed resolution. A new provision provides that the school district shall file a response within ten days unless the district within 15 days notifies the state hearing officer that it is challenging the sufficiency of the parent's due process complaint notice. The state hearing officer has five more days to make a finding. In addition to the obvious delay, of particular concern is that the complexity of filing for due process may have a chilling effect on parents.

4. **Resolution session:** Parents must go through a mandatory "resolution session" before due process. The school district will convene a meeting with the parents and relevant members of the IEP team within 15 days of when the school district receives the parent's due process complaint. The school district has 30 days from the time the complaint is filed to resolve the complaint to the satisfaction of the parents, after which a due process hearing can occur. This provision may encourage school systems to wait until a due process complaint is filed before trying to resolve issues. Attorney's fees are not reimbursed for work related to the resolution session.

5. **Attorney's fees:** Parent's attorneys may be responsible for paying the school system attorney's fees if a cause of action in a due process hearing or court action is determined to be frivolous, unreasonable, or without foundation. Parents may be responsible for the school system's attorney fees if a cause of action was presented for any improper purpose, such as to harass or to cause unnecessary delay or needless increase in the cost of litigation.

Obviously, parents should not file frivolous or improper causes of action, but it is important that school districts not use these changes in the law to intimidate parents. This could have a chilling effect on parents obtaining legal representation and filing valid complaints to improve their children's education.

6. **Qualifications for hearing officers:** A positive change is that there are now explicit qualification requirements for hearing officers.

## Discipline

1. **Stay put:** The right of a student with a disability to "stay put" in his/her current educational placement pending an appeal is eliminated for alleged violations of the school code that may result in a removal from the student's current educational placement for more than ten days. Previously the law only denied "stay-put" rights to students with disabilities involved in drugs, weapons, or other dangerous behavior or activity. The right to "stay put" while a parent challenges the manifestation determination or proposed placement is a critical element to ensuring a student's continued free appropriate public education in the least restrictive environment. Moving back and forth between the current placement and an interim alternative educational setting during an appeal can have a significant negative impact on achievement for children who already have difficulty adjusting to transitions. Parents must remain vigilant and ensure that their children continue to be provided the educational programming and services they need to make progress toward meeting their IEP goals. If this progress is negatively affected, the school may recommend a change to a more restrictive setting for the future. In addition, for purposes of reporting adequate yearly progress (AYP) under the *No Child Left Behind Act*, individual schools do not have to count children who are transferred to alternative settings and are, therefore, not in the same school for the full academic year. This could create an incentive for disciplinary actions against students with disabilities.

2. **Services to be received in interim alternative educational setting:** A child is entitled to receive programming and services necessary to enable him or her to receive a free appropriate public education consistent with section 612(a)(1) during the period in which he/she is in an interim alternative

417

education setting. Under IDEA 2004, the student must be provided services to enable him or her to continue to participate in the general education curriculum and to progress toward meeting the goals in the IEP. The new provision replaced language requiring that a child in an interim alternative educational setting receive services and modifications, including those described in the student's current IEP which will enable the child to meet the goals in the IEP. The change in language cannot be interpreted as diluting any of these services that are consistent with the definition of FAPE because a student with a disability must continue to receive FAPE during the period of removal from his/her current educational placement.

3. **Manifestation determination review:** Before IDEA 2004, the burden was on the school district to show that the behavior resulting in a disciplinary action was not a manifestation of the child's disability before being allowed to apply the same disciplinary procedures as they use for non-disabled children. The burden of proof for the manifestation determination review has now been shifted to the parents who have to prove that the behavior was caused by or had a direct and substantial relationship to the disability. The language requiring the IEP team to consider whether the disability impaired the child's ability to control or to understand the impact and consequences of the behavior has been deleted. The language that gave the school an incentive to address behavior appropriately by requiring the IEP team to consider whether the IEP was appropriate has also been deleted. Because the amendments to IDEA make it easier for schools to remove children for non-dangerous, non-weapon, non-drug related behaviors, and place the burden on parents to prove the connection between behavior and disability, parents will need to pay careful attention to the behavioral needs of their child in developing the IEP. Even if the child has not previously been subjected to disciplinary exclusion, parents may need to anticipate, to consider and spell out any concerns they may have about their child's possible emotional and behavioral responses particularly when they are not provided the supports and services they may need.

4. **Special circumstances:** Since 1997, IDEA had expressly authorized schools to unilaterally remove children to an interim alternative educational setting for as long as 45 days for offenses involving drugs and weapons—even if the behavior was

a manifestation of the student's disability. In addition, a hearing officer could make the same decision if it was determined based on a preponderance of the evidence that keeping the child in his/her current placement was substantially likely to result in injury to the child or others. Although school authorities have always had the authority to respond to an emergency and to unilaterally remove any student with or without a disability who is causing serious bodily injury to another, now schools can also unilaterally remove children for 45 days for "inflicting serious bodily injury." This term is defined as involving a substantial risk of death; extreme physical pain; protracted and obvious disfigurement; or protracted loss or impairment of the function of a bodily member, organ, or mental faculty. The hearing officer in determining whether to remove a child because maintaining his/her current placement is substantially likely to result in injury to self or others is no longer required to consider whether the school district's proposed change in placement is based on a preponderance of the evidence. In addition, the amended statute no longer requires the hearing officer to consider whether the school has made reasonable efforts to minimize the risk of harm, including the use of supplementary aids and services. These changes, to the degree they have the effect of punishing the child even if proper supports could have prevented the problem, arguably violate Section 504 of the Rehabilitation Act.

5. **Forty-five day limit:** The 45 calendar day limit on the removal for these offenses has been changed to 45 school days, which is significantly longer (now nine instead of six weeks of school at a critical time when students with disabilities are being held accountable for meeting high state standards.)

6. **Functional behavioral assessments:** The requirement for functional behavioral assessments and behavioral intervention plans are maintained in the discipline provisions

7. **Case-by-case determination:** A paragraph has been added to the discipline provisions, which states that school personnel can consider any unique circumstances on a case-by-case basis when determining whether to change the placement of a child with a disability who violates a school code of conduct. This is a good provision for parents to quote when they are having trouble proving that their child's behavior is a manifestation of the disability. It serves to remind the school personnel that common sense should prevail and all circumstances should be considered.

419

Chapter 38

# Tips for Teaching Students with ASD

## Chapter Contents

## Section 38.1

# *Instructional Approaches to Teaching Students with ASD*

This section begins with "Creating successful educational experiences improves motivation and learning," by Patrick F. Heick, PhD, BCBA. © 2010 May Institute (www.mayinstitute.org). Reprinted with permission. It continues with "What is generalization and why is it important for individuals with autism and other special needs?" by Teka J. Harris, MA, BCBA. © 2010 May Institute (www.mayinstitute.org). Reprinted with permission.

## *Creating Successful Educational Experiences Improves Motivation and Learning*

Educators often encounter students who become frustrated when asked to do challenging academic work. In some situations, this frustration may be the result of the mismatch between the student's skill level and the difficulty level of the assigned task. As a consequence, these students are likely to shut down and refuse to continue with an assignment. Unfortunately, teachers may unintentionally reinforce this escape behavior by allowing noncompliance, thereby ensuring it will occur again in similar situations.

Similarly, parents are likely to experience times when their children refuse to cooperate with a request to participate in an activity. Children who are successful in avoiding undesirable tasks—whether completing a chore or finishing homework—are likely to try these escape tactics again.

### *What can teachers and parents do to get children to cooperate?*

One potential solution involves a strategy called behavioral momentum. Researchers in the fields of psychology and education have shown that, in order to increase the likelihood that children will follow instructions they normally do not follow, it is often effective to give instructions they are likely to follow first, and then praise them when they comply. Then, immediately after offering praise, present instructions they are less likely to follow. This strategy greatly increases the likelihood of compliance.

According to this strategy, children who are unwilling to take out the trash but are willing to walk the dog would be more likely to take out the trash if they were asked to do so immediately after being praised for walking the dog. Likewise, students who are rewarded for completing simple math equations are more likely to comply when asked to attempt harder problems.

Another powerful and easy-to-implement strategy to help students learn new, fact-based information is called folding-in. This strategy, similar to using flash cards, attempts to build momentum and success by carefully interspersing known information with unknown information. Researchers have shown that learning is enhanced when new information is taught using a 30/70 ratio of unknown material to known material. With this method, students learning new material feel successful because they have mastered much of the material, and are never asked to learn more than 30% of what is presented.

This strategy can be used to successfully teach students of all ages different kinds of fact-based information—everything from letter and word recognition to chemical equations. The trick to this technique is frequent repetition of unknown and known information at the 30/70 ratio to ensure ongoing success and, subsequently, to promote a willingness to continue the learning process. Because successful implementation of this strategy ultimately leads to increased information known (and less unknown), teachers and parents need to continually monitor the process, adding more unknown information as necessary.

Teachers and parents may also want to reconsider the traditional flash card method of only drilling students with stacks of unknown information. When your student or child sits down to learn new words, math facts, or other information, remember to keep a healthy amount of known information in the mix to encourage ongoing effort with occasional success.

It is important to remember that motivation and learning are influenced by the success learners have with instructional demands. Setting up frequent opportunities for success and reinforcing children's efforts make it more likely that they will engage in more challenging tasks in the future.

## Generalization

### *What is generalization and why is it important for individuals with autism and other special needs?*

Generalization is the ability to complete a task, perform an activity, or display a behavior across settings with different people and at different times. The reason we are able to complete everyday tasks in a variety of situations and settings is that we have generalized the skills involved.

For example, most of us turn on lights, fasten jackets, and open doors without much thought or effort. These are tasks we can complete in a variety of ways. We might turn on a light by flipping a switch, pushing a button, or pulling a string. We can fasten our jackets with zippers, buttons, clasps, or Velcro. When we learned to do these things, we learned to manipulate a variety of materials to achieve the same result. We also learned to manipulate these materials in different settings. For example, opening the front door of your own home is very similar to opening the front door of someone else's home, a car door, or the door of the nearest fast food restaurant.

Generalization is a major goal for behavior analysts who work with individuals with special needs. It is important because it increases the likelihood that the learner will be successful at completing a task independently and not have to rely on the assistance of a certain teacher or materials only found in one teaching setting.

The importance of the generalization of skills is often overlooked. When someone learns new skills and behaviors, the expectation is that he or she will automatically generalize them. However, educators and analysts who work with children and adults with learning deficits and other challenges must not only teach new skills, but also employ additional strategies to increase the likelihood that their students will be able to generalize those skills.

Teachers and analysts should use a variety of materials during training sessions. For instance, when teaching an adult to operate a washing machine, it is a good idea to give him or her opportunities not only to operate the washing machine at home, but also at different locations such as at someone else's house or at a laundromat. He or she should learn to operate a microwave that requires the turn of a dial, as well as one requiring the push of a button.

Another consideration for teaching generalization is the format of the training session. Initially, teaching sessions should be very controlled and structured. Once the student has mastered the skill, however, generalization can become the goal, and the training sessions can become looser. This might mean varying the duration of the sessions, scheduling the sessions at different times of day, using different teachers, and changing the wording of the instructions given.

A reward schedule is also crucial when teaching generalization. It is always important to reward correct responses, especially when teaching a new skill or behavior. But after a skill or behavior has been learned, the frequency at which rewards are given can be decreased. A teacher might initially give a child learning sign language access to a preferred item, such as an edible treat or a small toy, each time he or she demonstrates a sign correctly. However, once he or she has learned the signs, the reward might be given only after he or she demonstrates two or three consecutive signs correctly.

As a clinician working with adults with special needs, I frequently encounter situations in which generalization is a necessity. We sometimes need to replace the appliances in our community-based group homes, and the residents must learn to operate new ones. There are also times when a substitute teacher is present or when the training session must be postponed or shortened due to unexpected events.

Teaching generalization skills to children and adults with special needs ensures their success despite changing circumstances. It provides these individuals with more ways to achieve desired outcomes and more opportunities to be successful in many different settings, thereby increasing their independence and self-confidence.

## Section 38.2

# *Teaching High-Functioning Students with ASD*

Note: In this section, the three terms, autism, Asperger syndrome, and other pervasive developmental disorders, will be referenced as AS, or the spectrum.

**Talents:** Many students on the spectrum demonstrate exceptional abilities in a vast array of skills and talents. These can include but are not limited to the following:

- Exceptional memory
- Mathematical skills
- Calendar projections
- Computers
- Music
- Exceptionally early and advanced reading skills (hyperlexia)
- Poetry
- Writing stories and general writing skills
- Spelling, punctuation, and grammar
- Imitations of people or animals
- Painting, sculpture, and other forms of visual arts
- Chemistry
- Physics

Sometimes the interests and/or talents of the individual may become quite specific and somewhat obsessive. Some examples are: cats, dogs, whales, llamas and other animals or plants; history (especially a certain period in history); 1950s stop lights; 1940s airplanes; a subway system in a particular city; maps; cattle branding squeeze machines; Thomas the Tank Engine; The Little Mermaid; Lego toys; dinosaurs; and sports.

Other students may not evidence exceptional skills in easily observed skills. Many are highly skilled in some areas and poorly skilled in others. Another group may have areas of exceptional skill they cannot or do not display to an instructor. Whenever these talents or interests seem obsessive, use them to widen the students learning adventures into other subjects.

Before teaching communication skills to individuals on the spectrum, be sure that your abilities to communicate with them on their terms are properly developed. If you want them to speak and communicate and behave in neuro-typical ways, be sure you give your best effort to understand their communication and behavior and keep that in mind when interacting with them. This does not mean, for example, that you should flap when they flap. Rather you should try to understand what causes them to flap or what feeling the flapping expresses—joy, excitement, frustration, boredom. If they repeat phrases, are they expressing concern, frustration, confusion, or an attempt at humor? When you communicate with them, speak normally, but do not use more words than necessary. Be clear. Emphasize what is most important in what you are saying.

While these considerations are meant to facilitate your interactions and successes with the AS student, all students are unique individuals. Each will have varying sets of talents and challenges.

## Areas of Challenge

1. Many people with AS have trouble with organizational skills, regardless of their intelligence or age. Even a straight "A" student with autism who has a photographic memory can be incapable of remembering to bring a pencil to class or of remembering a deadline for an assignment. In such cases, aid should be provided in the least restrictive way possible. Strategies could include having the student put a picture of a pencil on the cover of his notebook or reminders at the end of the day of assignments to be completed at home. Always praise the student when he remembers something he has previously forgotten. Never make disparaging comments or harp at him when he fails. A lecture on the subject will not help, and it will often make the problem worse. S/he may begin to believe he

427

cannot remember to do or bring these things. Two practical suggestions to help a student stay organized: Have him keep an agenda/day planner where s/he writes all daily homework assignments. (The teachers/assistants can also use this book to write short notes home.) Have him keep all of his loose papers in a trapper notebook or an accordion file with separated compartments (labeled for each class, a section for papers to come home, papers to return to school and blank paper, and so forth) so all papers can been seen organized one place.

2. Students on the spectrum are either hyper-organized or seem to have few or any organizational skills. A large number of students with AS seem to have either the neatest or the messiest desks or lockers in the school. The one with the neatest desk or locker is probably very insistent on sameness and may be very upset if someone disturbs the order he has created. This student is already highly organized—if not in the system you prefer, please respect that the student's organizational system is in his or her terms. The one with the messiest desk will need your help in frequent cleanups of the desk or locker so that he can find things. Simply remember that s/he is not making a conscious choice to be messy, s/he is most likely incapable of this organizational task without specific training. Train him or her in organizational skills using small, specific steps.

3. People on the spectrum can have problems with abstract and conceptual thinking. Some may eventually acquire a few or even many abstract skills, but others never will. Avoid abstract ideas when possible. When abstract concepts must be used, use visual cues, such as gestures, or written words to augment the abstract idea.

4. Many individuals on the spectrum show tremendous creativity and talent in such creative fields as music and art. While some may demonstrate a somewhat repetitive creativity, it is still uniquely generated by them and their intellect. Reading the profound poetry and experiencing the astounding artwork of many individuals on the spectrum—not to mention the incredible singing and acting talents of others—will convince you of their creative abilities. This does not indicate their capabilities in other academic or social areas, nor skills of daily living.

5. An increase in unusual or difficult behaviors probably indicates an increase in stress. Sometimes stress is caused by

feeling a loss of control. When this occurs, establishing a safe place or safe person may come in handy, because many times the stress will only be alleviated when the student physically removes himself from the stressful event or situation. If this occurs, a program should be set up to assist the student in re-entering and/or staying in the stressful situation.

6.  Do not take misbehaviors personally. The person with AS is not a manipulative, scheming person who is trying to make life difficult for you. Usually misbehavior is the result of efforts to survive experiences which may be confusing, disorienting, or frightening. People with AS are, by virtue of their handicap, egocentric and have extreme difficulty reading the reactions of others. Although they may use odd means to try to change their environment to make it tolerable, they are incapable of being manipulative.

7.  Most people on the spectrum use and interpret speech literally. Until you know the capabilities of the individual, you should avoid:

    -   idioms (save your breath, jump the gun, second thoughts, and so forth);

    -   double meanings (most jokes have double meanings);

    -   sarcasm, such as saying, "Great!" after he has just spilled a bottle of ketchup on the table;

    -   nicknames;

    -   cute names such as pal, buddy, wise guy, and so forth.

8.  Be as concrete as possible in all your interactions with these students. Remember that facial expression and other social cues may not work. Avoid asking questions such as, "Why did you do that?" Instead, say, "I didn't like the way you slammed your book on the desk when I said it was time for gym. Please put your book down on the desk quietly and get up to leave for gym." In answering essay questions that require a synthesis of information, AS individuals rarely know when they have said enough, or if they are properly addressing the core of the question.

9.  If the student does not seem to be able to learn a task, break it down into smaller steps, or present the task in several different ways (for example, visually, verbally, physically).

10. Avoid verbal overload. Be clear. Use shorter sentences if you perceive that the student is not fully understanding you. Although s/he probably has no hearing problem and may be paying attention, s/he may have a problem understanding your main point and identifying the important information.

11. Prepare the student for all environmental and/or routine changes, such as assembly, substitute teacher, rescheduling, and so forth. Use his written or verbal schedule to prepare him for change.

12. Positive behavioral supports can work, but if it is inflexibly used, it can encourage robot-like behavior, provide only a short-term behavior change, or result in more aggression. Use positive and chronologically age-appropriate behavior procedures.

13. Consistent treatment and expectations from everyone is vital.

14. Be aware that normal levels of auditory and visual input can be perceived by the student as too much or too little. For example, the hum of fluorescent lighting is extremely distracting for some people with AS. Consider environmental changes such as removing some of the visual clutter from the room or seating changes if the student seems distracted or upset by his classroom environment. Perhaps a seat in the front row would work, as this limits his vision of some of the visual clutter.

15. The overload and under-stimulation problems may occur in other senses, including tactile and olfactory stimuli. Avoid wearing strong perfumes and the touching of hands, and so forth, unless you know the student is not challenged by this.

16. If the student is not looking directly at you, do not assume s/he is not listening or is daydreaming. Some students on the spectrum have more reliable peripheral than frontal vision. When you speak, they tend to look at your mouth rather than your eyes. Your mouth is where the sound comes from. They seldom understand any communication you may want to give them with your eyes.

17. If your student on the spectrum uses repetitive verbal arguments and/or repetitive verbal questions, try requesting that he write down the question or argumentative statement. Then write down your reply. As the writing continues, the person with autism usually begins to calm down and stop

the repetitive activity. If that does not work, write down his repetitive verbal question or argument, and then ask him to formulate and write down a logical reply, or a reply he thinks you would make. This distracts him from the escalating verbal aspect of the argument or question and sometimes gives him a more socially acceptable way of expressing his frustration or anxiety. If the student does not read or write, try role playing the repetitive verbal question or argument, with you taking their part and them answering you. Continually responding in a logical manner or arguing back seldom stops this behavior. The subject of their argument or question is not always the subject that has upset them. The argument or question more often communicates a feeling of loss of control or uncertainty about someone or something in the environment. Individuals with autism often have trouble getting your points. If the repetitive verbal argument or question persists, consider the possibility that s/he is very concerned about the topic and does not know how to rephrase the question or comment to get the information s/he needs.

18.    In an effort to connect with your conversation, a student on the spectrum may seemingly go off on a tangent, talking about a topic that seems to have no connection to the classroom discussion. Because of his difficulty in generalizing information and concepts, he has perhaps focused on a single word or concept that was used in the discussion and began to talk about that word or concept in the context that he has experienced it before. (For example, in a discussion of Bowling Green, Kentucky, a student may start talking about his bowling scores, or an experience at the bowling alley.) Since it could be very difficult to discern what that past context could have been, simply redirect the student to the current discussion. Do not assume he is just daydreaming.

19.    Since these individuals experience various communication difficulties, do not rely on the student with AS to relay important messages to their parents about school events, assignments, school rules, and so forth unless you try it on an experimental basis with follow-up, or unless you are already certain that the student has mastered this skill. Even sending home a note for his parent may not work. The student may not remember to deliver the note or may lose it before reaching home. Phone calls or e-mails to the parent work best

until this skill can be developed. Frequent and accurate communication between the teacher and parent (or primary caregiver) is very important.

20.  If your class involves pairing off or choosing partners, either draw numbers or use some other arbitrary means of pairing. Or, ask an especially kind student if he or she would agree to choose the individual on the spectrum as a partner. This should be arranged before the pairing is done. The student with AS is most often the one left with no partner. This is unfortunate, as these students could benefit most from having a partner.

21.  Be aware that students with spectrum challenges are very socially naïve. This makes them perfect targets for bullying. Make sure that your school uses or establishes effective policies on bullying (zero tolerance) and uses active bullying prevention plans.

22.  Do not limit your expectations for the future of any student. Individuals with AS can and have achieved things far above the expectations of family, friends, and teachers. Just be aware that their struggles to achieve even the smallest goals may be far greater than you may assume.

# Chapter 39

# *Managing Challenging ASD Behavior*

## *Chapter Contents*

## Section 39.1

# *What to Do when Positive Reinforcement Is Not Working*

"What to do when positive reinforcement isn't working," by Patrick F. Heick, PhD, BCBA. © 2010 May Institute (www.mayinstitute.org). Reprinted with permission.

As an educator and clinician, I frequently encounter staff, parents, and teachers who use a variety of activities or items to reward or motivate their clients, children, or students. This strategy, termed positive reinforcement, can be very effective in supporting children and adults with autism spectrum disorders or other special needs to learn new skills. It can also help them maintain a desired level of performance of a skill they have already learned.

Positive reinforcement refers to the process of providing a reward to strengthen a particular behavior. The theory is that the rewards, often labeled reinforcers, increase the probability of a desired behavior being repeated in the future.

It is not unusual, however, that a potential reward or incentive does not appear to be initially reinforcing or loses its effectiveness over time. For example, a child may lose interest in receiving the same stickers for accuracy on math problems, and his performance may decline. If this is the case, there are several factors to consider.

First, notice the time between the occurrence of a particular behavior and the reward that follows. For a reward to be most effective, it should be delivered immediately following the behavior. The longer the delay between the behavior and the receipt of the reward, the less likely it will be effective.

It is also important to make sure that receiving the reward is based on demonstrating a particular behavior. This helps the individual learn that behaving in a certain way means that he or she will receive the desired reward. The reward should only be presented after the behavior occurs. If the reward is available independent of the behavior, or is presented inconsistently when first leaning a new skill, the behavior is less likely to be reinforced or strengthened.

Keep in mind that a reward can lose its effectiveness if it is over-used. This is relatively common and can be avoided by having a selection of desirable rewards available and making sure that the rewards are still desirable to the individual. As is the case with all of us, preferences change over time, and certain items that were once highly desirable may become unwanted or may even cause a negative response.

Lastly, staff, teachers, and parents should understand that their clients, students, and children all have different preferences. Items or activities that are highly desirable to some individuals may not be at all desirable to others. Therefore, expect differences in what is considered rewarding among different individuals, as well as over time.

Using positive reinforcement effectively allows staff, parents, and teachers to help individuals of all ages and abilities learn and maintain appropriate and adaptive behavior. As a result, these individuals will experience more success with the tasks they undertake and more satisfaction in their day-to-day interactions with other people.

Section 39.2

# *Practical Strategies for Responding to Challenging Behaviors*

Excerpted from "Challenging Behavior and Autism; A Guide for Transportation Personnel," © 2007 Jocelyn Taylor, MS, CCC, SLP. Reprinted with permission.

Editor's Note: While this information is specific to helping children with autism when they react with challenging behavior on a bus, the considerations, suggestions, and interventions may be helpful in a variety of situations.

Challenging behavior on the bus is common in children with autism. Once these challenging behaviors become established, they can be resistant to change. Some methods that work for influencing the behavior of other children may not be effective in the autism population. However, interventions that consider unique cognitive styles, communication styles, and sensory needs have been shown to be helpful. In other words, understanding the child's characteristics and then using the correct strategies to calm and comfort the student with autism can make a large difference in behaviors on the school bus.

### *Why do children with autism have difficulties riding the school bus?*

The core impairments that underlie autism may affect your student's behavior on the school bus. Understanding the link between the core impairment and behavior will help you to find practical strategies that deal with specific issues.

### *Response to Tantrums*

When behavior affects school bus safety, intervention is needed. If transportation personnel are dealing with temper tantrums on the school bus on a frequent basis, the student's education team should meet to determine what is triggering the tantrum and how to remove or avoid the triggers. As a general rule, strategies that are used in

**Table 39.1.** Core Impairment: Social Interaction and Relating to Others

| Core Impairment<br>The difficulty with... | Behavior<br>May result in... |
| --- | --- |
| Enjoying contact with people | Becoming stressed and upset on the school bus when physical contact occurs<br>Reducing motivation to ride the bus<br>Not following directions in order to please the driver or the attendant |
| The ability to understand how people feel | Appearing insensitive or causing offence<br>Not knowing how to react to others<br>Not understanding that other students may need a quiet bus ride |
| Understanding people's reactions | Being confused about the intention of the school bus attendant<br>Being confused about the message behind people's words<br>Understanding that other students may become frightened by tantrums or outbursts |
| Social situations | Confusion about how to board the bus<br>Confusion about emergency situations<br>Not knowing how to stay in the seat belt<br>Passing the time on the bus in inappropriate ways |

**Table 39.2.** Core Impairment: Communication

| Core Impairment<br>The difficulty with... | Behavior<br>May result in... |
| --- | --- |
| Expressing needs | Not being able to tell the bus attendant what is wanted<br>Not knowing how or when to ask for help<br>Expressing fear or worry in inappropriate ways<br>Not letting the adult know that the student does not understand what is expected |
| Understanding what people say | Non-compliance to school bus rules<br>Fear of a change in routine<br>Confusion in general<br>Not understanding what people want<br>Not understanding why a request was made |
| Interpreting people's body language | Not understanding when the transportation aide is joking or is serious<br>Not recognizing a threat from another student<br>Not recognizing when adults are reaching the end of their rope |

the classroom should be used on the school bus. Once the student's explosion is in full force, you want to use a short-term strategy that is effective and causes no harm. You want to do the following:

**Keep the damage to a minimum:** Make the environment as safe as possible. If feasible, move objects that could be thrown. Watch for structures against which the student could hurt himself. Get others out of harm's way, clear the area (this also may reduce the chance that the tantrum may be rewarded by the reaction and attention of others). Establish at what point the driver needs to stop.

**Get help:** Help from untrained personnel may make the situation worse, so discuss how you plan to handle the situation. Establish and get agreement on who is going to make decisions and be in charge during the incident. Have an emergency plan with input from the school and parents.

**Table 39.3.** Core Impairment: Flexibility of Thinking and Behavior

| Core Impairment The difficulty with... | Behavior May result in... |
|---|---|
| Sensory processing | Intolerance when the bus gets too noisy, hot, or bumpy Intolerance for loud instructions from the school bus attendant Intolerance for a restraint system Intolerance for vinyl seats, smells, or sun streaming in the window |
| Routine changes | The student becoming upset • When the bus is late or has to take an alternate route • When an alternate bus is used (the number on the bus is different or the seats are not the usual color) • When a substitute driver or attendant is present • During an evacuation drill • During an emergency that changes the normal routine • Going on a field trip |
| Having repetitive patterns of play | Needing to hold or play with a comforting item during the bus ride Needing to sit in the same seat every day |
| Having rituals and obsessions | The student getting upset if someone is in his seat Needing to sit near a particular bus-mate Needing the transportation staff to use the same greeting each day |
| Imagination | Not predicting the consequences of refusing to click the seat belt or following directions Not predicting the reaction of others |

**Use a low-key response:** If there is no immediate danger, the adults should stay out of the way—keep your distance. At this point, unless you have been made aware of calming strategies by the parents or the school that work for the student, doing nothing is the best choice.

**Intervene physically:** There are legal and ethical restrictions on adults in the transportation system. It is important to act in accordance with the school's policy and stated behavior plan. These general guidelines are good considerations:

- Do not intervene physically unless there is immediate danger or risk of injury to the student, you, or other students.

- Contain the situation using other methods before reverting to physical intervening.

- The purpose of physical intervention is to ensure physical safety not to punish or cause pain. Physical punishment is against the law and can cause psychological harm to the student.

- The amount of physical force should be in reasonable proportion to the risk of danger.

- Attempt to calm the child, either with known strategies for that child or by giving the child distance, before using physical force.

- Allow the child time to gain control.

**Allow the student to recover:** Things may take a while to get back to normal. The child is susceptible to another explosion if not given the chance to calm to a level of control. During the recovery phase, do the following:

- Give the student space, don't move in too quickly. This will allow you to calm down as well.

- After an explosive tantrum, the child will remain anxious. Part of getting back to normal includes putting small amounts of structure in place and rebuilding relationships. Find behaviors for which you can praise the student.

- Reintroduce demands slowing and calmly. You don't want to trigger another tantrum but if you don't reintroduce demands, then the student's tantrum worked. Before reintroducing demands again, wait until the student has calmed down. Scale down your demand and allow some kind of compromise. Make it easy for the student to go along with your request by increasing praise.

- Talk it through with the student if the language skills are present. If the student is non-verbal, ask the school for their method of communication. The ideal is to help the student take responsibility for self-control without blaming or triggering another tantrum. Helping the child to see one small thing that he could have done differently may help him to manage himself better in the future.

- Get support. Working with students who have tantrums and other challenging behaviors can be stressful. Do not underestimate your need for emotional support.

## Other Challenging Behaviors such as Aggression and Masturbation

### Prevention

The most effective way to deal with challenging behaviors such as aggression or masturbation is preventing the behavior in the first place. Effective prevention techniques include the following:

- Avoid the settings and triggers that lead to the challenging behavior. For example, seating the student near the front of the bus, keeping his hands busy with motivating activities and having the student wear clothing such as overalls, makes it more difficult for the student to put his hand down his pants.

- Alter settings and triggers by using higher levels of structure, clearer expectations, and advance reminders of rewards for desired behavior.

- Look at the settings where the problem does not occur. For example: Is the student calmer during the first part of the bus ride? Does the student feel more secure around particular adults or holding particular items? Once the successful settings are identified, duplicate those settings as much as possible.

### Teach New Skills and Behavior

Teach a new behavior that can take the place of an undesired behavior. Ask: Instead of screaming, what can the student do? Instead of throwing things, what can the student do? Instead of masturbating, what can the student do? The goal is to find a replacement behavior that is equally motivating. Systematically teaching the student to enjoy the new activity may be necessary. For example, a student was slapping people in order to try to interact with them. Obviously, this was not an effective method of engaging people in a positive manner. The staff was able to turn the slap into a stroke which was much more acceptable and enjoyable.

## When Behaviors Get Serious

- Be sure the student's behavior is not triggered by inadvertent, well-meaning adult practices.

- Do not act independently. Consult with parents and the appropriate persons in your school district.

- Be sure you are following the prescribed behavior plan.

- Have a reasonable bottom line for behavior that creates an unsafe situation—know when to stop the school bus and call for help. Keep in mind that stopping the school bus in an unscheduled manner may make the behavior worse. Plan how to support the student with information about what is happening and why.

Chapter 40

# Social Interaction Education for Students with ASD

## Chapter Contents

## Section 40.1

# *Understanding Special Interests and Social Interactions of Children with ASD*

Excerpted from "Dinosaurs 24/7: Understanding the Special Interests of Children with Asperger's Syndrome," by Mary Ann Winter-Messiers, Maitrise; and Cynthia M. Herr, PhD. Reprinted with permission from the Interactive Autism Network (IAN) Community (www.iancommunity.org), © 2007 Kennedy Krieger Institute.

What do a quirky lawyer, a child lost during a museum field trip, a family who needs a new home, a boy who witnessed the murder of his parents, a doctor who bonds with a mysterious young patient, an 18-year-old woman dealing with the sensory chaos of New York City, and an out-of-control toddler have in common? All were featured in prime time television programs in 2006, fictional or reality-based, which centered on a character with Asperger syndrome. *Boston Legal*, *Without a Trace*, *Extreme Makeover Home Edition*, *Cold Case*, *House*, *All My Children*, and *Supernanny* each ran episodes in 2006 focusing on Asperger syndrome. *The Apprentice*, *Numbers*, the Discovery Channel, the *Jane Pauley Show*, *ER*, and *The Closer* also featured programs on this syndrome. Christian Clemenson, the actor who plays a gifted lawyer with Asperger syndrome on *Boston Legal*, won an Emmy for Best Guest Actor in a Drama Series this year. In October, comedian Jon Stewart hosted a Comedy Central Benefit for Autism Education at New York's Beacon Theatre.

Clearly, the media and the prime time public are spellbound by Asperger syndrome. Some programs presented factual representations, others wildly fictional, but the theme draws viewers, especially when the storyline includes the unusual special interest of the central character. While television producers benefit from this attractive topic, however, thousands of real families live every minute of their lives caring for their children with Asperger syndrome. One of the most fascinating aspects of Asperger syndrome is the special interest areas in which over 90% of individuals with Asperger syndrome engage.[1]

Little research has been conducted into the special interests of children and youth with Asperger syndrome. Although parents, educators, and experts in the field of Asperger's seem well aware of the existence of these special interests, our review of the literature indicates that no one has researched the origin and development of such interests in children and youth with the syndrome. [2,3,4,5,6,7] Nor has anyone explored the effect of special interests on the social, communication, and emotional skills and deficits of children and youth with Asperger's, or how special interests might be integrated most effectively into school, home, and community.

The purpose of our exploratory study was to evaluate the impact of special interest areas (SIAs) on children and youth with Asperger's, as well as on their families.[8] The lead author and her graduate students began this study in January 2005 with a methodical search of the existing literature on the special interests of individuals with Asperger's. The research team then identified a research question, designed an appropriate study, and obtained university and school district approval to conduct the study. We defined SIAs as those passions that capture the mind, heart, time, and attention of individuals with Asperger's, providing the lens through which they view the world.[9]

During the summer of 2005, the research team conducted the study and gathered both qualitative and quantitative data from the study participants and their parents/guardians. The research team then spent the fall and winter of 2005 analyzing the data they had obtained. Various members of the research team presented the results of the study at two national conferences: the National Council for Exceptional Children conference in Salt Lake City, Utah in April, 2006 and the National Autism Society of America conference in Providence, Rhode Island in July, 2006.

### What did we learn?

We organized our findings into the following areas: (a) categories of SIAs, (b) the fusion of SIAs and identity, (c) gender differences in SIAs, (d) parents' knowledge about and feelings towards SIAs, (e) peers' perceptions of SIAs and how those perceptions negatively affect children and youth with Asperger's, and (f) the impact of SIAs on classic Asperger's deficits.

## Categories of SIAs

In the limited research concerning the special interests of individuals with Asperger's, Attwood,[12] Gillberg,[13] and Myles and Adreon[14] all noted that special interests vary widely. We found this in our research also. We identified 22 SIAs which we categorized into eight interest themes.

These included classic SIAs as well as unusual ones. The eight themes were transportation, music, animals, sports, video games, motion pictures, woodworking, and art. Table 40.1 lists the SIAs of all participants.

Although seven of the boys in our study identified video games as their SIA, further analysis of the interviews revealed that often the boys hid their true SIAs in order to gain social acceptance from their peers. Participants often used video games or other popular interests as a social bridge, even if these interests were not their true SIAs. We labeled this practice the masking of special interests because we found that participants used this technique to hide perceived socially unacceptable SIAs from their peers while still interacting with them. For example, Tom said that video games were his SIA, but later revealed his passion for woodworking.[15] Peter revealed his masking process when he told us, "Uh, I'm a gamer, uh, but my favorite video game, the only one I am actually good at, would be First Person Shooters...But the truth is, I like frogs...frogs frogs frogs frogs! I have, like, so many frogs at both my mom and dad's houses and I'm not going to ever sell them or give them away or stuff like that. If I was going to sell them, which I'm not, I'd be rich! Really, really, rich!"[16]

**Table 40.1.** Participants' Primary Special Interest Areas

| General Theme | Interest Area |
|---|---|
| Transportation | airplanes, cars, trains, trucks |
| Music | composing, drumming, rap music, saxophone |
| Animals | frogs, goats, horses |
| Sports | swimming, video games, role playing games (RPGs) |
| Motion pictures | Disney, Star Wars, Vampires |
| Woodworking | |
| Art | Anime, cartooning, manga, sculpting |

Note: Although N=23 in our study, the interests do not total 23 because two participants shared the same special interest.

## The Fusion of SIAs and Identity

It was clear from our data that participants' positive self-images were inextricably woven into their SIAs. The participants strongly identified with their SIAs and saw themselves defined by their SIAs. SIAs are critically important to children and youth with Asperger's. Though participants' self-images apart from their SIAs were strongly negative, we found that when they were involved in activities related to their SIAs, they felt more positive about themselves. They demonstrated expertise in their SIAs, control over their knowledge and involvement in their SIAs, and increased self-confidence. One participant, Ryan, confided, "I think I've got a lot more understanding on how things work than most people. I've got a corner in the back of my brain that allows me to perfectly simulate almost anything."[17] Steve told us, "I'm the main customer at a place called Hollywood Video. I am a movie whiz!"[18]

## Gender Differences in SIAs

Our female participants validated the research of Cohen[19] on the interests of girls with Asperger's in which she found that the most popular interests among her participants were art, primarily drawing and cartooning, and animals. The interests of the two girls in our study were manga and horses. Sarah, one of the two girls in our study, firmly stated "I'm an animal person. [People] can sense that I am an animal person."[20]

## Parents' Knowledge of and Feelings Toward SIAs

Most parents who completed a survey were very aware of their children's SIAs, and were able to correctly identify them. Parents saw the purpose of SIAs as having fun, relaxing, avoiding doing another task, avoiding thinking about something else, calming down, and reducing stress or anxiety. Parents acknowledged their children's expertise in their SIAs. Nearly all the parents surveyed correctly identified their children's SIAs. Most children and youth participants reported that their interactions with their parents concerning their SIAs were positive.

Parents' primary concerns regarding their children's SIAs were that they were socially unacceptable, not age-appropriate, and would not lead to college or careers. A grandmother lamented "once he is 'in' a game—there is no further participation with life in general—he rambles on and on about what he cares about, or things [about] himself. No interest shown in others."[21] One parent shared, "[His SIA] keeps him from learning new possibilities."[22] One boy's mother also expressed her concern for his future. "Can he really do this as a career?"[23] Sixteen of the[18] parent respondents said that they regularly interpreted their children's SIAs for family, friends, and teachers, explaining why their children were so involved in their SIAs. Fourteen parents stated that their children's SIAs had a positive impact on their families.

Parents expressed a wide range of emotions concerning their children's SIAs. These included the five most common positive feelings in our survey data: pride, humor, fascination, pleasure, and enthusiasm. For example, Brock's mother stated, "My son inspires my respect and admiration for all he knows and his amazing brain."[24] Marcus's mother affirmed, "It's part of what makes him special!"[25] Justin's grandmother wrote, "I'm glad to see if Justin has an interest he can go far with. If he chooses a scientific study he could be a genius."[26]

Parents also experienced negative emotions about their children's SIAs. The three most common were boredom, frustration, and embarrassment. Justin's grandmother expressed her weariness with Justin's SIA when she wrote simply, "This world is all about Justin."[27] One parent expressed her frustration, writing "It's tiring for others to listen to [him talk about his SIA] after a while; it's limiting for him, too."[28] Another parent agreed. "It's obsessive and gets old," she wrote.[29]

Some children and youth expressed frustration with their parents, too. Peter confided, "My Dad...did not really accept that I am, um, a gamer." When asked what he thought his parents thought his SIA was, he replied, "I don't think they've really got a clue. They'd probably think the video games 'cause they're always tellin' me to get off my butt and go do somethin'."[30]

## Peers' Perceptions of SIAs

Participants expressed reluctance to tell others about their SIAs due to rejection from their peers. Participants also noted that they were frustrated at being misunderstood by others. Their SIAs were often seen as socially unacceptable, and their peers lacked understanding and interest in the participants' SIAs. Charlie wanted to clarify, "I also make dragons, not just dinosaurs, everyone needs to know what they are—dragons, dragons, dragons!"[31] Brock admitted, "I just wish they'd think planes were cool."[32]

Brock also revealed his feeling of peer rejection, as well as his desire to be the expert, when he told one interviewer, "I wish [kids at school] would accept planes and, uh, not always pretend to throw up about it. I just wish they knew as much about it as I do, maybe even...no, maybe not even more."[33]

Participants clearly wanted to be recognized as experts, and accepted by their peers. "Well I first like tell 'em I'm talented, but then I like wanna prove, I mean prove, that I can do it."[34] Another participant stated, "Yeah...wulll...apparently, like, when I make something very good, then they'll be impressed."[35]

Many participants, such as Brock, revealed social awareness in their cautious dealings with peers, testing the waters before revealing their SIAs. "First, I usually don't talk about it... and if I have a really good friend... they might come over to my house and then they'll see all these planes around and they'll tell me that planes are a really cool thing... and then I'll know."[36] Justin told us, "Video games used to be at the top of my list. Now I always put girls at the top of my list. If it's a girl, I'll hang back, observe, see what kinda things she likes and I'll move in slow and steady. One could say that I like to buy lunch for pretty girls."[37]

Owen was willing to be flexible in talking with peers, saying "If they don't look interested I change the subject. I say, 'Hey, I can change my voice.'"[38] Steve, however, had learned self-preservation by backing off when teased by peers. "I don't really wish other people would know about it."[39] Charlie confided, "They wouldn't, like, care anyway."[40]

## The Impact of SIAs on Classic Asperger's Deficits

We discovered that SIAs had some very positive effects on some of the classic deficits of children and youth with Asperger's. Traditionally, children and youth with Asperger's exhibit deficits in the areas of language, social communication, emotions, and problems with sensory stimuli and fine motor activities. However, we found that these deficits were diminished when participants were engaged in their SIAs.[41]

As we interviewed participants and later listened to the taped interviews, we noticed distinct changes in the participants' speech whenever they talked about their SIAs. Some participants began to show significantly more enthusiasm and emotion when asked about their SIAs. In some participants, we noted that their speech was much clearer and they used more advanced vocabulary when talking about their SIAs. For example, when responding to general questions, Charlie repeatedly gave answers such as "Uh, I don't think so, I just, whatever," consisting of simple one or two syllable words with no clear content. When asked about his favorite thing to play with, however, his speech pattern changed instantly as he confidently replied, "My favorite is a Yu-Gi-Oh™ card that combines with three blue-eyed white dragons, and due to polymerization it forms those three into a three-headed dragon."[42]

Our team also observed improvement in body language, particularly an increase in eye contact and expressive gestures that accompanied speech. Further, we noticed a remarkable decrease in self-stimulation, distraction, and body movement in and around the tables and the participants' chairs.

All of our participants enthusiastically talked at length about their SIAs. The participants noted that they saw nothing unusual or extraordinary about their SIAs. Participants shared that they felt positive emotions when actively engaged in their SIAs, including enthusiasm, pride, and happiness. Danny could barely contain his joy in repeatedly telling the interviewers, "I was born to like...Walt Disney. Walt Disney is my life. Disney has been my most happiest hope in my whole life."[43] Nate, whose SIA was musical composition, proudly told the interviewers, "My parents think I'm an unbelievable, amazing drummer."[44] Convinced of his successful future in composing music scores for film, Nate confidently declared, "The reason I wanna move back there [to Hollywood] is, I wanna be a composer and, and just take over John William's job, get into that job, and compose Harry Potter, The Terminal...just, before I do that, I have to learn the notes." Nate described how the music made him feel. "I like composing music for movies so that I have a good feeling...I like feeling sad, happy, scared, sneaky."[45]

Individuals with Asperger's often find intense smells, loud sounds, or personal touch highly unpleasant.[46] Rising to these sensory challenges, our participants persevered for hours at a time when involved in their SIAs in spite of intense stimulation from model airplane glue, modeling clay, horse manure, goat odors, sawdust, sweat, sticky or dirty hands, and the bright lights, rapid movements, and loud, startling sounds of video games.

Though children and youth with Asperger's typically have acknowledged difficulties in tying shoelaces, fastening buttons, and handwriting, [47,48] our participants spoke not only of their advanced fine motor skills, but of extreme perseverance and patience in the fine motor skills that their SIAs required such as drawing, building, sculpting, creating models, playing keyboards, using video controllers, and playing musical instruments.

SIAs clearly serve a very positive purpose for children and youth with Asperger's. SIAs are vital to their well-being; they are viewed by children and youth not as a hobby or leisure activity or interest, but as an integral part of who they are. In their special interest, these children and youth acquire clear focus, a way to organize the world, a social approach, and a way to interpret life. SIAs are not taken lightly by children and youth with Asperger's, and neither should they be taken lightly by parents and teachers.

## How Can Parents and Teachers Get the Most Out of Children's SIAs?

SIAs can be powerful motivators for children and youth with Asperger's. Parents can take advantage of the strong connection their children have with their SIAs by using them to motivate or to reinforce children for completing or trying less desirable activities such as chores or to entice children to engage in social activities with the family. For example, a child with an SIA in horses might earn a horseback riding lesson for keeping her room clean for a week, or a student with an SIA in aviation might earn a trip to the local airport after helping his parents wash the family car.

SIAs provide children with Asperger's with a way to relax, de-stress, and cope with the world. Children and youth with Asperger's often arrive home after school tired and stressed after a day of working hard to stay calm and focused at school. Allowing a child to spend some time engaging in her SIA after school can help reduce her stress level so that the child can then participate more willingly in the family's evening activities.

In order to facilitate communication and encourage interaction between the child with Asperger's and his family, parents could arrange outings focused on the child's SIA or arrange for friends who share an interest in the child's SIA to participate with the family in an activity focused on the child's SIA. Parents could encourage a child to participate in a community organization that is related to his/her SIA as a way of increasing the child's socialization skills. For example, a youth who is interested in farm animals might join a local 4-H group and learn how to raise and care for a lamb, cow, or pig. A child with an SIA in trains could join a local model railroad group and learn about and share his/her own expertise about trains.

In the Asperger's community, many adults have developed careers based on their personal SIAs. These individuals can be a source of encouragement for parents, children with Asperger syndrome, and educators alike. For example, Dr. Temple Grandin is an associate professor of animal science at Colorado State University. Her passion for cattle has prepared the way for her career as an expert designer and consultant in humane cattle management and slaughter techniques.[49] Gilles Trehin, a young French man who created the fictitious city of Urville, has published a complete book of intricate drawings of Urville as he has imagined it since the age of 12.[50] Dr. Dawn Prince-Hughes, adjunct professor of anthropology at Western Washington University, has turned her identification with and passion for gorillas into a profession as a consultant and educator about their history, culture, and needs.[51]

Parents could use a child's SIA to motivate the child to cooperate with necessary daily living activities such as going to the dentist, shopping for groceries, or getting a haircut. Following such stressful events with free time to engage in the child's SIA may encourage the child to behave appropriately in order to hasten access to the SIA.

Because SIAs are such a vital element in the self-image and motivation of children and youth with Asperger's, it is imperative that they be welcomed and encouraged at school. From our data we learned how deeply participants and parents feel about educators respecting their insights concerning making room for SIAs at school. We also learned how strongly the participants wanted teachers to incorporate their preferred methods of gathering information, particularly reading, into the curricula. We cannot afford to ignore students' SIAs, or withhold engagement with them as punishment for misbehavior. With little additional effort, teachers can integrate SIAs into all core academic areas, including English, reading, writing, spelling, math, science, speech, and history. Students with Asperger's are much more likely to demonstrate their true levels of ability in academic assignments when SIAs can be included in the assignments. For example, students can be encouraged to practice reading skills by reading books about their SIAs. Teachers, with parents' help, can embed areas of special interests into assignments such as math problems that use examples from a child's SIA in order to motivate the child to practice solving math story problems.

For a middle school or high school student with Asperger's, an opportunity to shadow a professional in a field related to the student's SIA could promote a career interest for the student. For example, the student who is an expert on Disney films might shadow or interview a character animator to learn how animated movies are created and what kind of training is required for a career in film-making.

Students can also benefit from simplified versions of their SIAs to deal with negative emotions, reduce anxiety, and calm themselves in stressful situations. Students identify with their SIAs; therefore, a favorite small airplane, stuffed frog, photograph of a prized goat, sheet music of a revered composer, cover from a preferred DVD or video, or recent anime drawing may help the child in calming himself and reducing disruptive anxiety-driven self-stimulation or other behaviors. We must see SIAs for the gold mine they are in helping our students progress toward their academic, social, emotional, communication, and behavioral goals.

Unquestionably, making the shift to inviting SIAs into the academic arena requires effort on the part of parents and teachers. They must each be willing to think creatively to find ways in which to insert the SIA effectively and appropriately into the curriculum. Parents and teachers must be flexible, looking beyond the strict limits of the lesson plans and assignments to ask, "Is it our goal that Samantha write about summer vacation, or is it that she learn to write, even if she chooses to write about carnivorous plants?" Teachers must partner with parents, seeking their input on their children's SIAs, their ideas for how to integrate the SIAs into the curricula, and even their practical help in modifying assignments to incorporate the SIAs. Parents can integrate SIAs into countless areas of their children's home and community lives, increasing children's motivation, interest, and cooperation.

**Table 40.2.** Examples of the Integration of the Solar System as SIA into Core Upper Elementary School Curriculum

| Academic Areas | Solar System-Integrated Assignments |
|---|---|
| Reading | Read three chapters that interest you in *Astronomy: The Solar System and Beyond* by Michael A. Seeds.[52] |
| Writing | Have you ever dreamed of discovering a planet or a galaxy? Imagine you found one. Name it after yourself and write a newspaper article announcing your discovery to the world. Where did you find it? How did you discover it? How will your discovery change astronomy? |
| Spelling | Read Chapter 3, Astronomical Tools, in *Astronomy: The Solar System and Beyond*, above. List your favorite tools, such as "optical telescope," and learn to spell them. You might want to draw pictures of them, too. |
| History | Nicolaus Copernicus, a Polish astronomer, lived in 1473–1543. He was a brilliant scientist, but he paid a high price for his belief that the earth rotated around the sun. *Read Copernicus: Founder of Modern Astronomy (Great Minds of Science)*[53] by Catherine M. Andronik to find out what so enraged his critics. Think about this: if you had been Copernicus, do you think you would have changed your theory? |
| Speech | Dress as and present the passion and work of Charles Messier, French astronomer born in 1730. Explain to your audience what is meant by the "Messier Number." |
| Math | Find out how far each of the eight planets in our solar system are from earth. Now calculate how far they are from each other. Which one is furthest from any other planet? Which two are closest together? What is the average distance of all the planets from the earth? |
| Science | Just what is Halley's Comet, and who was Halley? Go to the library to find out exactly what a comet is and why Halley's Comet is so important. How do comets differ from stars? Will Halley's Comet come through again in your lifetime? |
| Art | Choose your favorite Messier Deep Space Object and make it come alive with paint, clay, fabric, recycled objects, or another medium that you choose. |
| Internet Skills | Where in the world is the Kuiper Belt? When does NASA plan to go there? What do the Oort Cloud and some really cold bodies have in common? To find out, research NASA's amazing website at solarsystem.nasa.gov/planets/index.cfm. Surfing NASA's site or other federal or university websites, find an astronomer and write him or her with your most burning questions about the stars. |

453

Children with Asperger syndrome can achieve far beyond expectations when they are allowed to be involved in their SIAs. Educators and parents must embrace SIAs as a means to an end, not an end in themselves. Over fifty years ago, Hans Asperger (1991/1944) already knew what we are just coming to see: special interests are the key to fulfillment and maximized potential in children and youth with Asperger syndrome. We can find reason to hope for significant and meaningful futures for children with Asperger's in his stirring words that call so clearly to us today:

"Able autistic individuals can rise to eminent positions and perform with such outstanding success that one may even conclude that only such people are capable of certain achievements. It is as if they had compensatory ability to counter-balance their deficiencies. Their unswerving determination and penetrating intellectual powers, part of their spontaneous and original mental activity, their narrowness and single-mindedness, as manifested in their special interests, can be immensely valuable and can lead to outstanding achievements in their chosen areas."[54]

## References

1. Attwood, T. (2003). Understanding and managing circumscribed interests. In M. Prior (Ed.), *Learning and behavior problems in Asperger Syndrome* (pp 126–147). New York: Guilford Press.

2. Attwood, T. (1998). *Asperger's syndrome: A guide for parents and professionals*. Philadelphia, PA: Jessica Kingsley.

3. Gillberg, C. (1991). Clinical and neurobiological aspects of Asperger syndrome in six family studies. In U. Frith (Ed.) *Autism and Asperger syndrome*. New York: Cambridge University Press.

4. Kanner, L. (1973). *Childhood psychosis: Initial studies and new insights*. Washington, DC: Winston.

5. Klin, A., Volkmar, F.R., and Sparrow, S. (2000). *Asperger syndrome*. New York: Guilford Press.

6. Myles, B.S., and Adreon, D. (2001). *Asperger Syndrome and adolescence: Practical solutions for school success*. Shawnee Mission, KS: Autism Asperger.

7. Myles, B.S., and Simpson, R.L. (2003) *Asperger syndrome: A guide for educators and parents*. Austin, TX: Pro-Ed.

8.  Winter-Messiers, M.A. (in press). *Toilet brushes and tarantulas: Understanding the origin and development of the special interest areas of children and youth with Asperger's syndrome.*

9.  Winter-Messiers, M. A. (2007). From Tarantulas to Toilet Brushes: Understanding the Special Interest Areas of Children and Youth with Asperger Syndrome. *Remedial and Special Education, (28)*3, 140–152.

10. Ibid.

11. Winter-Messiers, M. A., et al. How Far Can Brian Ride the Daylight 4449 Express? A Strength-Based Model of Asperger Syndrome Based on Special Interest Areas. *Focus on Autism and Other Developmental Disabilities, (22)*2, 67–79.

12. Attwood, T. (1998). *Asperger's syndrome: A guide for parents and profession*als. Philadelphia, PA: Jessica Kingsley.

13. Gillberg, C. (1991). Clinical and neurobiological aspects of Asperger syndrome in six family studies. In U. Frith (Ed.) *Autism and Asperger syndrome*. New York: Cambridge University Press.

14. Myles, B.S., and Adreon, D. (2001). *Asperger Syndrome and adolescence: Practical solutions for school success*. Shawnee Mission, KS: Autism Asperger.

15. "Tom"—personal communication, July 19, 2005.

16. "Peter"—personal communication, July 26, 2005.

17. "Ryan"—personal communication, July 26, 2005.

18. "Steve"—personal communication, July 20, 2005.

19. Cohen, M. (2003). *Understanding the unique social challenges of females with Asperger's syndrome*. Retrieved March 24, 2003, from www.autismsrc.org/whatsnew/ASA presentation_files/frame.htm.

20. "Sarah"—personal communication, July 26, 2005.

21. "Grandmother of a child with Asperger's"—personal communication, July 28, 2005.

22. "Parent of a child with Asperger's"—personal communication, July 23, 2005.

23. "Mother of a child with Asperger's"—personal communication, July 14, 2005.

24. "Brock's mother"—personal communication, July 25, 2005.

25. "Marcus' mother"—personal communication, July 24, 2005

26. "Justin's Grandmother"—personal communication, July 28, 2005.

27. Ibid.

28. "Parent of a child with Asperger's"—personal communication, July 27, 2005.

29. "Parent of a child with Asperger's"—personal communication, July 26, 2005.

30. "Peter"—personal communication, July 26, 2005.

31. "Charlie"—personal communication, July 20, 2005.

32. "Brock"—personal communication, August 5, 2005.

33. Ibid.

34. "Charlie"—personal communication, July 20, 2005.

35. "Child with Asperger's"—personal communication, July 20, 2005.

36. "Brock"—personal communication, August 5, 2005.

37. "Justin"—personal communication, July 26, 2005.

38. "Owen"—personal communication, July 26, 2005.

39. "Steve"—personal communication, July 20, 2005.

40. "Charlie"—personal communication, July 20, 2005.

41. Winter-Messiers, M.A., Herr, C. M., Wood, C. E., et al. (in press). *How far can Brian ride the Daylight 4449 Express? A strength-based model of Asperger's syndrome based on special interest areas.*

42. "Charlie"—personal communication, July 20, 2005.

43. "Nate"—personal communication, July 19, 2005.

44. "Nate"—personal communication, July 26, 2005.

45. Ibid.

46. Myles, B.S., Tapscott-Cook, K., Miller, N.E., and Rinner, L. (2002). *Asperger's syndrome and sensory issues: Practical solutions for making sense of the world.* Shawnee Mission, KS: Autism Asperger.

47. Attwood, T. (1998). *Asperger's syndrome: A guide for parents and professionals*. Philadelphia, PA: Jessica Kingsley.

48. Myles, B.S., and Simpson, R.L. (2003) *Asperger syndrome: A guide for educators and parents*. Austin, TX: Pro-Ed.

49. Grandin, T. (1996). *Thinking in pictures: And other reports from my life with autism*. New York: Vintage.

50. Trehin, G. (2006). *Urville*. Philadelphia: Jessica Kingsley.

51. Prince-Hughes, D. (2005). *Songs of the gorilla nation: My journey through autism*. New York: Three Rivers Press.

52. Seeds, M.A. (2002). *Astronomy: The solar system and beyond (with InfoTrac and the sky CD-ROM)* (3rd ed.). Belmont, CA: Brooks Cole.

53 Andronik, C.M. (2006). *Copernicus: Founder of modern astronomy (Great minds of science)*. Berkeley Heights, NJ: Enslow.

54. Asperger, H. (1991). Die 'autistischen psychopathen' im Kindersalter. In U. Frith (Ed. and Trans.) *Autism and Asperger Syndrome* (pp. 37-92). New York: Cambridge University Press. (Original work published in 1944).

## Section 40.2

# *Outcomes of School-Based Social Skill Interventions for Children on the Autism Spectrum*

"The Collective Outcomes of School-Based Social Skill Interventions for Children on the Autism Spectrum," by Scott Bellini, PhD. © 2007 Indiana Resource Center for Autism. Reprinted with permission.

Social skill interventions are only minimally effective for children with autism spectrum disorders according to a recent study conducted by researchers at the Indiana Resource Center for Autism (IRCA) (Bellini, Peters, Benner, and Hopf, 2007). The study was published in the journal *Remedial and Special Education*. The researchers conducted a meta-analysis of 55 published research studies investigating school based social skill interventions for children and adolescents on the autism spectrum. A meta-analysis involves synthesizing the collective outcomes of every study performed on a particular topic. The reviewed studies included a total of 147 students with an autism spectrum disorder ranging from preschool to secondary school. Specifically, social skill interventions produced low treatment effects and low generalization effects across persons, settings, and play stimuli. Moderate maintenance effects were observed suggesting that when gains were made via social skill interventions, the gains were maintained after the intervention is withdrawn. The low treatment effects observed in the present study are consistent with the results of previous social skill intervention meta-analyses on other populations of children (Gresham, Sugai, and Horner, 2001; Mathur, Kavale, Quinn, Forness and Rutherford, 1998; Quin, Kavale, Mathur, Rutherford and Forness, 1999).

In addition, similar intervention, maintenance, and generalization effects were observed between interventions targeting collateral skills (for example: play skills, joint attention, and language skills) and interventions targeting specific social behaviors (such as, social initiations, social responses, and duration of interaction). There were no significant differences between the outcomes of studies that implemented group interventions and studies that implemented individual interventions.

An important finding of the study was that students receiving social skills programming in their typical classroom setting had substantially more favorable treatment outcomes than did students who received services in a pull-out setting

The results of the meta-analyses, though certainly hard to swallow, shed some light on factors that lead to more beneficial social outcomes for children with autism spectrum disorders (ASD) and other populations of children. For instance, by synthesizing the results of this and other meta-analyses, we are better able to determine the ingredients of effective social skills instruction, and thus, make recommendations for programming. They are as follows:

1. Increase the dosage of social skill interventions.

2. Provide instruction within the child's natural setting.

3. Match the intervention strategy with the type of skill deficit.

4. Ensure intervention fidelity.

## Dosage

Gresham et al. (2001) recommended that social skill interventions should be implemented more intensely and frequently than the level presently delivered to children with social skill deficits. Though the researchers did not recommend a specific dosage, they stated that 30 hours of instruction, spread over 10–12 weeks is insufficient. The low intervention effects observed in the present meta-analysis may be attributed to the low level of instructional intensity provided in the reviewed studies, which was considerably lower than the 30+ hours recommended. Children with ASD exhibit significant social skill deficits that may potentially lead to academic, behavioral, and emotional difficulties. As such, the recommendation to increase instructional intensity is particularly salient for this population of children. School personnel should look for opportunities to teach and reinforce social skills as frequently as possible throughout the school day, and not just in pull-out settings.

## Intervention Setting

Gresham et al. (2001) noted that the weak outcomes of social skill interventions can be attributed to the fact that these interventions often take place in "contrived, restricted, and decontextualized" (p. 340) settings, such as resource rooms or other pull-out settings. The results of the present meta-analysis support this assertion. That is, maintenance and generalization effects were significantly lower for interventions that were implemented in pull-out settings. In contrast, interventions that were implemented in the child's typical classroom setting produced higher maintenance effects and higher generalization effects across persons, settings, and play stimuli. Furthermore, in addition to higher maintenance and generalization effects, the results of the present study also suggest that interventions implemented in the child's typical classroom produce substantially higher intervention effects. This finding has important implications for school-based social skill interventions. Teachers and other school personnel should place a premium on selecting social skill interventions that can be reasonably implemented within multiple naturalistic settings. This is particularly important for children with ASD, who may have considerable difficulties transferring skills from one setting to another.

## Matching Strategy with Type of Skill Deficit

Gresham et al. (2001) asserted that a key component of effective social skills programming is the ability of the interventionist to match the intervention strategy with the type of skill deficit: performance deficit or skill acquisition deficit. A performance deficit refers to a skill or behavior that is present, but not demonstrated or performed, whereas, a skill acquisition deficit refers to the absence of a particular skill or behavior. Of the 55 studies included in the present meta-analysis, only one considered the type of skill deficit exhibited by the participants, prior to implementing the intervention. School personnel should make an intensive effort to systematically match the intervention strategy to the type of skill deficits exhibited by the child, as this information guides the selection of effective strategies. For instance, if the child lacks the skills necessary to join in an interaction with peers, a strategy should be selected that promotes skill acquisition. In contrast, if the child has the skills to join in an activity but regularly fails to do so, a strategy should be selected that enhances performance of the existing skill.

## Intervention Fidelity

Only 14 of the studies in the present meta-analysis measured intervention fidelity (for example, whether the intervention was implemented as intended). Gresham et al. (2001) concluded that the failure of studies to provide intervention fidelity data makes it extremely difficult to conclude whether a social skill intervention was ineffective because of an ineffectual intervention strategy, or because the strategy was implemented poorly. Poor intervention fidelity may significantly diminish the outcomes of the social skill intervention, and diminish our ability to make decisions regarding the effects of individual strategies. Poor intervention fidelity may also be the result of poorly trained personnel. Presently, few educators and therapists receive training in social skills interventions as part of their undergraduate and graduate school training. As such, this places the onus on school districts to provide professional development opportunities for school personnel responsible for implementing social skill interventions.

**Results of this study** indicate that now more than ever, our field and, more important, children with ASD, are in desperate need of effective social skill programming. Not just easy to implement social skills programming, but *effective* social skills programming. The results of the meta-analyses, though certainly not positive, shed some light on factors that lead to more beneficial social outcomes for children with ASD and other populations of children. By synthesizing the results of meta-analyses, we are better able to determine the components of effective social skills instruction, and thus, develop more effective programming.

## *References*

Bellini, S., Peters, J., Benner, L., and Hopf, A. (2007). A meta-analysis of school-based social skill interventions for children with autism spectrum disorders. *Remedial and Special Education, 28*, 153–162.

Gresham, F. M., Sugai, G., and Horner, R. H. (2001).outcomes of social skills training for students with high-incidence disabilities. *Teaching Exceptional Children, 67*, 331–344.

Mathur, S. R., Kavale, K. A., Quinn, M. M., Forness, S. R., and Rutherford, R. B. (1998). Social skills interventions with students with emotional and behavioral problems. A quantitative synthesis of single subject research. *Behavioral Disorders, 23*, 193–201.

Quinn, M. M., Kavale, K. A., Mathur, S. R., Rutherford Jr., R. B., and Forness, S. R. (1999). A meta-analysis of social skills interventions for students with emotional and behavioral disorders. *Journal of Emotional and Behavioral Disorders, 7*, 54–64.

## Section 40.3

# *Computer-Based Training May Improve Social Interactions*

Excerpted from "Recovery Act Grant Aims to Teach Kids with Autism How to Better Express Themselves," National institute of Mental Health (NIMH), November 12, 2009.

## *Computer-Based Training in Creating and Responding to Facial Expressions May Improve Social Interactions*

Most children with autism spectrum disorders (ASD) seem to have trouble engaging in everyday social interactions. They may seem to have no reaction to other people or may respond atypically when others show anger or affection. Their own facial expressions, tone of voice, and body language may not match what they are saying, making it difficult for others to respond appropriately. Such barriers to communication can isolate children with ASD from their peers.

To help overcome these barriers, the National Institutes of Health (NIH) awarded a Challenge grant on behalf of the National Institute of Mental Health (NIMH) to support the development of a new training program that incorporates two existing computer programs. One program, called *Let's Face It!* helps children with ASD recognize facial expressions of others and understand the corresponding emotions. The other program, called the *Computer Expression Recognition Toolbox*, detects a user's facial expression in real-time, based on 37 different facial expression dimensions (for example, widening one's eyes, raising the inner or outer corners of one's eyebrows, wrinkling one's nose, etc.) and their intensity.

In the new study, Marian Bartlett, PhD, of the University of California–San Diego, and colleagues will use the two programs as a basis for developing and testing a new computer-assisted program to train children with ASD how to respond to facial expressions of others and how to produce facial expressions conveying particular emotions to others. The researchers will also characterize facial expression production in children who do not have ASD, which can provide important information for research on the normal development of motor skills for social communication.

# Chapter 41

# *Teaching Lifetime Goals to Children and Adults with ASD*

All children and adults need to accomplish goals that result in safe and productive lives. Here are some guidelines for identifying and addressing essential life goals.

## *1. Use Only Safe Behavior*

Target the elimination of dangerous or potentially dangerous behavior.

- The criteria for institutionalization against your will and choice is: danger to self, danger to others.
- Behavior could be misunderstood, viewed as a criminal, victimized.
- Children and adults with autism spectrum disorders (ASD) can be put in the corrections system or in jail.
- Teach alternate behaviors for the person to use instead of the dangerous ones.

Be sure to teach:

- crossing the street with someone or knowing when to move forward into the street with someone else,

- moving away from danger,

- asking a trusted adult before doing something a stranger says to do,

- not to enter other people's homes without permission,

- to stay away from bodies of water when they are alone.

List behaviors that the child or adult uses that are dangerous or could become dangerous. List alternate behaviors that should be learned.

## 2. Taking Complete Care of Her or His Own Body

Everyone needs to be independent in the bathroom to the greatest extent possible for these reasons:

- one may not have as many job opportunities if have to be taken to the toilet,

- others usually prefer to live with someone who can toilet or bathe on their own (with the exception of physical disabilities),

- being clean and smelling good makes us more acceptable in society (appearance is important), and the

- potential for sexual abuse is very high among people with disabilities and caring for oneself helps to reduce that potential by having private activities done when alone.

Be sure to teach:

- rules regarding privacy for self and others,

- as much independence as possible in the bathroom and while dressing.

What skills in self-care does the child or adult need to acquire? Be specific.

## 3. Touching Others and Being Touched Appropriately

Who to hug, touch, kiss, and continue to talk to, or follow including:

- "circle of friends" concept can be used to teach many different concepts, including concepts of touching;

- need to recognize different ways that they be subtly told to go away or stop touching the other person;

- need to be able to take "no" for an answer;
- need to be able to tell "no" and get away and seek help quickly;
- need to learn who to touch, how and when;
- need to learn who can touch them, how and when.

Be sure to teach:

- what to do if you are not sure if someone should touch you or you should touch them, how to seek help or go to a safe place;
- how to move away from someone who does not want your attention;
- how to move away from someone bothering you and you need to get help.

What behavior and skills related to touching, being touched and showing interest in others does the child or adult need to learn?

## 4. Respectful Use of Property

How to touch or use other's property and knowing how to ask first:

- asking can be verbal, gestural, printed, and so forth, it does not depend on speech;
- need to learn how to tell "my" things from someone else's, perhaps with a visual reminder at first;
- need to know how to use property properly and put it back in good condition.

Be sure to teach:

- some way to ask before taking something that belongs to someone else;
- some way to know the difference between your property and someone else's;
- treating things with respect and care;
- replacing what you broke or destroyed.

How does the child or adult currently react to the property of others? Does s/he understand the underlying concept of property/possessions? What behaviors and skills does the child or adult need to learn in this area?

## 5. Knowing Two Different Responses to Give When People Tell You Yes or No

Suggestions include:

- won't always develop automatically, but can be learned;
- use charts, social stories, choice-making charts, decision trees and videos;
- teach physical coping skills (deep breathing, stretching, walking, singing);
- practice in many environments;
- practice for new social situations that may arise in the future.

Be sure to teach:

- who to talk with to help you cope after receiving an undesired answer,
- how to move away and do something else when someone tells you "no" and remain calm.

How does the child or adult respond when someone says either yes or no when the child or adult wants to hear the other answer? What kind of coping/communication skills does the child or adult need to learn in this area?

## 6. Knowing from Whom to Get Help, and How and When

Important guidelines include:

- the need to be taught efficient and effective ways of getting safe, adult assistance in all settings;
- teaching in each situation many different times until they get the concept or provide them with the information if the concept never develops;
- creating rules (first ask a person with the store uniform or a name tag, for example);
- having a system of identification that every child or adult carries. Teach when and how to give that to authority or helpers;
- teaching each child or adult to carry a current list of all medications (amounts, types and times administered) being taken;

- needing to know how to get help from authority figures or police officers, how to respond to their commands including how to remain calm while being questioned or physically searched by an officer.

Be sure to teach:

- the signs that mean the child or adult needs help;
- a way the children or adults can tell their name and address to persons in authority, tell that they need help that does not depend only on speech;
- an efficient way to and give information upon request by authority figures;
- whom to call to help them if they are having problems;
- how to decide who is safe to approach to ask for help in many environments.

Note: Do not depend on the child or adult's ability to speak in a crisis. Everyone's ability to use speech and language decreases under stressful conditions. Use something written, taped on a tape or compact disk (CD) player, and/or carried in a wallet or purse.

What does the child or adult do when s/he needs help in public? How does s/he identify who can help them? How does s/he ask for help? What skills does the child or adult need to learn in this area?

## 7. Learn to Identify Internal States and Express Them

- Describe feelings or sensations in terms of intensity and level of ability to cope.
- A problem coping is not a tantrum: language to describe is important here.
- Need to become aware when they may be ill or uncomfortable and need medical help, and be able to communicate it to others.
- Need to have a plan to avoid upsetting stimuli and find safe places in all environments for when they become overwhelmed.

Be sure to teach:

- pointing or other symbol for "something hurts inside;"
- how to cover ears, dim lights, and so forth to increase comfort level (Repeated exposure to something that you cannot tolerate does not make you able to tolerate it.);

- how to move away from a disliked stimulus instead of moving towards it;

- words, signs, or symbols to use (Practice using these signals during a time of low or no stress. Then apply it during emotional/ highly stimulating situations.);

- watch for situations and provide words/symbols for "You feel... (best guess)." "You need to.." (Be sure to provide rewards when individuals talk about internal states.);

- refer to the book *How Does Your Engine Run* by Williams and Shellenberger to teach self-regulation and self-understanding.

How does the child or adult identify internal states and communicate about them? What skill(s) does the child or adult need to learn in this area?

## 8. Learning to Express Empathy, Sympathy, and Caring

- Friendships become more intimate and meaningful as people share their feelings with one another; it is important to express feelings appropriately to the right person and be a good listener.

- While a person may be competent at a job, s/he will not be well-liked if s/he appears cold or uncaring. Negative perceptions can affect success on the job and in social settings.

- Peers, school friends, and workmates expect others to be sensitive to their feelings and needs.

- Being a team player involves understanding and valuing the thoughts and feelings of others; this is a highly valued trait in education, sports, and business cultures.

Be sure to teach:

- that others have and express feelings "just like me;"

- that sometimes people feel the same things I do at the same time;

- that sometimes people are feeling a different feeling than me at the same time;

- that others like it when we care about their feelings;

- physical signs of emotion in others (body language, facial expression) and correct responses;

- danger signs when someone is angry and could get out of control and how to move away from that person;

- specific ways to show empathy and learn to comfort, such as offering a tissue to someone who is crying or getting them a glass of water;

- the boundaries and rules of expression of feelings—what can be shared, with whom, and when.

How does the child or adult show that he understands the feelings of others? What behavior and skills related to empathy, recognizing, and responding to the feelings of others does the child or adult need to learn?

## 9. Giving Negative Feedback—Protesting, Refusing, Disagreeing

While many people can learn to follow a sequence of events or a plan, they do not know how to appropriately express negative things such as:

- I don't want to _____.

- I don't like ____.

- I disagree with you.

- I think you are wrong.

- I won't_____.

Be sure to teach:

- how to identify the feeling when negativity is building up;

- to find a way to name and express the negative thought or feeling in a way that is not harmful;

- to choose and practice options for handling emotion in negative situations (practice in advance in supportive environments);

- how to choose words that let someone know that you do not like what they are doing or saying, but you still like them.

In what situations is expressing negative feelings, protesting or refusing a problem for the child or adult? What skills does the child or adult need to learn to express negative feelings appropriately?

## 10. Making Plan B—Fixing Situations and Dealing with the Unexpected

- There will always be unexpected occurrences.

- People with ASD do not automatically learn how to change their minds or change plans.

- Situations in which a new plan might be needed should be thought about in advance and practiced in supportive environments and then in the actual places those skills might be needed.

- These skills must be systematically taught, not just talked about.

Be sure to teach:

- What "unexpected" feels like while it is happening.

- How to stop and say, "This is something unexpected."

- How to consider several options that could fix the problem.

- To think about the options, and then choose one.

- To anticipate the "unexpected" and invent their own options in advance.

- That we can choose another option and we are still okay when something unexpected happens.

In what situation does the child or adult fall apart when something unexpected happens? What routines does the child or adult have that cannot be changed without upset? What skill(s) does the child or adult need to learn to be able to cope with the unexpected?

# Chapter 42

# *Secondary School Experiences of Students with ASD*

This chapter provides a national picture of the secondary school experiences of students with autism who received special education services under the auspices of school districts at the time they were initially sampled for the *National Longitudinal Transition Study-2* (NLTS2). Students were identified by their school districts as having autism as a primary disability. Criteria for identification as a student with autism differ from state to state, resulting in wide variation among students in the autism disability category. The variation in criteria used and the resulting variation in the ability of students included in the autism category suggest that this category includes those identified with autism spectrum disorder (ASD) and conditions such as Asperger syndrome and pervasive developmental disorder

This survey found that secondary school students with autism take a range of courses in a given semester, with many taking academic, vocational, and other types of courses, such as life skills. Most take classes in both general and special education settings, although they are more likely to take courses in a special than a general education setting.

The curriculum used to instruct the majority of students with autism who are in general education academic classes often is modified to some degree. Reports of most other teacher-directed aspects of the class, such as instructional groupings, materials used, and instructional experiences outside the classroom, are largely the same for students with autism as for their classmates.

Excerpted from "Facts from NLTS2: Secondary School Experiences of Students with Autism," U.S. Department of Education, April 2007.

This similarity of teacher-directed experiences of students with autism and their peers in general education academic classes contrasts sharply with the differences between the groups in their participation in those classes. Students with autism are consistently reported to be less likely to participate in their general education academic classes than are their classmates.

In addition to academic subjects in general education settings, students with autism take general education vocational classes. Similar to experiences in general education academic courses, many students with autism in general education vocational classes experience the same instructional practices as the class as a whole.

Almost nine in ten secondary students with autism take at least one non-vocational special education course in a semester. The use of a general education curriculum without modification is rare in such classes; the large majority of students with autism receive a curriculum with some degree of modification or specialization, or they have no curriculum at all. Students are more likely to receive individual or small group instruction in special education than in general education classes. A variety of instructional materials and equipment are used in non-vocational special education classes, augmented by instructional activities that occur outside the classroom. More than half of those with autism participate in class discussions, respond orally to questions, and work with a peer or group at least sometimes in their non-vocational special education courses.

Almost all secondary students with autism are reported to receive some type of accommodation, modification, support, technology aid, or related service. Additional time to complete assignments and tests and modified tests and assignments are among the more frequent types of accommodations. Instructional support often is provided through monitoring of students' progress by special education teachers and individual help from teacher aides, instructional assistants, or personal aides. Technology aids are less frequently provided than other types of supports and services. In addition to the accommodations and supports they receive in their classes, students with autism receive a variety of related services, addressing a wide range of needs and functional issues. Speech-language pathology services are the most frequently received type of service. Almost half of secondary students with autism have a case manager provided from or through their school to help coordinate and oversee services.

# Chapter 43

# *Preparing for Postsecondary Education*

As a student with a disability, you need to be well informed about your rights and responsibilities as well as the responsibilities postsecondary schools have toward you. You will have responsibilities as a postsecondary student that you do not have as a high school student. Office for Civil Rights (OCR) strongly encourages you to know your responsibilities and those of postsecondary schools under Section 504 and Title II. Doing so will improve your opportunity to succeed as you enter postsecondary education.

## *As a student with a disability leaving high school and entering postsecondary education, will I see differences in my rights and how they are addressed?*

Yes. Section 504 and Title II protect elementary, secondary and postsecondary students from discrimination. Nevertheless, several of the requirements that apply through high school are different from the requirements that apply beyond high school.

## *Do I have to inform a postsecondary school that I have a disability?*

No. However, if you want the school to provide an academic adjustment, you must identify yourself as having a disability. Likewise, you should let

This chapter includes text excerpted from "Students with Disabilities Preparing for Postsecondary Education: Know Your Rights and Responsibilities," U.S. Department of Education, September 2007. The complete document is available online at http://www2.ed.gov/about/offices/list/ocr/transition.html.

the school know about your disability if you want to ensure that you are assigned to accessible facilities. In any event, your disclosure of a disability is always voluntary.

### What academic adjustments must a postsecondary school provide?

The appropriate academic adjustment must be determined based on your disability and individual needs. Academic adjustments may include auxiliary aids and modifications to academic requirements as are necessary to ensure equal educational opportunity. In providing an academic adjustment, your postsecondary school is not required to lower or effect substantial modifications to essential requirements.

### If I want an academic adjustment, what must I do?

You must inform the school that you have a disability and need an academic adjustment. Your postsecondary school may require you to follow reasonable procedures to request an academic adjustment. You are responsible for knowing and following these procedures.

### Do I have to prove that I have a disability to obtain an academic adjustment?

Generally, yes. Your school will probably require you to provide documentation that shows you have a current disability and need an academic adjustment. You may need a new evaluation in order to provide the required documentation. Neither your high school nor your postsecondary school is required to conduct or pay for a new evaluation to document your disability and need for an academic adjustment.

### May a postsecondary school charge me for providing an academic adjustment?

No. Furthermore, it may not charge students with disabilities more for participating in its programs or activities than it charges students who do not have disabilities.

### What can I do if I believe the school is discriminating against me?

Contact the Section 504 coordinator, Americans with Disabilities Act (ADA) coordinator, or Disability Services coordinator who coordinates the school's compliance with Section 504 or Title II or both laws. The school must also have grievance procedures that must include steps to ensure that you may raise your concerns fully and fairly and must provide for the prompt and equitable resolution of complaints.

## *Know Your Rights*

Students with disabilities who know their rights and responsibilities are much better equipped to succeed in postsecondary school. Work with the staff at your school because they, too, want you to succeed. Seek the support of family, friends, and fellow students, including those with disabilities. Know your talents and capitalize on them, and believe in yourself as you embrace new educational challenges.

# Part Seven

# Living with Autism Spectrum Disorder and Transitioning to Adulthood

# Chapter 44

# *Safety in the Home*

Most parents and caregivers would view safety as a significant concern regarding their children in the home environment. Modifications such as placing gates in stairwells and doorways, covering electrical outlets, and using childproof locks on cabinets are some of the things many parents do to ensure safety. In response to these concerns, the Autism Society has partnered with law enforcement and a preparedness consultant to create disaster preparedness tips and a *Safe and Sound* packet.

For parents of "typical" children, such safety precautions are usually necessary for the first few years of childhood, after which the child develops, matures, and no longer requires the use of modifications. However, for parents of children on the autism spectrum, it is sometimes a different story. There are a myriad of additional issues to consider when addressing the safety of the individual with autism, family members, and the home environment—often throughout the life of the individual with autism spectrum disorder (ASD).

Consider the many behaviors an individual with autism may engage in that could be unsafe: throwing utensils, breaking plates and cups, sweeping items off surfaces, dumping drawers and bins, and climbing out of or breaking windows. Or, consider what can happen when natural curiosity and household appliances converge: putting items in appliances,

This chapter begins with "Safety in the Home," © 2008 The Autism Society (www.autism-society.org). Reprinted with permission. It concludes with "Disaster Preparedness Tips for Families Affected by Autism," © 2008 The Autism Society (www.autism-society.org). Reprinted with permission.

flushing things down the sink or toilet, touching burners, turning on hot faucets, inserting items into electrical sockets, chewing on wires, and crawling in a washer or dryer. Finally, consider the potential dangers that can result from playing with matches, lighters, or fire.

Often children with autism who display such behavioral concerns do not understand the ramifications of their actions, which at best can be bothersome and at worst can be devastatingly tragic. Therefore, it becomes incumbent upon the caregivers in the home to provide both a safe environment and ways to teach their children to be safe.

There are several environmental and safety modifications that can be made in the home as well as steps that can be taken to prevent unsafe or inappropriate behaviors. The following suggestions have been found to be helpful in preventing dangerous behaviors and ensuring a safer environment. The suggestions range from using locks for security or limiting access to the individual, to labeling every functional item and area in the home with photographs or symbols to assist in communication.

Sometimes parents balk initially at the idea of having to place locks on doors or cabinets, place alarms outside a child's bedroom, or label the house with photos or cards. They often say: "This is not a classroom." However, your home is indeed a natural learning environment, just like a classroom.

Establish priority areas for modification. Modify the most important areas first—such as the individual's bedroom, bathroom, leisure areas, kitchen, and back yard—since these are the primary areas of interaction for many children. When getting started, think about the room(s) in which the child spends the most time; for some children, it would be a recreation/family room, whereas for others it might be the bedroom or kitchen. In addition, consider the behaviors to be modified and the relationship of those behaviors to the environment. Behavior modification works to alter an individual's behavior through positive and negative reinforcement. Remember that behaviors always serve some purpose, and in order to alter a particular behavior it must first be understood. If the individual likes to put things in the toilet or run hot water in the bath, modifications should begin in the bathroom. If the child runs out of the house, modifications should begin with securing exterior doors with locks.

**Arrange the furniture appropriately:** Arrange the furniture in a way that "makes sense" for the activities the individual is expected to do. That is, if the individual will be doing "seated" activities, ensure that there are clear table surfaces and appropriate chairs. If the child frequently runs out of a room via a predictable path, arrange the furniture and close doors so that he or she is unable to escape. Limit the need for excessive movement and/or transition. Move furniture away from shelves or places where the child may climb. Keep furniture surfaces clear (if the individual is a "sweeper") and place items out of reach on shelves or bins, or lock things away. In addition, use gates or barriers to provide safety from falling down steps or to limit access to certain areas in the home.

**Use locks where appropriate:** It is important to place locks on exterior doors that provide entry or departure to and from the home. For individuals who run away or leave the home without supervision (also referred to as "elopement"), having locks on the doors can prevent them from leaving. Place locks on interior doors and cabinets where the individual should not have free access.

Some parents feel more secure when their child is locked in his or her bedroom at night to prevent "middle of the night" wandering. If you choose to put locks on the doors, use locks that you are able to open, such as a lock with a keyhole/key, a hook-and-eye lock, or a slide-bolt. Some parents place the lock key above the door frame of the room to have quick and easy access. If a button-knob lock is used on the outside of the door, make sure that the child does not lock you into the room with him or her. It is imperative that you have immediate access to any room where the door is locked in the event of fire or other emergency.

Regarding locks on cabinets and drawers, use safety locks (often plastic devices) to secure items that may be unsafe for the individual. Many parents place these locks on bathroom and kitchen cabinets to prevent access to items in the cabinets.

**Safeguard your windows:** If your child likes to climb out of windows, place locks on them. Hardware stores carry special locks for just this purpose. If your child breaks glass or pounds windows, replace the glass panes with Plexiglas to prevent injury. Some parents have had to also place wooden boards over windows to prevent injury or elopement.

**Make electrical outlets and appliances safe:** Cover or remove electrical outlets and access to electrical appliances. Use plastic knob covers (also available at hardware stores) for doors, faucets, ovens, and stove burners. Lock the door to the room or rooms with the washer or dryer, appliances, or power tools to limit access. Ensure that all wiring for appliances and electronics is concealed in a way that the child cannot play with the wires. Individuals on the autism spectrum often have a curious interest in how things work, but that can be coupled with a pervasive "unawareness" of dangerous situations—a potentially powerful combination when it comes to electrical materials.

**Lock dangerous items away:** Secure items that are dangerous if ingested, such as detergents, chemicals, cleaning supplies, pesticides, medications, and small items that a child may mouth or chew. It is easy for an individual with autism to confuse a bottle of yellow cleaning fluid with juice based upon appearance or to pour/spill liquids out of a bottle (some of which may be poisonous or toxic). Also, pills that look like candy can easily be eaten by mistake. Place such items out of reach or in cabinets with locks. Keep the poison control phone number in a permanent place that is clearly in view.

Secure items and materials that are dangerous or unsafe if used without supervision such as sharp objects and utensils (scissors, knives, razor blades). When unsupervised, many children like to cut things (clothing, curtains, wires, books, and so forth) into pieces with scissors or knives. If necessary, use scissors that have blunted ends (child-safety scissors), and be sure to provide supervision when the child is involved in cutting activities. In addition, secure items that need to be limited (for example: candy, video games, lighters, matches, televisions, digital video disc [DVD] player, toilet tank covers) with a lock or ties.

**Label everyday items:** Place visual labels (symbols, photos, words, textures) on functional items, rooms, cabinets, drawers, bins, closets, and anything that has relevance for the child. By labeling the environment, a child with ASD may better understand what is expected and may be less likely to engage in undesirable behaviors. In addition, if the child understands the function of an item (such as a piece of furniture), he/she is more likely to use it for its intended purpose. For example, by placing visual labels on the bed for sleeping, the child may be less likely to view the bed as a trampoline. Placing labels on drawers and closets may reduce power struggles over asking your child to put things away because he/she will know where to put them.

**Organize everyday items:** Organize functional items in see-through plastic bins or boxes with visual labels (symbols, photos, words, textures) so the child can see and use the receptacles. Place the bins on shelves or in places that the child can easily see and access. Once again, the better the organization, order, and structure in the environment, the more likely it will reduce the frustration level of a child on the autism spectrum, and the less likely he or she will be to engage in appropriate behaviors.

**Institute appropriate seating:** Ensuring that the individual is seated properly at a table or work station can help prevent behavioral problems, such as throwing objects, knocking over furniture, self-stimulatory behaviors, and acts of aggression. For example, some children need to be seated in chairs with arms or a wrap-around style desk when doing work. Others may need to be seated in a place where they cannot easily escape from the table, such as against the wall or in a corner. In addition, a proper sitting posture (body at a right angle and feet flat on the floor) will help facilitate good learning and/or eating behaviors.

**Use visual signs:** Use dividers, tape boundaries, and signs as needed for setting expectations and limits. For example, the use of stop signs on doors, drawers, furniture, and appliances has helped some children understand that these items or areas are off limits. For children who climb on high surfaces or enter areas that they should not, stop signs will let them know that what they are doing is dangerous. Using color tape to designate boundaries on carpets, floors, or walls can help to visually remind children where their bodies need to remain.

**Secure eating utensils and place settings:** When using utensils during mealtimes, consider tying utensils to nylon string and attaching them to the chair or leg of the table. This way if the child throws the utensils, they will remain attached to the string. There have been children who have "unintentionally" thrown forks across the table and injured other family members. If the child throws or sweeps plates, bowls, and cups, secure them with adhesive Velcro and attach them to a secure placement. Use plastic or rubber plates, bowls, and cups to prevent shattering of breakable items.

**Safeguard bath items/toys:** Consider keeping bath toys in a bag or bin away from the tub and unavailable until bathing or hair washing are completed. This will help the child focus on bathing and prevent power struggles while in the tub. You do not want a child flailing around while in a slippery bathtub since he, she, or you could be injured. When the child is finished bathing or hair washing, you can then give access to tub toys. Keep bath items (soap, washcloth, shampoo, sponges) together in a plastic bin or rubber bag and accessible. Replace open-lip bottles with pump dispensers so the child will not empty or ingest the contents.

**Remember fire safety:** Regarding fire safety, it is important to keep lighters and matches out of reach or locked up. Place safety covers over gas stoves and oven knobs so that a child cannot turn them on. Always supervise children closely when there is an active fire in the fireplace or when there is a barbecue with open flames. Many community fire departments can provide stickers (called tot finders) for bedroom windows of children, so that in the event of a fire, the firefighters can locate a child's bedroom quickly. While it may be difficult to teach an individual on the autism spectrum about the dangerous nature of fire, it may be possible to teach him or her about how to behave when it comes to fire safety.

Developing social stories (with photographs, pictures, words) about smoke detectors, fire drills, fire alarms, touching fire, and so forth, and reading the stories to the child on a regular basis is the place to begin. (A social story is a short, personalized story that explains the subtle cues in social situations and breaks down a situation or task into easy-to-follow steps). In addition to social stories, the use of visuals (photos, pictures) can assist the child in understanding what they are not supposed to do and/ or what they are expected to do. For example, a "no touching the oven burners" sign could consist of a photograph of the oven burners with a bright red "no" symbol or stop sign over the photograph to visually depict the rule for the child.

**Consider identification options:** It is important that your child has proper identification in the event that he or she runs away or gets lost and is unable to communicate effectively. Once a child with ASD becomes mobile, he or she may decide to walk out of the home without supervision. Children on the autism spectrum often like to be outside and in motion, so leaving the home to go outside is common. Once outside the home, the child is then vulnerable and may be unable to get home or communicate where they live.

If the child will tolerate wearing a medical identification (ID) bracelet or necklace, get one (they can be found your local drug store). However, many children with autism do not like to wear jewelry, so the next best option is to place iron-on labels into each garment. Some children can be taught to carry and provide an identification card from a wallet or fanny pack and can learn to show their identification cards if they are not able to verbalize the information to another person. Some parents have also used specially designed tracking devices, perimeter systems, or service dogs for children on the spectrum who are known to elope.

**Introduce intervention techniques to teach safety:** In addition to the physical modifications to your home, you will want to introduce behavior modification techniques to teach your child how to be safe and act appropriately. There are a myriad of augmentative behavioral interventions that can be employed to do this. Examples of these interventions would be: social stories, activity schedules, visual rules, signs and charts, peer and adult modeling, reinforcement for safe and appropriate behavior, and consistent consequences for unsafe or inappropriate behavior.

Once general safety, good judgment, competence, and understanding of what is expected can be demonstrated, many of the environmental modifications can be faded over time. Introducing the home modifications and intervention techniques mentioned will not only help to keep your child and your family out of harm's way, they will also help ensure that your child is ready and able to learn and, ultimately, better able to reach his or her full potential.

**Resources:** Most of the items and products (safety knobs for appliances, locks, and so forth) mentioned, can be purchased from hardware stores, department stores, and children's stores in your community. You can also contact your fire department to see whether they have locator stickers or other materials to foster fire safety.

## Disaster Preparedness Tips for Families Affected by Autism

With the help of renowned emergency preparedness expert Dennis Debbaudt, who has a son with autism, and Autism Society Board Member Ruth Elaine Hane, the Autism Society—with support from NASCAR driver and Autism Society friend Jamie McMurray—is committed to helping families with special needs prepare for emergencies. During any emergency, whether it be weather-related or man-made, we want those in the autism community to be prepared.

Should you have access to a video recorder or camera, it is strongly recommended that you videotape your property and important possessions. Then, send copies of those photos or videos to a friend or family member in another location for safe keeping.

### Tip #1: Practice Calm

Parents and care providers need to project a demeanor of calm during a disaster or emergency, even if we're not. Children and adults on the spectrum may sense your emotional state—and mimic it. Practice for and prepare to project a sense of calm.

## *Tip #2: Prepare for Immediate Needs before Disaster*

Be ready to evacuate. Have a plan for getting you and your loved ones out of your home or building (ask family or friends for assistance, if necessary). Also, plan two evacuation routes because some roads may be closed or blocked in a disaster.

Create a self-help network of relatives, friends or co-workers to assist in an emergency. If you think you may need assistance in a disaster, discuss needs with relatives, friends, and co-workers and ask for their help. Give a key to a trusted neighbor or friend who may be able to assist you in a disaster.

Contact your local emergency information management office now. Many local emergency management offices maintain registers of people with disabilities so they can be located and assisted quickly in a disaster. For a list of state offices and agencies, visit www.fema.gov/about/contact/statedr.shtm.

Wearing a medical alert tag or bracelet to identify your disability may help in case of an emergency.

If you have a severe speech, language, or hearing disability, do the following:

1.  When you dial 911, tap space bar to indicate TDD call.

2.  Store a writing pad and pencils to communicate with others.

3.  Keep a flashlight handy to signal whereabouts to other people and for illumination to aid in communication.

4.  Remind friends that you cannot completely hear warnings or emergency instructions. Ask them to be your source of emergency information as it comes over their radio.

5.  If you have a service dog, be aware that the dog may become confused or disoriented in an emergency. Store extra food, water, and supplies for your dog (as well as yourself). Plan to take care of your pets in advance, particularly if sheltering is necessary, so you can concentrate on the rest of the family.

Have a disaster supply kit prepared that you can use at home or in an evacuation setting. Kits should include these items:

1.  Flashlight with extra batteries

2.  Portable, battery-operated radio and extra batteries

3.  First aid kit and manual

4.  Emergency food and water for at least two days (per person)

5. Manual can opener

6. Essential medicines for three to seven days

7. Cash and credit cards (withdraw cash in advance if possible)

8. Sturdy shoes

Also, in case of evacuation, pack a safety and comfort kit, which can include the following:

1. Blanket

2. Pillow

3. Folding chair

4. Sleeping bag or cot

5. Personal hygiene items

6. Identification and valuable documents (insurance, birth and marriage certificates, and special-needs forms)

7. Change of clothes

8. "Comfort" items such as a compact disk (CD) player and CDs (with extra batteries) or a DVD player and DVDs

9. Ear plugs or eye shades

10. Storage boxes to store small items (could be plastic with fitted lids)

11. A drawing of the building layout and map of the area to give an orientation of where you are in relation to your home

12. An identification (ID) bracelet and autism information cards to explain behaviors to others

Some of these helpful tips are provided in part by FEMA's report, "Disaster Preparedness for People with Disabilities." To view the FEMA report in its entirety, go to www.fema.gov/library/viewRecord. do?id=1442.

### *Tip #3: If Disaster Strikes*

Look for items that may have broken or been displaced that could cause a hazard, particularly electrical lines.

Beware of carbon monoxide poisoning. People have died or been poisoned by carbon monoxide in times of disaster due to the use of generators, grills, camp stoves, or other gasoline, propane, natural gas or charcoal-burning devices inside the home, basement, garage or camper or even outside near an open window. The Centers for Disease Control and Prevention (CDC) warns that you should never use these devices inside.

# Chapter 45

# *Ensuring Support at Home*

## Chapter Contents

# Section 45.1

# *Family Support Models*

## *Why Family Support Is Important*

There are an estimated 500,000 to 1,000,000 individuals living with autism in the United States at this time. From this, an assumption can be made that there are somewhere between 2–6 million immediate family members of people with autism and innumerable extended family members living with or around them. Each one of these individuals may, at different times in their lives, experience a significant degree of stress associated with meeting the complex and idiosyncratic challenges of having a family member with autism. In order to address this need, systems of family support need to be available, individualized, flexible, and relevant to the needs of individual families at a given point in time. The benefits, if we do this, are significant and include the following:

- Family functioning is less disrupted.

- The preservation of intact families is supported.

- Educational benefits accrue to the child with autism spectrum disorder (ASD).

- There are reductions in the use of crisis models of support.

- There is the potential for long-term cost savings as we shift from a crisis intervention model of family support to one based upon preventing crises in the first place.

## *A Functional Definition of Family Support*

From an applied behavioral analysis (ABA) perspective, the term support needs to be viewed in the same functional manner as is the term reinforcement. Just as something can be called a reinforcer only if it increases behavior, parent support interventions should only be considered support if they reduce parental stress and/or increase adaptation. In other words, what is support to one may be stress to another.

## Models of Family Support

### Parent Training

Parent training is generally regarded as integral to successful adaptation (for example: Koegel and Koegel, 1995) to the birth of a child with autism but, over time, some of the initial benefits may wane. Some of the challenges that may impact the support component of parent training may include the following:

- Failure to attend to issues of role clarity and potential conflicts (being a parent versus being a therapist).

- The development of a disproportionate sharing of training responsibilities between both parents so that one parent, (often the mother) is forced to adopt a senior trainer position.

- Home and family issues often grow in complexity as individual's age and brief parent training sessions may be insufficient to address these new challenges.

- Training needs to be specifically tailored to each individual family's situation and, as such, may require greater resources than may be available.

### Parent Support Groups

Parent support groups may provide attendees with several benefits including, "1) alleviating loneliness and isolation [and] 2) providing information" (Seligman and Darling, 1989, p. 44). However, challenges to support component of such groups may include:

- restricted access to the group for either or both parents due to such things as distance or lack of competent childcare;

- the costs associated with accessing specialized child care;

- the diversity of needs reported by families of children with autism may make it difficult for any one family's needs to be met;

- the competence of the facilitator may vary from group to group.

However, some recent reports (for example, Hsiung, 2000; Wellman, Haase, Witte and Hampton, 2000) indicate that access to the internet and online support groups may help reduce the impact of some of these challenges.

## Respite Services

Respite services are designed to provide families a regularly scheduled break (respite) from the demands of being primary caretaker for their child with a developmental disability (Abelson, 1999). When consistently available and provided by trained staff, respite services can provide some much needed support. Potential challenges to the support component of respite, however, may include these:

- Restricted access to respite services particularly for more rural families.

- The availability of staff trained to meet the complex needs of learners with autism, particularly in the context of a given family's home, is generally low.

- Questions persist regarding the perceived high turnover of respite staff.

- There are varying degrees of comfort with a service (for example, having someone in your home) itself.

- Funding for respite varies from state to state and, at times, from county to county to within a state.

## Integrated Models of Family Support

Integrated models of family support (for example, Turnbull and Turnbull, 1997) endeavor to provide services as a function of family characteristics, interactions, functions, and life cycle. Under this model, families are able to choose from a variety of supports (in or out of home respite, family training, support groups, monetary vouchers, and so forth) that best meet their needs at a given point in time. While limitations such as cost or availability may be significant, the ability of families to choose from a menu of individual services based upon their perception of need would appear to be congruent with our previous, functional definition of support resulting in decreased stress and increased accommodation, satisfaction and happiness.

## Section 45.2

# *Grandparents Play Key Role in Lives of Children with ASD*

April 6, 2010, the Interactive Autism Network (IAN), www.ianproject .org, the nation's largest online autism research project, announced results of the *Grandparents of Children with Autism Spectrum Disorders Survey*, finding that nearly one-third of grandparents who participated were the first to raise concerns about their grandchild's development. Since its launch in 2007, the IAN Project has helped to accelerate the pace of autism research by gathering valuable information online from individuals on the autism spectrum and their parents. The launch of the October 2009 survey was the first time that the IAN Project has collected information from grandparents. The *IAN Research Report: Grandparents of Children with ASD–Part 1*, and the subsequent report that will be released later in the month, demonstrate the substantial impact having a grandchild on the spectrum has on grandparents' lives, as well as the contributions they make through early detection— which is crucial to early diagnosis and intervention, child care, and financial support.

"It became clear that grandparents—a population largely overlooked by policymakers and researchers—had valuable insights to share when they came to us asking how they could participate in the IAN Project," said Dr. Paul Law, Director of the IAN Project at the Kennedy Krieger Institute in Baltimore, Maryland. "These survey results show that experiences are remarkably diverse, but one thing is clear: grandparents often play a major part in their grandchild's life and experience their own stresses and triumphs in these families."

In just eight weeks, more than 2,600 grandparents completed the survey. The findings highlighted summarize the compelling results from the *Research Report* released April 6, 2010 as well as Part 2 of the report.

493

## The Grandparents and Their Families

Grandparents represented a wide age range, although most were between the ages of 55 and 74.

- Family relationships: Nearly 90% felt that the experience of facing their grandchild's situation together had brought them and their adult child—the grandchild's parent—closer, although many worried for their adult child raising a child on the autism spectrum.

- Support and coping: Of those who were married or in a committed relationship, 92% said they felt their spouse or partner supported them always, or most of the time. The majority of grandparents reported that they had adjusted to their grandchild's diagnosis and were doing very or fairly well.

- Genetics in autism: Approximately 15% of grandparents had two or more grandchildren on the spectrum. Of those with more than one grandchild with ASD, two-thirds reported that their grandchildren were siblings, while the other third reported their grandchildren with ASD were cousins.

## Grandparents as Caregivers

Many grandparents played a major role in raising concerns about their grandchild's development.

- Fully 30% said they were the first to raise concerns about their grandchild, while another 49% said they had supported others who began to raise concerns.

- Grandparents often play a major role in helping care for a grandchild with ASD: Nearly 11% reported living in the same household as their grandchild, with another 46% living within 24 miles. In addition, of those who were traditional grandparents (not their grandchild's custodial parent), 14% said they and their grandchild's family had moved closer to each other so they could help the grandchild's family "manage all that is involved with his or her ASD," while 7% said they had actually combined households for the same reason.

- 71% said they played some role in treatment decisions for their grandchild.

- More than 15% were providing transportation for their affected grandchild to or from appointments or school at least once per week.

- More than 31% said they provided some direct child care at least once per week.

## Proactive Grandparents

- Participating grandparents kept themselves very well informed about ASDs; 99% said they "read or do research to better understand autism spectrum disorders" because of their grandchild's diagnosis.

- Grandparents were very active in advocating for their grandchildren on the autism spectrum, with nearly 50% taking part in autism walks or fundraisers, 33% involved in political advocacy, and 31% attending conferences or workshops on autism.

## Financial Impact

A significant majority of grandparents reported contributing to their grandchild's general or special financial needs.

- More than 22% reported going without something they had hoped for in order to provide for their grandchild's financial needs. In fact, 18% had become primary babysitter so their adult child could work, 11% had raided retirement funds, and 8% had borrowed money.

- Nearly 60% had made sacrifices not provided in response choices, such as working more hours or taking on a second job, providing respite care, or leaving funds in a special needs trust.

- About 25% of grandparents reported spending up to $99 per month to meet their grandchild's autism-related needs, while 30% paid even higher amounts. There were some grandparents spending more than $500 per month.

"It is hoped that the results of this survey will help researchers, policymakers, and advocates learn about the experiences and opinions of grandparents of children with an ASD, and advance efforts to advocate for improved services and resources," said Dr. Law.

# Chapter 46

# *Depression, Parenting, and ASD*

It is not easy to be the parent of a child on the autism spectrum. There are joyous moments, but there is no denying the challenges parents face, and the toll these take. Parents worry themselves sick, fight for services, sacrifice careers, sink into debt, and rage at the injustice of it all. Parents grieve.

Researchers have tried to understand the strain involved, and its effects. They have studied depression and anxiety, as well as stress and coping, in the parents of children with disabilities. If we can understand what stresses have the most negative impact on families, we can move to address them. If we can figure out what psychiatric issues run in families, we can be ready to intervene sooner rather than later, helping both parents and children at risk to function better and lead more satisfying lives.

## *Stress and Well-Being*

Most parents of children with disabilities or chronic health problems suffer a great deal of stress. There is evidence, however, that parents of children on the autism spectrum suffer the most stress of all.

This chapter includes "Relieving Parental Stress and Depression: How Helping Parents Helps Children," by Connie Anderson, PhD. Reprinted with permission from the interactive Autism Network (IAN) Community (www.iancommunity. org), © 2010 Kennedy Krieger Institute. To view this article with references, visit http://www.iancommunity.org/cs/articles/parental_depression. Also, Tables 46.1 and 46.2 under the section titled "Mothers, Fathers, and Depression," are reprinted with permission from the Interactive Autism Network (IAN) Community (www .iancommunity.org), © 2009 Kennedy Krieger Institute.

There are several reasons why the stress of those parenting children with an autism spectrum disorder (ASD) is so high. All parents of children with disabilities must cope with grief, worries about the future, and the struggle to find and obtain appropriate services. Parents of children with ASDs face some additional stressors. First, they often live with uncertainty about what caused their child's autism, as well as possible guilt (no matter how undeserved) over whether they did or failed to do something that led to their child's ASD.

Second, the core disability associated with ASDs is a social one. Most parents hope for a warm and loving relationship with their child. It is bewildering to find you have a baby who does not like to be held, or a child who will not look into your eyes. Parents adapt, learning to love the way their child loves, but usually not without having passed through some confusion and pain.

Third, no matter what their specific ASD diagnosis or intelligence quotient (IQ), children on the autism spectrum often have problem behaviors, from refusal to sleep, to intense and frequent tantrums, to extreme rigidity. These behaviors can make living with them day-to-day very trying and lead to another variety of guilt: the kind you experience when you are not feeling loving toward a difficult child. In addition, such behaviors strain the entire family, impacting sibling relationships and marriages.

A number of studies have specifically linked the troublesome behaviors of children on the autism spectrum to high levels of parental stress. Such stress is not only damaging in its own right, but also has been linked to higher rates of depression.

## Depression

When a child is diagnosed with an autism spectrum disorder, grief and worry are natural reactions. Parents struggle to learn everything they can about autism as quickly as possible, forced to make major decisions with far from perfect knowledge while navigating complex education and healthcare bureaucracies. Some suffer periods of sadness in addition to periods of stress. Some may feel more than sadness. They may actually become clinically depressed.

Everyone feels down now and then, and parents of children with ASDs may feel down more often than most. Clinical depression is more than feeling down, however. It is not "the blues" but a diagnosable medical condition. A major depressive episode, as defined by the psychiatric bible—*The Diagnostic and Statistical Manual of Mental Disorders, Fourth Edition (DSM-IV)*—must include at least five of the following symptoms:

1. Depressed mood most of the day, nearly every day, as indicated by either subjective report (feels sad or empty) or observation made by others (appears tearful).

2. Markedly diminished interest or pleasure in all, or almost all, activities most of the day, nearly every day (as indicated by either subjective account or observation made by others).

3. Significant weight loss when not dieting or weight gain (such as, a change of more than 5% of body weight in a month), or decrease or increase in appetite nearly every day.

4. Insomnia or hypersomnia nearly every day. (In other words, a person doesn't sleep, or sleeps far more than usual.)

5. Psychomotor agitation or retardation nearly every day (observable by others, not merely subjective feelings of restlessness or being slowed down).

6. Fatigue or loss of energy nearly every day.

7. Feelings of worthlessness or excessive or inappropriate guilt (which may be delusional) nearly every day (not merely self-reproach or guilt about being sick).

8. Diminished ability to think or concentrate, or indecisiveness, nearly every day (either by subjective account or as observed by others).

9. Recurrent thoughts of death (not just fear of dying), recurrent suicidal ideation without a specific plan, or a suicide attempt, or a specific plan for committing suicide.

All of a person's symptoms must have been present during the same two-week period and must represent a change from previous functioning. At least one of the symptoms must be depressed mood or loss of interest or pleasure.

The important thing to note is that a psychiatrist will not give a diagnosis of depression to a person who just feels low. Beyond the mood issue, there are physical components: trouble sleeping or sleeping constantly, restlessness or lethargy, increased or decreased appetite, and fatigue.

### Stress and Depression: Connections

Researchers are trying to learn which parents of children with ASD are sad and stressed, and which suffer from true clinical depression.

They are also exploring how stress and depression may be related. Some of the connections are as follows:

**Depression and stress are both believed to be impacted by neurobiological factors,** such as neurotransmitters that are not working properly. Anti-depressant medications can help by intervening in this process that has gone wrong.

**Depression and stress are both known to be influenced by attitudes and ways of thinking and living that are associated with resilience,** that is, with being able to keep managing through high levels of stress. These include optimism and humor, the ability to accept a situation and move on, a tendency to cope by taking action (as opposed to falling into a passive, resigned state), spiritual belief, altruism, and advocacy. Cognitive-behavioral therapy is an example of a treatment that helps people change their way of thinking to fight depression. Empowering people helps them, too, as they can become less passive and more active in trying to better their situation.

**Depression and stress may share a genetic basis.** Recent scientific studies show that a naturally occurring variation of a specific gene is linked to stress and depression. Individuals with this gene seem to experience stressful life events more intensely than people with a different variation of the gene. They are also more likely to suffer symptoms of depression. This is evidence of a gene-by-environment interaction. Stressful events occur, but genetics influences how deeply their impact is felt and the likelihood that depression will follow.

Some researchers have actually found evidence of a possible genetic connection between major mood disorders and autism. Studies have found both parents of children with ASDs and the children with ASDs themselves are more prone to major depressive disorder than other parents and children. This may help to explain the very high figures for reported depression in parents of children with ASDs found by the IAN Project.

If such a connection is confirmed, it will be clear that there is some biological, genetic link between major mood disorders and at least some types of autism. This may lead to new insights about both types of disorder, and hopefully, to interventions. Meanwhile, those working with families will know they should be on the look out for mood disorders both in children with ASDs and in family members. Hopefully, intervention will then occur sooner rather than later, with better outcomes for all.

## Gender Differences—Moms and Dads

Researchers have found that mothers of children with autism, as compared with mothers of unaffected children or children with other disabilities, suffer the most from depressive symptoms. Fathers also suffer from such symptoms, but to a lesser extent than mothers. This may be due in part to a gender difference in how distress is expressed. The DSM-IV, for example, states that irritability can be a symptom of depression for children and adolescents. Some researchers are now suggesting that this irritability criterion might be valid for men, as well. Others claim that men tend to become depressed in reaction to different stressors than women do, with problems at work and divorce felt more keenly by men, and problems in their network of interpersonal relationships felt more keenly by women. (Note that having a child with a disability is more likely to disrupt a mother's relationships with relatives, friends, school personnel, and health-care representatives than it is to disrupt a father's job.) Still others theorize that there are many stressors that impact women more often than men, including sexual victimization, poverty, single parenthood, and the burdens of caring for the elderly, which may account for some of the difference.

Furthermore, research has shown that women in families with a child on the spectrum tend to bear the brunt of day-to-day burdens and domestic labor; end up responsible for managing the higher levels of conflict in these families (between autistic and non-autistic siblings, for example); and receive more blame from outsiders and their spouse for their child's behavior. Any of these could certainly detract from a caregiver's ability to cope.

## Chicken and Egg—Child Behavior and Parent Distress

Does a child's difficult behavior make parents depressed, or is it a parent's depression that adds to a child's difficulties? Thanks to the specter of the now-debunked refrigerator mother theory, this is a touchy question. The refrigerator mother theory blamed a mother's cold, rejecting stance toward her child for that child's autism. Wrote the producers of a documentary film on the subject: "If anything could be more devastating to a mother than having her child succumb to autism, it might be having to shoulder the blame for the affliction. That's what happened to a generation of mothers in the 1950s and '60s, when medical orthodoxy blamed autism on the mother's failure to bond with her child. Though wholly discredited today, the 'refrigerator mother' diagnosis condemned thousands of autistic children to questionable therapies, and their mothers to a long nightmare of self-doubt and guilt."

Mother-blaming is the last thing anyone wants to do now. On the other hand, there is no question that a parent in distress is not likely to parent as well as one who is feeling in balance and able to handle whatever may come. Maternal depression, for example, has been shown to be associated with psychosocial maladjustment among children with disabilities. Remaining calm and matter-of-fact while a child screams does not come easily to anyone, least of all to someone already feeling unable to cope. Yet screaming back will likely only escalate the situation, spinning a child with little ability to self-regulate further out of control.

Family systems theory describes the back-and-forth of the situation, how each person's distress impacts the others, and vice versa. Helping anyone in the system has the potential to help all. In other words, improve child behavior and Mom and Dad may become less stressed and better able to manage whatever may come. Decrease Mom's and Dad's stress or depression and they may be more able to manage their child's behavior in a firm and calm manner, helping the child to stay in better balance.

In fact, research has shown that teaching parents skills that help them to improve their child's behavior, or teaching them skills that help them cope through their own distress, is very helpful. Moreover, it appears that providing both types of interventions is more effective than providing either strategy alone.

It is important to note, however, that it is not only the coping skills of parents that need to be addressed. The development of better treatments that improve children's functioning will go a long way toward helping children and their families. The provision of appropriate services, including respite care, will help families. Improving the systems with which families must interact will help families. The better the programs offered by schools, state departments of disability, or health-care organizations, the less stress families will suffer when trying to obtain help for their children.

## *How Parents Are Doing Matters*

Sometimes you will hear a desperate parent say, "Forget about me. It doesn't matter how I feel. Just take care of my child." This sentiment is understandable, but it ignores that the family is a system, and that each person has an impact on the others. Decreasing the stress faced by parents of children with ASDs, and doing everything possible to improve their mental health and ability to cope, is a worthwhile goal. Helping parents helps children, too.

## Mothers, Fathers, and Depression

### *Why is this important?*

Parent mental health is important in ASD families for several reasons. For one thing, mental health status indicates how parents are faring as they cope with the stresses of having a child with an ASD. In addition, researchers are interested in genetic factors: do depression and ASDs run together in some families? Or is it the stress of having a child with an ASD that contributes to depression in mothers?

Table 46.1 shows that nearly half of the mothers taking part in IAN Research, at some time in their lives, have been diagnosed with or treated for depression.

**Table 46.1.** Mothers and Depression: Data from IAN Research: Have you ever been diagnosed with or received treatment for depression?

| | |
|---|---|
| Yes | 48% |
| No | 52% |

**Table 46.2.** Fathers and Depression: Data from IAN Research Have you ever been diagnosed with or received treatment for depression?

| | |
|---|---|
| Yes | 22% |
| No | 78% |

Table 46.2 shows that 22% of the fathers taking part in IAN Research, at some time in their lives, have been diagnosed with or treated for depression.

# Chapter 47

# *Toilet Training Children with ASD*

Teaching your child to use the toilet correctly can be a difficult task, whether they have autism or not. But if your child has autism, the process of developing a toilet routine can take longer, and involve its own particular challenges. This guide provides some useful steps that will hopefully make your toilet training a success.

There are many factors you need to take into consideration when deciding the right time to start toilet training. Choose a time when you have few engagements and are feeling relatively stress free. Concentrate on one behavior; it's very difficult to change two behaviors at once so tackle one issue at a time. Ideally, everyone working with your child will start toilet training at the same time and follow your agreed approach, so make sure your child's school/caregiver and so forth are aware of when you are starting the routine, the steps to be followed and the equipment needed. Your child may behave differently than normal during this time especially when the change of routine first takes place so it's a good idea to let everyone know why there could be a change in behavior.

Remember that independent toileting is the ultimate aim and may take many months but there will be many small steps and successes along the way.

---

Excerpted from "Toilet Training," © 2010 National Autistic Society (www.autism.org.uk). Reprinted with permission.

## Developing a Toileting Routine

Children with an autistic spectrum disorder (ASD) often like routine. You can build upon this desire for predictability to develop a successful toilet training routine. Teach as a whole routine from communicating need to using the toilet to drying hands, rather than just sitting on the toilet. Keep the sequence of behaviors the same every time and use visual cues to support the routine. Often when an activity is anticipated, less resistance occurs. There are some examples of visual supports on the Do 2 Learn website at www.dotolearn.com/picturecards/printcards/index.htm

The first sign that a child might be ready to start toilet training is when they start to become aware of needing to go to the toilet. This may be displayed by changes in behavior patterns, appearing distracted or fidgeting when they are wet or have soiled, or they may inform a parent/caregiver when they need changing. In terms of physical readiness, it is suggested that a good indicator would be whether a child is able to remain clean for one to two hours at a time. As well as physical factors associated with toilet training, there are social factors to consider. It is rare for a child with autism to have the social motivation to want to be like mummy/daddy/friend and use the toilet. Your child might not see the point in changing to use the toilet after using diapers for a number of years. Change can be very difficult for children with autism, so therefore, it is often easier not to use a potty as part of toilet training to avoid another change from potty to toilet.

When changing your child's diaper, do this where the toilet is so they can start relating toileting activities to the bathroom. Observe your child over a few days or a week to see when they do a wee or a poo. It is quite usual for a fairly regular pattern to emerge, especially if mealtimes and drinks are provided at about the same time every day. Identifying the times can help to establish when to take your child to the toilet with an increased likelihood of them doing a wee or poo leading to positive reinforcement. Show your child a photo or drawing of the toilet and say *"your child's name, toilet,"* take them into the toilet, follow your visual sequence for undressing, and sit your child on the toilet. Even if they do not open their bowel or bladder, continue to follow the visual sequence as if they had.

Continue to take your child at set times based on your observations of when they are most likely to go. If they wet themselves at another time, take them to the toilet as quickly as possible, and try to get them there so some of the wee goes into the toilet. Ignore the wetting and positively reinforce that the wee has gone into the toilet and continue the rest of the toileting routine. You will need to decide whether or not, and how, to praise your child for successfully following the toileting routine. Some children enjoy and respond to social praise (good boy, or a tickle), others respond better to an object. Some children find praise difficult and keeping a calm, structured routine with a preferred activity after toileting may work better. It's important to remember that all children are different and they will not all respond to the same teaching techniques—what works for one child may not work for another.

Having a visual sequence beside the toilet can help your child understand what is expected of them, for example: trousers down, pants down, sit on the toilet, wee/poo in the toilet, wipe (you may need to show how many squares of paper to take), pants up, trousers up, flush toilet, wash hands. Above the sink at eye level you would then have another picture routine for washing hands (see hand washing section). Make sure the pictures are very clear so there is no misunderstanding. For example, if you are teaching your son to stand and wee in the toilet, show an outline drawing of him standing and weeing in the toilet, if you are teaching sitting, show a picture of him sitting and weeing in the toilet.

## Dressing and Undressing

While toilet training, dress your child in clothes they can easily manage themselves: elasticized waist bands on trousers and skirts or dresses that are not too long. The clothing needs to be comfortable so beware of labels, tags, or seams that may rub. Thomas the Tank Engine or Barbie underwear can be a great motivator for some children to begin toilet training.

Your child may have to be taught how much they need to undress to use the toilet. Use clear pictures and language. "Backward chaining" can be an effective way to teach new skills. This involves breaking a skill down into smaller steps, teaching the last stage of the sequence first. So if you were teaching your child to pull up his trousers you would pull them up to his hips, and then he would pull them up to his waist. Next time you would pull then up to just under his hips, and he would pull them over his hips and waist. This is a particularly good way of teaching new skills as it raises your child's self-esteem as they have taken the final step of the task themselves to complete the sequence.

## Hand Washing

Teach hand washing as part of the whole toileting routine. Follow the same steps each time: sleeves up, tap on, wet hands, squirt soap, rub hands together, rinse hands, turn off tap, shake hands, dry hands. At first you may need to stand behind your child and physically prompt them, slowly withdrawing. Beware of using verbal prompts as your child can become dependent on these without you realizing. Have a laminated hand washing sequence at eye level above the sink to remind your child of the steps they need to take. The sequence can either be in photographs, pictures, or the written word—whatever is most suitable and motivating for your child. You may need to create a way of removing or covering over each symbol as the step is completed to show that it is finished and to move on to the next step.

You may wish to teach your child to use the cold tap only. Beware that if you teach them to use the hot tap independently at home when they go into other settings and wash their hands the water may be too hot and could burn them.

## Boys—Sit or Stand?

When deciding whether to teach a boy to sit or stand to urinate ask yourself the following questions:

- Can they distinguish between when they want to wee or poo?

- Do they have the co-ordination, focus and control needed to aim?

- If they learn by imitation, is there someone they can watch?

If the answer to any of these is yes, then they are probably able to be taught to stand to urinate. To start teaching them to aim, it can be useful to put a piece of cereal (preferably one they don't eat as this could lead to confusion) down the toilet so they have something to aim for and concentrate on.

## Bowel Control

Bowel control is usually learnt after bladder control—although all individuals are different and learn at their own rate and pattern. Some children with autism can find bowel movements very frightening and not understand what is happening, perhaps thinking that their insides are coming out. It can help to get a book with pictures from the library to explain the digestion process.

For others the feel of a full diaper can be comforting, the weight of the diaper can squeeze them or they may enjoy the sensory feeling. You could replace these feelings in other ways instead of withdrawing them completely with toilet training. Those that enjoy a feeling of a full diaper may like to be tightly wrapped in a heavy blanket, this can be timetabled in to their daily routine and they can be given a means of communication to request this activity. When teaching bowel control, sit your child on the toilet, keep the diaper on but with a hole cut in the bottom, slowly cut away the diaper each time until they are able to go without the diaper at all. To start with they will still have the feeling of a security around their waist which in turn will enable them to feel relaxed enough to poo on the toilet. Those that enjoy the sensory feeling can be provided with messy play activities such as gloop (cornflour and water mix), Playdough, or other messy play activities.

## *Habit Training*

Some children are toilet trained through habit. Habit training is effective for children who may: lack awareness, not understand the significance or meaning related to physical sensations, be limited by decreased or absent physical sensations or have unsuccessfully tried toilet training before. Habit training involves training the body to go at set times. Take your child to the toilet at set times throughout the day, every day. As before, keep a chart to discover the best time to take your child. While sitting on the toilet, it is very important your child feels relaxed enough to open their bladder or bowels. Having the tap running in the background can help enable your child to wee and blowing bubbles or blowing up a balloon can help your child to open their bowel. Sometimes having a toy to handle—not one which causes excitement—can be useful to both keep your child on the toilet and relax them. Keep certain toys or books for just when they are sitting on the toilet.

If your child lacks awareness or sensation, they may have to be taught a strategy before getting off the toilet to avoid accidentally weeing on the floor. You can start teaching this process by slowly counting to ten out loud when they have finished weeing before allowing them to get up or giving them a sand timer to look at before they get up. To help your child to independently manage their own toileting routine when they are older, you can buy watches which you can set to vibrate at certain times throughout the day. You can then teach your child when the watch vibrates they are to go to the toilet.

## *The Environment*

The bathroom needs to be a calm, relaxing, structured environment in order to encourage independence and success with the complete toileting routine. Structuring the bathroom and removing all distractions can help your child understand what is expected of them while in the toilet. Removing objects which are not associated with toileting such as toothbrushes, make-up, and laundry will help aid your child's understanding and avoid distractions. Think about making the bathroom as comfortable as possible, adding foot supports, side rails, reduced lighting, switching off the fan, and a smaller toilet seat can all help reduce anxieties.

Make sure everything in the bathroom is set up to encourage independence. Is everything in your bathroom at the right level for your child? Can they reach the soap and towel? Is the soap too highly scented for your child? Do you need to adapt the bathroom for safety reasons such as the temperature of the hot water? Some children are sensitive to the sound of the fan so it may be necessary to adjust the light setting so it doesn't automatically come on with the light.

Your child should be able to sit comfortably on the toilet with hips and knees flexed at a 90 degree angle and have feet flat on a secure object.

## Night Time

Once your child is mostly dry during the day you will then be able to start night-time toilet training. Have a set bedtime routine which does not change with weekends or holidays. Limit the amount your child eats and drinks before bed, having no fluid an hour before bedtime, but ensuring your child has enough fluid throughout the day. Take your child to the toilet before they go to bed. They then may need to be taken once during the night. You could fit this in with your routine by taking them before you go to bed. Then take them as soon as they wake. If they are unable to keep dry during the night, you may need to try different times in the night to take them—may be not when you go to bed but in the middle of the night. There are a number of different products available to protect bedding.

## Further Tips

- Giving a drink ten to 15 minutes before toileting can help increase the chances of your child successfully doing a wee on the toilet but avoid giving too much as this creates an unnatural routine.

- You will need to decide if you are going to teach your child to shut the door as part of the whole toileting routine or only in certain situations.

- Avoid using childlike terms for toileting as your child may find it difficult to change language later in life. It is not appropriate for a 20 year-old to say he is going for a pee-pee.

- When your child first learns to poo on the toilet it may be easier for them to wipe themselves with wet wipes rather than toilet paper.

- If your child has a fear of flushing the toilet, you may wish to remove this from the visual sequence and leave it until the end of the routine—after your child has dried their hands. They then may need to stand in the door way while you flush the toilet and gradually stand closer each time until they are able to flush for themselves. Playing calming music to drown out the noise of the flush or explaining with pictures what makes the noise when the toilet is flushed may also help.

- When your child is in a car ensure they have a protector to sit on to stop the car seat from being soiled by accidents. Avoid drinks before long car journeys.

- Be aware that some children will hold onto their wee or poo until they have their diaper put on, for example if they know they always have a diaper on before going in the car they may wait until it is put back to release their bowel or bladder.

- There is a range of absorbent pants and swimwear for older children available.

- While toilet training you will be spending more time than usual focusing on your child. If you have other children, you may need to put aside some extra time just for them.

- Once your child is toilet trained at home you will want to teach them to use toilets when out in the community. When visiting new places, show your child where the toilets are and use the same routine as you do at home. Use the same picture and toy or book they may have for toileting at home.

- Some children smear their poo. This is a very challenging behavior to come to terms with. There are a number of reasons your child may do this. Firstly, take them to your healthcare provider to make sure there are no physical factors as to why this is happening (being in pain). They may not have understood the process of wiping and you may need to teach them hand over hand. The toilet paper could be too harsh for their sensitive skin therefore using wet wipes may be easier for them. Some children enjoy the feel of smearing, so provide other acceptable activities which give the same feeling such as finger painting, gloop (corn-flour and water), or Playdough. Some children may see cleaning up after they have smeared as a reward particularly if they like water or receive lots of attention from their caregiver. Even if they are reprimanding them, it can still be seen a reinforcement. Use minimal interaction and alternative clean-up methods such as baby wipes or a tepid shower.

- If your child is learning to use the toilet in another setting as well as at home, such as school, send in any equipment you use at home, for example a toilet seat they may use to make the seat smaller. Also remember to send spare clothes, plastic bags to put any wet clothes in, and wet wipes. It is important that you have clear lines of communication during this time so having a home/school book to share concerns and successes is vital.

# Chapter 48

# *Transition to Adulthood for Individuals with ASD*

## *Chapter Contents*

# Section 48.1

# *Transition Plan*

Excerpted from "Life Journey Through Autism:
A Guide for Transition to Adulthood," © 2006 Organization for Autism
Research (www.researchautism.org). Reprinted with permission.

Transition planning allows you, your young adult with autism spectrum disorder (ASD), and his school system to begin planning for the road to graduation and beyond. The planning process introduces you and your young adult to services, activities, instruction, and support designed to provide him with the skills necessary to succeed post-high school. A good transition plan will include both long- and short-term goals, identify the necessary supports, and be very specific to the interests, abilities, and desires of your child.

While this process may seem overwhelming and even scary, starting early will allow you to take smaller, more manageable steps and help you and your son or daughter reach your goals successfully and, ideally, with less stress. Therefore, this chapter outlines the key steps of the process, the overarching goals of transition planning, and how to create a successful transition plan that takes into consideration all of your young adult's strengths and plans for the future.

This information will become part of your young adult's individual education plan (IEP) although it may be developed as a separate document called an individualized transition plan (ITP). In either case, it may include information on such areas as these:

- Vocational training and job sampling (similar to on-the-job training)

- Employment goals and a timeline for achieving them

- Goals in support of residential opportunities, including independent living

- Community participation goals, including social and leisure skills, travel training, purchasing skills, and personal care, to name a few

- Goals relevant to postsecondary education (college), when appropriate

- Coordination with state and private adult services agencies and providers

Long-term transition planning is an ongoing process that reflects the continuing development and changing needs of your young adult. You will work closely with your young adult and the transition planning team at his school to create this guiding plan of action.

## Planning to Plan—Reflecting and Gathering Information to Build Your Young Adult's Transition Plan

Start small, but think big. Before you begin the actual paperwork and planning with your young adult's school and IEP team to implement the transition plan, you can start planning on your own to lay a foundation for the entire process. This section will outline a three-step process to:

1. Facilitate thinking and brainstorming about your young adult's future (assessment)

2. Begin planning future goals (goal writing)

3. Understand realistic challenges to these plans (anticipating obstacles)

Various worksheets may help you with this process. Involve your child with ASD in the planning process as much as possible. Person-centered planning not only empowers the individual, but it also creates a more productive and effective transition plan in the long run.

**Step 1. Assessment:** As you begin the transition planning process, think about the big picture of your young adult's future:

- What do you want your child's life to look like five years, ten years, or 20 years from now?

- What do you not want your child's life to look like in five years, ten years, or 20 years from now?

- What will he require to get to one and avoid the other?

As a parent of a young adult with ASD, you may have struggled to adjust your expectations for the future you once dreamed of for your child. But realistic, concrete goals and expectations are the foundation of a successful transition plan. It is important not only to set goals that can be reached by your child, building one on the next, but also to be

515

sure to challenge your child's growth and leave room to be pleasantly surprised by all that your child can accomplish through this process.

Throughout this discussion (often called futures planning), the concept of future quality of life is central. Quality of life basically refers to how satisfied your child feels about his or her education, work, recreation, spiritual life, social connections, community living, health, and emotional well-being. You may not have specific ideas about all of these areas, but you should start imagining and thinking about what you would like for your young adult and what your child would like for him/herself as s/he transitions out of high school. At different times in this process, you will begin to find connections among all of these areas and start to identify realistic and attainable goals for your child. Although the concept of quality of life is often as much about the process as it is about the product, neither process nor product should be readily compromised as part of transition planning. Once you have this broad vision in mind, start brainstorming about some of the specifics, such as personal interests, strengths and challenges, past learning history, and the supports that will be necessary for your young adult along the way. These constitute the starting point of the transition plan. For overviews of two popular planning protocols, PATH (Planning Alternative Tomorrows with Hope) and MAPs (Making Action Plans), please see:

Falvey, M. A., Forest, M., Pearpoint, J., and Rosenberg, R. (2000). *All my life's a circle: Using the Tools: Circles, MAPs, and PATH*. Toronto, Canada: Inclusion Press.

Pearpoint, J., O'Brien, J., and Forest, M. (1998). *PATH: A workbook for planning alternative tomorrows with hope for schools, organizations, businesses and families*. Toronto, Canada: Inclusion Press.

**Personal interests:** As with any adolescent, your child with ASD may have strong, very strong in some cases, personal interests and hobbies. These preferences may be discovered by observing your young adult to see what makes him happy, what he does during downtime, or what items or activities motivate him. In addition, asking yourself or your son (as the central figure in this process) questions like the following can form another jumping off point for considering future educational and vocational options:

- Are there certain topics or activities of particular interest to your young adult?

- Are there certain topics, activities, or environmental conditions that your young adult does not like or has difficulty tolerating?

- What are your young adult's current academic or related strengths or talents?

- To what extent does your young adult's current skill set match the demands of desirable activities or environments?

- What are your young adult's dreams?

- What kind of support will your young adult require to achieve his goals after graduation?

- What are your hopes regarding this process?

- What are your fears regarding this process?

Systematically answering these questions will allow you to begin to see the connections between what your child is good at and interested in now, and what your child can do in the future. Everyone, including you, is more able and willing to work and excel at something that he likes to do, and your child with ASD is no exception. Tailoring transition planning to your child's personal interests will help keep him focused and engaged, while suggesting clear and meaningful next steps toward achieving his goals. You, your young adult, and the rest of the transition team can work together to document your child's personal interests and explore his connections to the transition goals.

**Strengths (capabilities) and weaknesses (challenges):** You are obviously well aware that there are certain areas in your child's life that he does better in and other areas that are more challenging to him. It is important to list all of your young adult's strengths and challenges, and then to look at them with a new eye. Consider the following:

- How can these areas be of benefit to your young adult as he transitions beyond high school?

- What are some areas in which a certain challenge may actually become a strength?

- How can you help your young adult best capitalize on a specific strength?

- To what extent do the identified challenges directly impact your child's potential in the workplace or other areas of adult life?

In real life, patterns of behavior previously considered to be potential challenges may actually help in the workplace—things like attention to detail may be especially valued at a quality assurance position, and punctuality is always valued in any workplace. If your young adult is overly interested in sci-fi movies, is there a way in which this can be translated into a strength? If so, how? Take a look at how specific capabilities and challenges that your young adult faces can be turned into assets in the workplace or school. Table 48.1 give examples.

**Table 48.1.** Marketing Characteristics as Employment Strengths

| Characteristics | Employment Strength |
| --- | --- |
| Nonverbal | May be less likely to verbally disrupt fellow coworkers |
| Limited social interest | May stay more focused on work and not waste time |
| Strong sensory preferences | May enjoy working in a quiet office |
| Is very schedule- or rule-bound | Comes to work on time, takes breaks at the right time, and returns from break on time |
| Appears ritualistic or compulsive | May offer excellent attention to detail and quality control |

Source: Holmes, A., and Douglas, J. (2005). *Meeting the needs of adults with autism*. Paper presented at the ASA National Conference, Nashville, TN.

**Building on experience:** Building from your child's strengths and challenges, it is useful to think about areas in which he has succeeded or been challenged in the past. The following questions may help in discovering those areas:

- What areas of instruction have engaged your young adult and been areas of success? What areas were challenging?

- What specific challenges did your young adult face in school and what was done to minimize them?

- What types of teacher-student interactions were most helpful to your young adult?

- What environmental conditions were most conducive to learning? What environmental conditions were most disruptive to learning?

- If there were challenging situations in the past, particularly in the community, how were they most beneficially resolved? What did you or others do that worked well, somewhat well, or not at all?

- Does your young adult do well in settings with minimal structure? What does he like about these less structured environments?

- If job experiences have already been provided, how did they go? What could have been done better?

Previous experiences, whether good or bad, are excellent sources of valuable information relevant to the transition planning process. These experiences can illuminate areas where your young adult is more likely to succeed or areas that may not work the best for him. This kind of knowledge is also extremely valuable to the transition planning process.

Aside from the learning value, previous work experience coupled with comprehensive, community-based instruction, makes it more likely that your young adult will have an easier time accessing employment in the future. If your child has not had any work experience, consider looking for opportunities now, early on in the transition process. If actual work experiences are not a possibility, you may want to consider having your son volunteer in an area of interest as this, too, can provide information on your child's interests, challenges, strengths, and weaknesses across a variety of tasks and environments. Finding such opportunities may not, at first glance, appear easy. However, by networking with friends, other parents, your employer, the businesses you frequent (local shops), and community services (houses of worship), you will probably find a number of opportunities just waiting to be discovered.

**Support structure:** Throughout the life of your child with ASD, a support network of teachers, counselors, friends, family, and others has been important and helpful. This support structure will continue to be important to both you and your young adult through the transition period and across new environments. However, because social relationships can be challenging for someone with ASD, this area requires some closer consideration and attention:

- What supports will be needed to encourage social interaction and relationships?

- Can you explore avenues for socializing, such as religious affiliation or other community activity?

- How well do people in the community (where he is most likely to work, shop, recreate, and so forth) know your son? What do they know about him?

- What supports, if any, are needed to structure time for recreation?

- Does your young adult have any special interests that others may share? Can these serve as the basis for a social relationship or friendship?

- Are there service organizations at a local high school or college that coordinate a buddy or mentor program in which same-age peers are paired with individuals with disabilities for social outings and activities?

- Keep in mind that many of the people involved in your young adult's support network leading up to graduation will not be there after graduation. Developing comprehensive and effective support networks is, almost by definition, an ongoing process.

### *Friendships and Relationships*

It is important for your child to be taught the difference between a stranger, friend, acquaintance, boy/girlfriend, or family member, and what types of interactions are appropriate with all of these different types of people.

Strategies:

- Have a discussion with your young adult about the people they encounter on a daily basis.

- Create flash cards with pictures on them and label them friend, stranger, acquaintance, etc., along with the roles and interactions associated with each.

- Develop an activity in which your child will sort and match various work cards/pictures to the appropriate social heading. For example: "Activities I do with my friends," versus "Activities I do with my family;" or, "Ways to greet people I know," versus "Ways to greet people I don't know."

- Talk about the different types of people they know and the appropriate way to act around each type.

- Teach your young adult that he has the right to say no, and ensure that the means to do so is available.

- Give your young adult different scenarios and ask him to role-play how he would interact with the other person. Consider videotaping these role-plays and using them later for video modeling.

- Develop a list of rules (a social story might work here), which may be useful to govern these interactions with different types of people.

- Provide the opportunity to use these new discrimination skills in the environments where they would be of most use (such as the mall).

Where possible, it is also important for your young adult to know how to make and keep friends. Strategies may include these:

- Discuss with your young adult what makes a good friend and what qualities they would like in a friendship.

- Discuss what qualities they bring to a friendship.

- Use examples of friendships from books or movies to help facilitate the discussion.

- Scripts of conversation starters or appropriate topics of discussion could be used.

- Brainstorm possible places to meet people who could be friends.

- Discuss different types of friends, such as acquaintances, coworkers, or closer friends.

- Stress that friendships take time to develop.

**Step 2. Writing overarching goals:** Later in the transition process, you will be asked to help determine—and write down—many specific objectives you want your young adult to achieve. But now is the time to think of the broad, overarching goals that qualitatively reflect the future you want for your young adult. You can think of this as a mission statement for the transition you envision.

These overarching goals should build from the information you gathered in the previous assessment regarding quality of life, personal interests, strengths and challenges, and past experience. You can record these goals, together with your child, to prioritize and articulate broad goals for career, education, living, relationships, recreation, health, and community. These goals will become more structured, with specific tasks and objectives, as you work together to create the transition IEP.

**Step 3. Anticipating obstacles:** A goal is not meant to be easy to accomplish, and it is not something that will only take a short amount of time to achieve. But each goal can be broken into smaller

521

steps for achievement. As you think of the skills, lessons, materials, and information you and your young adult need to move through the transition process successfully, obstacles may present themselves. For instance, as you created the list of goals for your child, did you think of any skills that he may need to be successful? Or resources that will help him accomplish them? Lack of any key ingredient may delay, if not stall, the transition process. So, if certain skills need development, such as effective communication techniques, toileting, table manners, cell phone use, or personal hygiene skills, now is the time to create a strategy to develop them. Other obstacles may appear along the way, but you are building a solid plan that can be revised and modified to accommodate the changing needs, desires, and skills of your young adult with ASD.

## The Transition Plan

**Characteristics of a good transition plan:** *The Individuals with Disabilities Education Act* (IDEA) specifies that transition planning is a coordinated set of activities for a student with a disability that is:

- outcome-oriented—a process with clear goals and measurable outcomes;
- student-centered—based on the specific skills that the student needs and reflective of the young adult's interests and preferences;
- broad-based—includes instruction and related services, community experiences, development of employment and post-school living objectives, and acquisition of daily living skills and vocational evaluation;
- a working document—outlines current and future goals, along with the specific strategies for achieving these goals, and changes over time.

**What the plan should include:** Your young adult's transition plan will be customized based on his needs. In particular, a solid transition plan will include many of the following elements:

- Assessment of your young adult's needs, interests, and abilities
- Statement of preferences for education, employment, and adult living

- Steps to be taken to support achievement of these goals

- Specific methods and resources to meet these goals, including accommodations, services, and/or skills related to the transition goals

- Instruction on academic, vocational, and living skills

- Identification of community experiences and skills related to future goals

- Exploration of service organizations or agencies to provide services and support

- Methods for evaluating success of transition activities (such as, a video portfolio)

**Additional logistical information in the plan:** In addition to stating the goals for your young adult, the transition plan should include logistical information on how the plan will be implemented and monitored, such as:

- a timeline for achieving goals;

- identified responsible people or agencies to help with these goals;

- clarification of how roles will be coordinated;

- a plan for identifying post-graduation services and supports, and obtaining the necessary funding.

**Writing measurable goals allows evaluation of success:** Ideally, all of the above goals should be measurable to ensure you have a precise way to identify when the goals have been accomplished. An example of a measurable transition goal follows:

- Overarching goal: The student will have an appropriate work environment post-high school.

- Measurable goal: Together with the school guidance counselor, transition coordinator, or vocational rehabilitation counselor, the student will explore options for employment post-high school. The student will complete a vocational assessment and participate in a minimum of one unpaid internship, volunteer experience, or after-school job in an area of his interest over the next six months. This participation is defined as a minimum of five hours/week for no less than 12 weeks. This will help the student determine further needs for vocational training.

## *Who is involved with the transition planning team?*

- You and your child with ASD and interested family members
- Your young adult's transition coordinator
- Your young adult's general education teachers, when applicable
- Your child's special education teachers
- Division of vocational rehabilitation (DVR) or administration on developmental disabilities (ADD) representative
- Administrators
- Psychologists
- Speech and language pathologists
- Other related service providers

### Optional and helpful team members:

- Advocacy organization representative
- Business education partnership representative
- Guidance counselor, when appropriate
- Residential services representative, when appropriate
- Mental health agency representative
- Postsecondary education representative, when applicable

Transition planning should help you and your young adult connect with the adult service system. Adult service organizations (including those listed) that may provide or pay for post-transition services need to be invited to participate in the development of ways of the IEP transition plan. If they are unable to attend, then the school must find alternative ways of involving them in planning any transition services they might pay for or provide. Each transition activity should include someone who consents to monitor the provision of that service as outlined in the IEP.

Guidance counselors, related service providers, vocational rehabilitation counselors, and administrators all have a potential voice in designing transition plans for students. These participants may vary, depending on the goals and needs of your young adult.

There is one major difference between transition planning and the IEP meetings you may be used to—it is required that your young adult with ASD be involved.

## Your Role as a Parent

As a parent, you play a very important role in the development of the transition plan. You will need to do the following:

- Be your child's primary advocate in the absence of his or her ability to do so.

- Provide unique and personal information about your child that is not reflected in the school's or agency's records.

- Ensure the transition plan is meaningful, practical, and useful for your individual child.

- Monitor transition planning in the IEP to ensure agreed-upon activities are implemented; frequent communication with your child and other IEP team members will help keep the plan a working document.

- Promote your young adult's independence, self-advocacy, and decision making.

- Plan for future financial and support needs, such as guardianship, estate planning, Supplemental Security Income (SSI), and related work incentives, along with other sources of financial support.

Source: Center for Innovations in Education [CISE] at the University of Missouri, Columbia. [1999]. *Fundamentals of transition.* Columbia, MO: Author. Available online at www.cise.missouri.edu/publications/funtra ns.

The IEP team relies on your knowledge of your child. Effective transition planning adopts an approach that is sensitive to the culture and context of the family, thus empowering your family's role in guiding your adult child with ASD.

Families must be notified ahead of time when an IEP meeting includes development of a transition plan. While many schools will send materials prior to the meeting to help you think about your vision for your child's future, other schools may not. You will have to initiate the process yourself.

## Implementing and Monitoring the Transition Plan

You will work with the transition team during a series of meetings to develop a comprehensive transition plan for your young adult. You should record important details during any planning meetings. Once the actual plan is completed by the team, it is a living, evolving document that should be reviewed and updated several times a year to ensure it reflects and meets all of your young adult's needs, and adequate progress is being made to that end. Each team member will be responsible for implementing the specific transition tasks, together with your child with ASD.

By creating a document with outcome-oriented goals that can be measured, you can more efficiently and effectively monitor your young adult's progress. It is important to work with the transition planning team to periodically update this plan as your young adult continues through school to ensure a successful transition to adulthood.

### *What to Do If You Do Not Agree with Transition Services Provided by the School*

Hopefully, the transition process will be a smooth, collaborative effort among all team members supporting your child with ASD. Nonetheless, it is important to know your rights as a parent if you cannot come to an agreement with the school regarding your child's education:

- You have the right to ask for an impartial hearing. A hearing may be held on any matter relating to the identification, evaluation, or placement of your child or the provision of a free appropriate public education (FAPE). Hearings are to be held by either the State Department of Education or the school personnel directly responsible for your child's education. To obtain a hearing, you should make a written request to the person who is responsible for the education program your child attends.

- If you believe the educational rights of your child are being violated by nonimplementation of the IEP, you should make a written request to the person who is responsible for the education program your child attends or your state's Department of Education. The IDEA affords parents procedural safeguards if agreement cannot be reached regarding the identification, evaluation, educational placement, or FAPE for your child. If you do not feel appropriate transition services are being provided, you may exercise your rights as explained in the Procedural Safeguards for Children and Parents, which can be obtained from your state or local districts.

## *Early Planning Leads to Success*

Planning for your young adult's future and exploring the world of postsecondary education or employment may seem daunting or even a distant prospect. However, starting to plan early and building particular life skills, postsecondary education, or employment goals into your young adult's transition plan/IEP will break the process into manageable steps and help engage an accessible, ongoing support system of transition team members.

# Section 48.2

# *Life Skills*

Excerpted from "Life Journey Through Autism: A Guide for Transition to Adulthood," © 2006 Organization for Autism Research (www.researchautism.org). Reprinted with permission.

This section discusses various residential options for adults with autism spectrum disorder (ASD). In addition, we discuss many of the life skills that may be particularly important to your young adult as s/he moves toward adulthood. Many of these skills can be addressed in the context of your young adult's transition plan. Early and adequate instruction and preparation in life skills is critical to ensure your young adult is prepared for the transition to adulthood.

## *Living Arrangements*

Adults with ASD can live in many different situations. Because there may be waiting lists, all require early planning and preparation. The following is a list of different types of common living situations, listed from most supportive to least supportive. You may have to create a specific opportunity that best fits your child's needs. For additional information on this topic, please go to the Centers for Independent Living website: www.ed.gov/programs/cil.

- Supervised group home living: Typically, three to six individuals live together in an agency-run home. These homes are often staffed by trained personnel who assist the residents with various aspects of living, depending on their needs. Daily organized activities are usually conducted outside the home.

- Adult foster care: Your young adult and possibly another individual could live with a family that has been recruited to assist them with daily living. An agency would oversee the recruitment of these foster caregivers, certify the home, and provide guidance and financial support to the foster family.

- Supervised apartment living: This may be a good choice if your young adult will need some assistance but would prefer to live in a larger apartment complex with neurotypical individuals. Usually, there is an agency staff person or service provider onsite to respond to emergencies and offer limited assistance based on your young adult's needs.

- Supported living: Your young adult would live with extra support in his own place or in your home. It can mean living with another person who has a disability or with a neurotypical individual. The level of care provided by the support person will vary, depending on the needs of your young adult. Needed services and supports are brought to the home instead of the person going out for them.

- Independent living: This is usually in an apartment that would be rented or owned by your young adult. Outside training and support will need to be provided to help your young adult learn to become independent, with an emphasis on the daily living skills mentioned in the next section.

## Life Skills Mastery

Throughout the transition process, you can continue helping your young adult master many of the life skills associated with independence in the community. Your young adult may have mastered some of these skills, but others may be more difficult and/or quite complex (for example, driving a car). As always, the best strategy is to prioritize the skills with the highest functional relevance (the ones s/he will actually use most often) as part of his or her transition plan.

**Personal care** includes a broad set of daily living skills ranging from personal grooming and hygiene to dressing, doing laundry, clothes shopping, and beyond. Help your young adult develop a daily routine inclusive of showering, shaving (if appropriate), applying deodorant, and so forth. Together with your young adult, you can develop and implement task-analyzed chains (steps) for each of these skills (such as: shampoo first, rinse, conditioner second, rinse, wash face with soap, and so forth). For dressing, start by helping your young adult pick out appropriate clothes (such as, by season or activity) for school the night before, and explain why certain types of clothing are more appropriate for certain environments. Then systematically fade yourself out of the process, thereby allowing your young adult to choose his own clothes and complete his grooming tasks without direct supervision. These are important steps toward independent living.

**Time management:** Many children with ASD have difficulty staying organized and managing their time effectively. From Velcro-fastened activity schedules to electronic personal digital assistants (PDAs), the tools are available to help your young adult organize his time more effectively and efficiently. Here are some key skills and tips that can help along the way:

- Break each day up into chunks: Assign various tasks for each time period. For example, your child may be in school from 8 a.m.–3 p.m. From 3–4 p.m., he may work on homework; from 4–5 p.m., update his schedule for the next day; from 5–6 p.m., help with dinner, and so on. By chunking the tasks, it will help your child stay organized and not get overwhelmed.

- Create an individualized activity schedule: You can help your child put together a "To Do" list of items, including homework, chores, and appointments, or leisure/recreation activities. Over time, allow your young adult to do this on his own and check his progress (self-monitoring).

- Use an organizer: a) A simple paper organizer that can be divided by tabs and include sections for lists, homework assignments, and a schedule of activities (Again, help your young adult establish a routine to check and update the organizer.); or, b) an electronic organizer or personal data assistant (PDA). If your young adult likes technology, this could be a fun way to learn about organization. Most organizers have calendars and places to create lists with pop-up reminders when a task should start. Help your child learn how to use these organizers. Create a routine to update the list and schedule every night. The development of simple time management and organizational skills will help make your young adult's transition to adulthood that much easier.

**Hobbies and recreation:** Many learners with ASD have certain areas of interest or specific topics that he or she really likes, for instance, math, Legos™, animals, machines, or a specific videotape/

529

DVD. As part of the transition planning process consider how individual interests might be used to help your son or daughter develop contacts outside of the classroom. Some interests (hobbies) have related organizations that meet socially—Yu Gi Oh!™ or Magic: the Gathering® clubs, science fiction clubs, computer/technology clubs, chess clubs, military history clubs, and so on. Introduce your young adult to these groups and encourage his participation. The ability to meet new people based upon a similar interest and expand his potential support system can be extremely helpful as your young adult gets older.

**Sexuality and relationships:** As your child matures, it is necessary to educate him about the changes in his body and feelings. Puberty can be a difficult time for most adolescents, and especially confusing and challenging for an individual with ASD. You and your family should decide on the best way to address these physical and emotional changes with your young adult with ASD, while keeping open and positive methods of communication. This is also an important time to address relationships with members of the opposite sex, as well as appropriate social skills related to friendship, dating, and the difference. As the parent, it is important to know what, if any, sexuality education is being provided by the school or any other support organization.

**Safety** is a very important topic. Interpersonally, your child may lack certain skills that would help him determine if a situation is safe. Discuss how to recognize and avoid potentially dangerous situations that may occur as your child matures, including advances from strangers. For learners whose verbal comprehension may be limited, discrimination training in the form of stranger/friend differential, good-touch/bad-touch®, or who can or cannot help you with your menstrual cycle remains important and can often be taught with a combination of picture discrimination and actual role-play instruction.

## Daily Living Skills

A variety of daily living skills increases in importance during the transition period. Start early and practice these skills so your young adult will be better able to take care of himself throughout adulthood. Remember, some of these skills may be specifically listed in his transition plan at school. This section lists various skill areas that may be helpful for your young adult to focus on during this time period.

## General Skills

**Phone skills** aid in safety and seeking help, teach basic social skills, increase independence, and may be necessary for a job.

Skill building steps include practicing what to say, how to ask who is calling, and writing down the information for a message; and, memorizing or programming important phone numbers into the phone to assist him with contacting people.

**Cleaning and maintaining a home** increases independence, reduces a caregiver's workload, develops possible job skills, and helps promote social inclusion.

Skill building steps include demonstrating the different types of cleaning products for different areas, such as floors, bathroom, toilet, and other areas; emphasizing safety; and showing your child the appropriate tools to use with them, such as paper towels, sponges, and gloves. If appropriate, read the directions together. Start your child shadowing you and watching as you clean the house. Next, assign a small job to your child that will be his responsibility.

**Laundry and clothing skills** increase independence and teach responsibility for his own appearance.

Skill building steps include providing instruction on sorting clothes into different types of loads, explaining the measuring of detergent and use of the washing machine and dryer, demonstrating how to iron, and providing supervised practice.

## Money Management

**Banking services** allow your child to make more of his own decisions and decrease others' ability to take advantage of your child.

Skill building steps include setting up a simple checking account and/or savings account for your child to really help with mastering the skills of paying bills, saving money, and budgeting resources. Arrange a visit to a local bank and meet with a customer service representative with your child to discuss the different banking options and how to access them. Discuss what a checking account is and how it can be used to pay bills and keep track of transactions. Show your child how to write a check and how to record checks in a ledger; a simple "cheat sheet" inserted into a checkbook can also be a useful reminder for your child about how to write checks.

**Budgeting** increases independence and allows your child to make more of his own decisions.

Skill building steps include helping your child understand the weekly expenses that he may incur, such as for food, clothes, school supplies, and maybe entertainment. Helping your child determine the appropriate amount to spend in each expense category and then monitor his spending accordingly. Set up a monthly meeting with your child to review his accounts and budget, update them as needed, and monitor his spending and acquisition of these important skills.

**Credit cards** increase independence, provide financial security in an emergency, and help to build credit rating and expand future financial options.

Skill building steps include explaining how credit cards work, making sure to cover the finance charges and minimum monthly payments. If you feel a credit card may be useful for your child, get one with a low limit, such as $500, and help your child monitor his spending and bill paying.

## Transportation

**Public transport** use increases independence and provides increased opportunities for work and recreation.

Skill building steps include reviewing the train or bus schedules to help your child determine the appropriate time and route to get him to the designated destination. Review maps of the routes, as well as where your home is located, to orientate your child to the area. Quiz your child to see if he has mastered how to determine the appropriate method of transportation to a location. Discuss the cost for using public transportation, as well as how to plan enough time to get to a certain location on time. Give your child a map and a tip sheet with directions, along with important phone numbers to call if needed.

**Driving** increases independence and provides increased opportunities for work and recreation.

Skill building steps include getting driving lessons from a driving school or a rehabilitation center that caters to the needs of individuals with disabilities. Highlight other important safety rules, such as not talking on the phone when driving or changing the radio station. Keep important directions in a file in the glove compartment

## Health

Various health-related skills, such as fitness, nutrition, and managing doctor's appointments, will help your child as an adult.

**Exercise** reduces stress, provides opportunities for social interaction, and increases fitness and health.

Skill building steps include finding an activity, such as running, weightlifting, rowing, or other fun outdoor activities, that may give your child a fitness outlet and also a way to meet people. Try recreation centers in your area that may also have classes or activities of interest to your child. Help your child access these services and appreciate them early so that he will more readily use them as an adult.

**Nutrition and cooking skills** serve as key daily living skills.

Skill building steps include asking your child to help out in the kitchen. Assign small tasks, such as measuring or slicing, and work on recipes together as you prepare lunch or dinner. Compile a list of your child's favorite meals, with detailed recipe guidelines. Show your child basic cooking techniques and how to use appliances; allow him to practice and maybe take notes. As cooking lessons progress, use cookbooks offering step-by-step, illustrated instructions. Highlight positive nutrition habits, and provide your child with a list of appropriate types of food and amounts to eat each day (such as how many vegetable or fruit servings, meat servings, dairy servings). Create a weekly menu plan to help your child plan nutritious meals, along with a detailed shopping list. Make meal preparation a family experience, sharing the techniques with everyone in your family and also sharing responsibilities.

**Appointment keeping and time management** helps to manage doctor's appointments.

Skill building steps include explaining which doctors help with which services, such as the dentist, psychologist, occupational therapist, pediatrician, or other providers your child regularly visits. Give your child a calendar, and begin helping him manage and keep track of appointments. Have your child compile a list of relevant questions for the doctor before any appointment; help him make sure questions are answered once there. Create a toolkit, including calendar, notebook, and list of phone numbers of providers.

## Conclusion

There are many life skills that will help your child with ASD as s/he becomes an adult. Preparation and practice are key to learning these skills. You may also have other topics that you want to ensure your young adult has mastered before graduating. Remember to work with your young adult's transition planning team to include the specific challenges or skills on his plan. By building these skills into the transition planning process, the team will help you assemble the appropriate resources to ensure these goals are met for a successful transition.

# Section 48.3

# *Legal and Financial Planning and Assistance*

Excerpted from "Life Journey Through Autism: A Guide for
Transition to Adulthood," © 2006 Organization for Autism Research
(www.researchautism.org). Reprinted with permission.

Planning for your young adult's future doesn't end after transition.
While it may be difficult to think about a future when you are not
around to care for your young adult with autism spectrum disorder
(ASD), it is important to begin taking the necessary steps to secure the
accommodations and services he will need after your death.

At the beginning of the transition planning process, you brain-
stormed your adulthood goals for your young adult with ASD, including
quality of life issues, residential issues, and education and vocation
goals. As you begin planning farther into the future, you will need to
address and compose legal documents that articulate lifestyle, financial, and other requirements for your young adult's care.

**People involved:** Begin by identifying key people who can assist in
the process. This should include, when possible, your family, your young
adult with autism, an attorney, a financial advisor, caseworkers, medical practitioners, teachers, therapists, and anyone involved in providing
services to your young adult. In some cases, a professional known as
a Lifetime Assistance Planner can be contracted with to act as a team
advisor to make sure that all parts of the plan are coordinated and
complete. Usually, however, this role falls to the parent, the transition
coordinator, or the student. To locate a Lifetime Assistance Planner,
search in your local yellow pages or on the internet for a Chartered
Lifetime Assistance Planner (ChLAP).

**Developing a lifestyle plan:** Lifestyle planning is a way that the
family records what they want for the future of their loved ones. This
plan can be developed as a letter of intent written by you, the parent
or caregiver, and can provide information on your young adult with
ASD. This letter can include medical and treatment history, current
ability levels, and your hopes and goals for the future. Some topics this
letter should cover include the following:

- Bathing and dressing preferences, including the type and level of assistance that may be provided and by whom

- Preferences with regard to music, movies, and related activities

- Dietary needs and preferences

- Environmental preferences (for example, does not like fluorescent lighting)

- Personal or idiosyncratic preferences (for example, prefers a specific coffee mug)

- Medication guidance

- Any and all lifestyle options that will ensure quality, dignity, and security throughout his adult life

The letter of intent is not a legal document, but it provides important context to guide the future care of your child. Emotionally, it records your feelings about the future as well as your young adult's goals. Practically, it provides detailed information on medical and behavioral history, effective interventions and supports, your young adult's strengths and challenges, and specific care instructions. Some families even videotape daily tasks to illustrate key instructions. A detailed letter will help provide excellent insights for future caregivers and a smooth transition. Start your letter of intent now, and revise and update it, as needed, to ensure that it remains an appropriate resource for your young adult with ASD.

## Legal Planning

Most of all, preparing for the future means establishing the legal protections to ensure your wishes are specifically carried out in the best interests of your young adult with ASD. Find a lawyer who specializes in special needs and/or disabilities to help you create legal documents tailored to your family. He or she will use appropriate language and methods to provide for your young adult with ASD. The basic documents you should consider creating are a will and a special needs trust (SNT).

**Will:** After your death, a will provides specific, detailed plans for your estate and the care of your young adult. If you do not have a will, then the state will usually divide your property and assets equally among your family members, including your young adult with ASD. Because certain government benefits have financial eligibility requirements, leaving your estate to your young adult with ASD may make him ineligible to receive these resources. Therefore, it is essential to prepare your will and estate to maximize the benefits and protections for your young adult with ASD, ensuring financial stability and continued care. A lawyer can help you put the necessary arrangements into place.

**Guardianship:** Your will can establish a guardian for your child with ASD. This person, such as a family member or other trusted individual, can be named in your will and can serve to help manage the affairs of your child as he gets older. If your child is an adult (age 18 or older) when you pass away, there are different types of guardianships that may be appropriate, depending on the needs of your child. For example, a guardian can be charged with managing the financial and medical affairs for your child, making decisions on his behalf.

**Special needs trust (SNT):** Another legal protection would be an SNT. An SNT is a way to provide financial support to your child with ASD to maintain a good quality of life, while allowing him to remain eligible for certain government benefits. An SNT is managed by a trustee, who you appoint on behalf of your child with ASD. Because there are strict rules regarding trusts and government benefits, it is important to work with an experienced lawyer who is familiar with estate planning for individuals with disabilities. There are a number of agencies that may be able to help you establish an SNT. Do your own research, consider getting referrals from other families who have already gone through the process, and always consult with an attorney to ensure compliance with all relevant federal and state regulations.

## Financial Planning

Consider the financial resources necessary to support your now adult child after your death. You can begin by creating a detailed budget of expenses that includes everything from housing to personal needs, both currently and in the future. This will give you an idea of how much money will be needed to care for your young adult and a goal for building a trust fund. Next, you must begin thinking about how to cover the costs and/or fund the trust. There are a number of different resources to consider, including stocks, mutual funds, individual retirement accounts (IRA), 401(k)s, real estate, home equity, life insurance, and others. Don't forget to include the government benefits, such as social security, that your child may receive. A financial planner can be a very useful person to guide you through this process, especially one who specializes in special needs issues.

536

**Stepwise preparation process:** The following is a stepwise plan to consider and protect the special needs of people with disabilities:

1. Prepare a life plan. Decide what you want for your young adult regarding residential needs, employment, education, social activities, medical and dental care, religion, and final arrangements. You can use many of your goals from transition planning as part of this plan.

2. Write a lifestyle plan and letter of intent. Write down the goals you have for your young adult's future. Include information regarding care providers and assistants, attending physicians, dentists, medicine, functioning abilities, types of activities enjoyed, daily living skills, bereavement counseling, end of life care, and rights and values. An accompanying videotape may help clarify your specific desires in any of these areas.

3. Determine finances. Determine your young adult's future expenses. Determine the resources you will need to cover the costs. Don't forget to include savings, life insurance, disability income, social security, and other government benefits.

4. Prepare legal documents. Choose a qualified attorney to assist in preparing wills, trusts, powers of attorney, guardianships, living wills, and other planning needs.

5. Consider an special needs trust (SNT). An SNT holds assets for the benefit of your young adult with ASD and uses the income to provide for his supplemental needs. If drafted properly, assets are not considered income, so government benefits are not jeopardized. Appoint a trustee to administer this trust.

6. Use a life plan binder. Place all documents in a single binder and notify caregivers and family where they can find it.

7. Hold a meeting. Give copies of relevant documents and instructions to family and caregivers. Review everyone's responsibilities.

8. Review your plan. At least once a year, review and update the plan. Modify legal documents as necessary.

Source: The 10-step process was developed by Barton Stevens, ChLAP, founder and Executive Director of Life Planning Services in Phoenix, AZ.

## Conclusion

Planning your estate can be a poignant, challenging, and sometimes daunting process. Start early and take a step-by-step approach to create important documents for the future care of your young adult with ASD. You will also empower yourself and your family by taking control of the process and making sure it takes into account the best interests of you and your young adult with ASD. Remember, a solid future plan should be detailed enough to provide the following:

- Lifetime supervision and care
- Supplementary funds to help ensure a comfortable lifestyle
- Ongoing access to government benefits
- Dignified final arrangements for your young adult
- A basis for avoiding family conflict

## Some Final Comments

Adults with ASD continue to exist outside the societal mainstream in numbers far greater than is appropriate. Among the many reasons for this under-involvement, the continued failure to adequately and appropriately plan for the transition to adulthood is perhaps the most within our immediate ability to correct. Transition planning is not about what is probable, but what is possible. Effective transition planning involves high expectations, a bit of risk, tremendous cooperation, and significant effort on the part of the young adult, his family and teachers, school administrators, community members, and adult service providers. But the outcome, a job coupled with true quality of life, would appear to be worth the effort. As you begin to think about the future for your child, some things to keep in mind include these:

- It is easy to be successful when you set the bar low, so think big and have high expectations.
- Start planning early, certainly no later than age 16 years.
- To the maximum extent possible, work cooperatively with all involved in the process to the benefit of the young adult with ASD.
- Remember that transition planning is a process, and first drafts of ITPs are rarely the final draft.

- Keep your eyes on the prize of your long-term transition goals for employment, living, and/or postsecondary education. Frame all your discussions with reference to those desired outcomes.

- Involve extended family and friends in the process, particularly in the area of employment, as they may have contacts and resources you do not.

- With reference to community skills, remember to teach where the skills are most likely to be used. It is more effective to teach grocery shopping at an actual supermarket than it is to teach it in the classroom.

- Identify the level of risk with which you are comfortable, and then work to maximize independence within that framework. (For example, while you may be uncomfortable with him crossing the supermarket parking lot without close supervision, he may not need the same intensity of supervision in the supermarket.) As the young adult gains greater independence across tasks and environments, reassess your acceptable level of risk.

- Remember, you are a critical part of this process no matter what title you have (parent, speech pathologist, transition specialist, and so forth).

- Good, effective transition planning is effortful and time consuming. Sadly, there are no known shortcuts; however, when it is done well, the outcomes are well worth the effort.

Section 48.4

# *Transition Models for Youth with Mental Health Needs*

Excerpted from "Successful Transition for Youth with Mental Health Needs: A Guide for Workforce Professionals," National Collaborative on Workforce and Disability for Youth (www.ncwd -youth.info), May 2009.

The transition from adolescence to adulthood is a challenging time. It is a time in which the young person is called upon to make complex decisions about schooling, work, finances, and personal relationships. For the more than three million young adults (ages 18–26) diagnosed with serious mental health conditions, this phase of life poses even greater challenges.

Youth with mental health needs often face unemployment, underemployment, and discrimination when they enter the workforce. Statistics show that youth with mental health needs, diagnosed or undiagnosed, are over-represented in foster care, the juvenile justice system, and among school disciplinary cases and high school dropouts.

The absence of a coordinated system of service delivery also presents significant challenges for youth and young adults with mental health needs as they age out of youth services. Through partnerships with service agencies and organizations in their communities, youth service professionals can assist youth in preparing for the adult world.

## *Mental Health Recovery Models*

The following mental health recovery service delivery models offer promising ways to provide an effective, integrated, self-directed system of care for young adults with mental health needs:

**Transition to Independence Process (TIP):** The TIP approach is an evidence-based program model that stresses the importance of providing access to appropriate services, engaging young adults in their own future planning process, and utilizing services that focus on each individual's strengths.

**Assertive Community Treatment (ACT):** This community-based, multi-disciplinary approach was developed in the 1980s to provide treatment, rehabilitation, and support services to persons with severe and persistent mental illness. Using the ACT approach, cases are managed by a multi-disciplinary team, providing services directly to an individual that are tailored to meet his or her specific needs.

**Systems of Care (SOC):** The SOC approach is characterized by multi-agency sharing of resources and responsibilities and by the full participation of professionals, families, and youth as active partners in planning, funding, implementing, and evaluating services and system outcomes. The SOC approach facilitates cross-agency coordination of services, regardless of where or how children and families enter the system.

## Systems Factors that Affect a Program's Success

A program's—and its client's—success are affected by several system-wide factors. All programs emphasized cross-systems collaboration and used multiple mechanisms to achieve it, including advisory boards, memoranda of understanding, and use of unique funding sources. Dimensions of cross-system collaboration include: local collaboration and service alignment that creates networks of care; identifying, accessing, and leveraging funding streams; and states' capacity for systems change.

## Summary

Youth and young adults with mental health needs face major barriers as they attempt to make their way in the adult world. Through thoughtful systems, change at the local and state levels, and the adoption of promising new program models promoting collaborative networks of care, more youth and young adults with mental health needs can become self-sufficient adults who experience personal and employment success.

# Chapter 49

# *Finding Appropriate and Affordable Housing*

Many states and local areas have policies and practices that enable individuals, with support from family and friends, to exercise control over their supports and services and, occasionally, the budget of Medicaid funds allocated for their services. Exercising participant direction over services and funding usually includes developing a person-centered plan, developing a budget and spending plan, serving as the employer of record (recruiting, hiring, supervising and scheduling support staff), identifying and purchasing needed goods and services, and working with a support team which may include a case manager, support broker, fiscal intermediary, and family and friends.

## What We're Doing

We are studying the impact of the policies and practices associated with participant direction on individuals and their families. We are discovering what roles and responsibilities various people have and how individuals, families, and agencies implement participant-directed service models. There are many "islands of excellence" throughout the country; however, good ideas and best practices are not shared easily

---

with others. We are gathering examples of the best practices encountered in our research so that others can learn from the experiences of those working in this innovative field.

## Accessing Affordable and Appropriate Housing

### Financial

- Look for a local Center for Independent Living in the government section of the phone book. These organizations often have housing specialists who can assist you in obtaining information about resources for purchasing or renting a home or apartment in your community.

- Get as much information as possible from your local Department of Housing and Urban Development (HUD) public housing agency/authority (PHA). Put the individual's name on the Section 8 Housing list. Ask if there is more than one housing list, for example one for project-based housing and another for tenant-based. Also, ask what happens if your name comes to the top of the list before being ready for a new living situation. Often, individuals can turn the voucher down once or twice before moving back to the bottom of the list.

- Begin looking for housing even before the individual is issued a Section 8 Housing voucher. It is difficult to find rental housing in some communities that accept Section 8 vouchers. Few states require owners of rental property to take vouchers.

- Ask your PHA if they provide assistance with housing searches or a list of rental properties that accept vouchers.

### Neighborhood

- Consider what kind of neighborhood would be best for the individual needing housing. Drive through the neighborhood you are considering at different times during the day and evening to see what activities are occurring. Also, observe the amount of traffic in the neighborhood.

- Consider transportation needs. Where will you need to be going? Places to consider include grocery shopping, recreational activities, dining, work, laundromat.

- If you rely on public transportation, determine the time schedule and routes that support getting to required destinations. Also, check out the proximity of the public transportation and if a busy street will have to be crossed.

## Housing Type/Design

- Determine what type of housing setting is desired, such as an apartment, condominium, single family dwelling.

- If the individual requires a housemate, look for a house/apartment that provides adequate private space for roommates. Having a private place for housemates to retreat to is important. Also, take into account the amount of parking space available for personal assistants or housemates.

- Does the individual have special considerations for weather? For example, if you live in an area prone to tornadoes, look for a house/apartment with a basement or safe space. If you live in an area that receives significant snow fall, who will do snow removal?

- When choosing a single family home, keep in mind the amount of yard and external house maintenance that will be required.

## How do I implement participant direction of funding and supports and services in my state or area?

1. Every state offers a different array of services or programs. Some states have statewide programs. Others make it available only in certain areas, or to a limited number of people. To find out if your state offers participant direction through a demonstration project (like the one funded by the Robert Wood Johnson Foundation) or through the new Independence Plus Initiative, check with your state's Developmental Disability Council. If participant direction is not available, you might want to bring together a task force to work toward making it available in your state.

2. If it is available in your state, find out if participant direction is available in your local area by contacting your local developmental disability organization (if you don't know whom to call, ask your state Developmental Disability Council). Some local agencies choose not to offer participant direction as an option. Sometimes a person has to already be receiving funding through a Home and Community-Based Services (HCBS) Waiver before they can transition to participant direction of

their funding and supports and services. Many local agencies as well as states have long waiting lists for funding.

3. If participant direction is available, find out if it is fully implemented in your area. Does it include both employer authority and budget authority? Are there support brokers? Are there fiscal intermediaries? Are there people who can conduct dynamic, person-centered planning sessions?

4. Locate information or materials on person-centered planning, fiscal intermediaries, and support brokers.

5. If participant direction is not fully in place, it might be more difficult to implement. If this is the case, you might ask yourself the following questions:

   • Do I have the time and energy to set up a person-centered planning team, oversee individualized budgets, and coordinate with support providers? In other words, can I do this without a support broker?

   • Does the individual with the developmental disability have a support system that is stable and committed to his or her needs? High-school friends, for example, may not work well in person-centered planning team because many move away or lose touch.

6. State or local agencies will have different procedures for applying and implementing participant direction. However, here are some of the steps you might follow:

   • Convene a team to develop a person-centered plan. Team members might be family members, close friends, a support broker, and representatives from service agencies. Identify a facilitator to lead the meetings and a support broker to help identify and manage the human supports. The support broker might also be able to facilitate the person-centered planning meeting.

   • First, focus on the vision the person and his/her allies have for his/her life. Decide what lifestyle supports are required to achieve this preferred lifestyle. This might be thought of in terms of living arrangements, work or other preferred day-time activities, and social and community activities.

   • Marshall financial resources. These might be low-income housing supports or vouchers, day services funds, residential rates, personal assistance funds. Different programs call them different things. The amount of these funds and how that amount is determined varies from state to state. Add whatever income is available from employment.

- Identify a fiscal intermediary to manage your funds.

- Identify the human supports needed, such as housemates, behavior specialists, job coaches, personal assistants, or mentors. Once these people are identified by role, the team can look at the budget and determine how much they can afford to pay support people.

- Develop a budget based on support needs. Some funds must be targeted for certain expenses. For example, Medicaid can't pay for transportation expenses, but Social Security Insurance (SSI) can.

- Revisit the plan frequently. The team (the person—or their representative, you, the fiscal intermediary, and support broker) will have to file reports with the state and local agencies.

## Finding and Retaining Personal Assistants and Housemates

- Create a profile of the "ideal" personal assistant (PA) or housemate.

- Think about the people who the client enjoys most being around. What are the characteristics/traits of these people that make them a good match for this individual?

- Add to the list the attributes that are important to you, such as creative problem-solving, good communication skills, patience.

- Consider the type of support that will need to be provided and what requirements this will entail.

- Be creative about where you advertise the position, but always keep in mind the ideal profile you created and where you might have the greatest chance of finding such a person.

- Ask current PA's and/or housemates to recommend people they think would be compatible support persons.

- Offer wages that are as high as possible. Providing adequate wages and benefits (such as vacations, health insurance) reduces turnover of support persons.

- Before hiring, provide opportunities for potential PA's and/or housemates to spend time with the person needing services to determine compatibility.

- When offering a candidate a position, make clear what restrictions the PA and housemates must agree to. For example, will you allow smoking, overnight guests, or drinking alcoholic beverages?

- Spend time with the person needing services and his/her roommates in informal situations. Take them out for dinner periodically to show appreciation.

Chapter 50

# *Adult Autism and Employment*

## *Chapter Contents*

# Section 50.1

# *Choosing Vocation and Employment*

Excerpted from "Life Journey Through Autism: A Guide for
Transition to Adulthood," © 2006 Organization for Autism Research
(www.researchautism.org). Reprinted with permission.

Whether a job provides financial support, personal fulfillment, social opportunities, or some combination of these, it is a very important component of adult life. In fact, what one does for a living is often regarded as a defining feature of that person and his role in society. Finding the right employment match for a student with an autism spectrum disorder (ASD) may be challenging, but the rewards can also be great in terms of personal satisfaction in a job well done and as an active, participating, well-regarded member of society.

*Individual with Disabilities Education Act* (IDEA) federal special education law requires that school districts help students with disabilities make the transition from school to work and life as an adult. Although IDEA mandates services and programs while your young adult is in school, there are no federally mandated programs or services for individuals once they leave the school system. This means that your adolescent will need to make the most of this transition period to develop his life skills and prepare for entering the work force. A broad timeline is presented here (NICHCY, 1999).

**Early in high school or middle school,** with support from both you and the transition team, your child with ASD should do the following:

- Learn more about the wide variety of careers that exist.

- Take part in vocational assessment activities in the community through job sampling at the actual places of employment.

- Have the opportunity to learn, by practice and exposure, what his work preferences might be.

- Identify training needs and effective strategies to address deficits.

- Be provided with sufficient opportunity to develop basic competencies in independence, self-monitoring, travel training, and life outside the classroom.

**While in high school,** your young adult, you, and the transition team should do the following:

- Develop effective disclosure strategies relative to your son's abilities and needs.

- Identify critical skill deficits that may impede the transition to post-21 life and provide individualized instruction to minimize the deficits.

- If applicable, learn the basics of the interview process and practice being interviewed.

- Learn more about school-to-work programs in the community, which offer opportunities for training and employment through job sampling, youth apprenticeships, cooperative education, tech-prep, mentorships, independent study, and internships.

- Become involved in early work experiences, particularly those emphasizing work-based or on-the-job learning experiences, including volunteering, job sampling (for example, trying out a job for several hours or days), internship programs, and summer jobs.

- Identify transportation options for getting to and from work, as well as other community-based options; determine to what extent your young adult will need to develop the skills related to using public transportation.

- Reassess interests and capabilities based on real-world experiences and redefine goals as necessary.

- Identify gaps in knowledge or skills that need to be addressed.

- Contact the Division of Vocational Rehabilitation (DVR) or Administration on Developmental Disabilities (ADD) agency and/or the Social Security Administration before age 16 to determine eligibility for services or benefits post-graduation.

**Finding a job:** As you are considering a work environment for your young adult with ASD, it will be important to consider both his likes and interests, and also what impact his disability will have on employment. You can use the information you gathered during earlier assessments to help pinpoint where your young adult's interests and a career might intersect. This section will discuss other things to consider when finding a job for your young adult.

**Vocational education is one option:**

- Be aware that vocational training may be included as part of the transition services.

- Vocational education is an organized program that prepares individuals for paid or unpaid employment.

- Vocational training is a long-term project that begins by developing student awareness of possible career choices and positive work attitudes very early in the transition process.

- Vocational training is provided by your state's DVR or by school-based vocational programs. Speak to your child's guidance counselor to find out who to call to arrange these services for your child with ASD.

## What kinds of jobs are available for individuals with ASD?

The employment available for an individual with ASD reflects the breadth of the entire job market. Generally, a job may belong to any of three categories that vary in the amount of support they offer the worker with a disability. Ranging from least to most supportive, these categories are competitive employment, supported employment, and secured or segregated employment—although not mutually exclusive, and an individual may find employment in more than one category.

**Competitive employment:** A full-time or part-time job with market wages and responsibilities is considered competitive. Usually, no long-term support is provided to the employee to help him learn the job or continue to perform the job. The majority of jobs are considered competitive employment, such as waiting on tables, cutting grass, fixing cars, teaching, computer programming, or writing guidebooks on transitions. Competitive employment is most often associated with individuals who are already fairly highly skilled, such as an adult with Asperger syndrome, but may be suitable for other individuals with greater challenges as a function of the task and the environment in which they are to work.

**Supported employment:** In supported employment, individuals with autism work in competitive jobs alongside neurotypical individuals.

One of the characteristics of this type of employment is that the person receives ongoing support services while on the job. The support is provided as long as the person holds the job, although the amount of supervision may be reduced over time as the person becomes able to do the job more independently. Examples of work environments allowing this type of support often include universities, hotels, restaurants, office buildings, or small businesses.

Entrepreneurial supports is a term for a new and particularly innovative type of supported employment. In this situation, a new business is created around the skills and interests of a very limited number of individuals. For example, a young adult who likes to destroy things he does not see as perfect could have entrepreneurial support developed for him where he would go to different offices and be their document shredder. For documents they want shredded, they could tear the corner (making it imperfect), and he could gladly feed it into the shredder. Through this program, he could be contracted with a number of offices; going to one or two offices a day to shred documents would be his job. Often, a Board is formed for this new organization that consists of family members, support personnel, community members, and, ideally, at least one member with experience running a for-profit business. This Board helps ensure the organization's success.

Supported employment, in whatever form it takes, can be funded through state developmental disabilities or vocational rehabilitation agencies, but families will have to advocate strongly that: (1) supported employment, by definition and statute, is intended for people with severe disabilities; and (2) individuals with ASD can, in fact, work if given the proper support, training, and attention to job match characteristics.

**Table 50.1.** Types of Employment

| Secured/Segregated | Supported | Competitive |
|---|---|---|
| Segregated | Community integration | Fully integrated into general work force |
| Focus on group learning | Ongoing job support | |
| Basic skills building | Wages and benefits | Requires special skills |
| Minimal compensation or unpaid | Place first, then train | Natural supports and natural consequences |
| Behavioral supports in place through job tenure | Flexible, wide-ranging supports in place that are personalized | Employment supports offered as needed |
| | Built-in "safety net" | |

Source: NICHCY, (1999). Technical Assistance Guide.

**Secured or segregated employment:** In secured or segregated employment, individuals with disabilities (not necessarily autism specific) work in a self-contained unit and are not integrated with workers without disabilities. This type of employment is generally supported by a combination of federal and/or state funds. Some typical tasks include collating, assembling, or packaging. While such programs remain available, critics argue that the sheltered workshop system is more often geared toward the fostering of dependence within a tightly supervised, non-therapeutic environment than toward encouraging independence in the community at large.

## Job Match

When searching for jobs for your young adult with ASD, it is important to consider the match between your child and a particular job's social, navigation, and production requirements. This job match is the extent to which a particular job meets an individual's needs in terms of challenge, interest, comfort, camaraderie, status, hours, pay, and benefits. Generally, as people move through the job market over time, they get closer and closer to an ideal job match.

Individuals on the spectrum may not be as motivated by money as their neurotypical coworkers are. So, for the majority of individuals with autism, their motivation to work will be directly related to the extent to which they enjoy the work they are being asked to do. A good match is of critical importance in these cases. When considering things that contribute to job match, they can be classified into physical and social components, as shown.

**Components of the physical job match:**

- Hours of employment
- Acceptable noise levels at the job site
- Pay, leave, and other benefits
- Acceptable activity levels
- Physical requirements of the job (such as lifting)
- Acceptable margin of error (quality control)
- Production requirements

**Components of the social job match:**

- Acceptable level of interaction with coworkers and supervisors

- Clear job expectations
- Grooming and hygiene requirements
- Demands on communication skills
- Personal space available
- Phone/vending machine/cafeteria
- Coworker training and support
- Community status

## Job Search

Look to see what employment options are currently available in your area. Networking among friends, colleagues, and acquaintances will often be your best job search strategy. Once opportunities are identified, find out what kinds of skills your young adult will need to be successful in those environments. Then, identify what supports your young adult might require to do this job. This exercise can be done in advance of an actual job search to start your thinking about these topics.

Think "job carving." Remember, the U.S. job market is both highly technical and generally complex, with most employees being required to handle multiple components of a given job. This complexity, however, can play to the advantage of adult learners with ASD through a process referred to as job carving (Nietupski, J. A., and Hamre-Nietupski, S., 2000). Job carving is a specialized job development process that recognizes and takes advantage of this complexity by carving separate tasks from more complex jobs and, subsequently, combining these tasks into a new job that meets both the needs of the adult learner and the potential employer. Please note that if the needs of both parties are not met, no job can be carved. Effective job carving requires direct knowledge of a potential employee's abilities, interests, and limitations, along with observational and negotiating skills.

**The range of possible jobs for individuals with autism** includes the following:

- Reshelving library books
- Factory assembly work
- Copy shop
- Janitor jobs

- Restocking shelves
- Computer programmer
- Math teacher
- Engineer
- Stocks and bonds analyst
- Book indexer
- Copyeditor
- Landscape designer
- Veterinary technician
- Biology teacher

If you are unable to find anything that seems appropriate for your young adult, you may have to craft something specific to match his interests and skills. You can engage the transition team at school to help with this effort.

## References

NICHCY, (1999). Technical Assistance Guide.

Nietupski, J. A., and Hamre-Nietupski, S. (2000). A systematic process for carving supported employment positions for people with severe disabilities, *Journal of Developmental and Physical Disabilities*, 12, 103–119.

# Section 50.2

# *Career Planning Issues*

Excerpted from "Adult Autism and Employment: A Guide for Vocational Rehabilitation Professionals," by Scott Standifer, PhD, Office of Disability Policy and Studies, School of Health Professions, University of Missouri. © 2009 University of Missouri. Reprinted with permission.

## *Problems with Job Coaches*

Job coaches who are unfamiliar with people with autism spectrum disorder (ASD) can make work adjustment significantly worse for a client and lead to loss of the job (James Emmett, 2009). Although much of the research literature recommends job coaching for people with ASD, many common job coaching activities are inappropriate for clients with ASD and should be avoided.

**Do not become embedded in the person's routine:** People with ASD usually value routine and often will begin building a routine and set of expectations from the first day on the job. If the job coach is a prominent part of the person's work environment at the start, the person will come to expect that job coach to be there, prompting them, every day. Attempts to fade the prompts out a week or two later will be very difficult and may cause the person to become frustrated or simply "lock up." The person will stand there waiting for the job coach's prompt.

**Be cautious with verbal prompts:** Spoken reminders and prompts seem to be especially noteworthy and salient to people with ASD. For some reason, a person is more likely to embed verbal prompts in their routine than non-verbal prompts. If the job coach is frequently stepping in to say things like "Now, be sure you check ..." or "The next step is ...," it will be much harder to remove those prompts later on without upsetting the person.

**Use "point prompts:"** Point prompts consist of touching the person gently on the shoulder to get their attention and then, without speaking, pointing to indicate the next step. These prompts are much less prominent to the person with ASD, less likely to be embedded in routines, and easier to fade out.

**Use modeling and visual prompts:** Demonstrate how to do something, without speaking. These also are less prominent to the person and easier to fade.

**Use environmental prompts.** These are diagrams, icons, visual markers (lines on the floor, colors on the floor, room partitions, and so forth) which help the person orient themselves in the schedule and work space. They might include reference sheets in a notebook or labels placed on tools. These prompts can support the person's routine and be left in place after the job coach leaves.

**Support "natural" prompts and resources:** Find out which co-workers or on-site support/training staff the person could use on a regular basis for questions or reminders. The job coach should support them in creating a system of appropriate prompts which can remain in place after he or she leaves. By acting as a consultant, advisor, and monitor for these natural supports, the job coach can stand back from the actual work activities and not become embedded in the person's routine.

## Other Career Planning Issues

**Routines and predictable schedules may be very important to the person**. However, endless repetition with no flexibility or variety may bore them. A good middle ground is a job with a relatively small set of job activities that can be scheduled beforehand so, even though each day may be slightly different, the person can know ahead of time what they will be doing. Part of the person's regular routine then becomes checking the schedule each day. This gives them better coping skills later on if the job tasks need to change in some way.

**If possible, try to match the individual's existing interests to the job.** They may have a very deep but narrow knowledge base which can be an asset in the right situation. However, this often is not possible. Alternatively, you might try to frame job tasks in terms of the person's topic of interest, using the language and categories of that topic as a metaphor, but be careful that they do not take it too literally.

**Assess how the person learns best.** Many people with ASD have strong visual skills and learn best with illustrations, demonstrations, and icons or physical symbols. Review what educational interventions, if any, the person had in school for suggestions.

**People with ASD are often very reliable workers,** with a strong sense of duty and doing what is right. They also may have a strong desire to get along with their coworkers, even if their social skills are not strong.

**The person may be good at solitary activities,** especially ones that require practice, endurance, visual accuracy, or repetition.

**The person may be very good at activities that involve attention to detail.**

**Jobs that involve a lot of waiting** or a lot of last minute changes in schedule or tasks might be a challenge.

**Jobs in noisy, busy, or cluttered environments could be a challenge.**

**Working directly with the public may be a challenge** for the person. Contact with a small set of co-workers may be better.

**The social aspects of work are common challenges** for people with autism and one of the main reasons they lose jobs.

**Supervisors and co-workers may need training** on how to interpret the person's normal behavior. It is important that co-workers not misinterpret the person's normal behavior as rudeness or lack of cooperation. They should also be aware that an increase in unusual or "difficult" behaviors may mean the person is feeling stress of some type. The person may need to retreat from the situation for a while to a safe place, coworkers may need to adjust the environment for the person, or a supervisor may need to find out if something at home is upsetting the person.

**Individuals with a fixation** on a particular topic, may retreat to talking about it when they are nervous, distressed, or do not know what to say or do. It may be a challenge for them to think of any other topic. To others this may seem like rudeness and self-centeredness. Coworkers and supervisors may need training to view this as a type of behavioral communication about the person's anxiety.

**Interviewing for a job may be a challenge.** For job-hunting situations, the person may prefer to concentrate on showing a portfolio of work or demonstrating work skills rather than depending on the social skills of interviewing. Alternatively, there may be a way of objectively rating the person's skill, such as a certification test or grade point average. This lets them sell their skills rather than their personality.

**Public transportation, such as a bus, may be very uncomfortable** for the person because of both social and sensory issues. A bicycle, car, or car-pooling situation may be better. It is also useful to plan for backup transportation in case something goes wrong one day with the main transportation. The person should schedule some practice runs of the backup transportation so it is not a new and stressful event. The person may want to schedule days to use the backup system on a regular basis to keep in practice. The person may need to have an instruction card or sheet at home to help them remember about the backup arrangement.

**Handling more than one project or activity at a time may be a challenge** for the person.

**Promotion from the initial job may be a challenge** later on, especially if the promotion puts them in a management position.

**Office meetings** can be challenging for the person, requiring additional supports:

- The social dynamics and skills of meetings are different from typical conversations.

- The person may have trouble understanding what others are thinking or feeling.

- Agendas may be difficult to understand.

- Discussions often deviate from agendas.

- The person may fixate on one aspect of the discussion ("Tomorrow is a holiday") and not process other topics ("We are facing budget cuts"), placing them out of sync with others in the meeting.

- The meeting interrupts the usual routine of the day.

**Possible meeting supports** might include the following:

- Social skills training on meetings (see social stories, comic book conversations)

- A co-worker to act as "mentor" or "translator" for the person during meetings

- Clear meeting agendas with a few main goals and objectives highlighted

- A slower pace for the meetings to allow processing time

- Summary follow-up notes on meetings

**Possible career options:** It is always best to talk with the person about their career preferences. This list is just for brainstorming and is not intended to be exclusive or complete.

- Data entry
- Engine repair
- Graphic arts
- Computer programming
- Proof reading
- Quality control
- Inventory stocking and control
- Mail room services
- Book keeping
- Banking
- Accounting
- Legal research
- Laboratory work
- Drafting, or other technical work
- Library services aid (many corporations have private libraries and librarians on staff)
- Website maintenance or design
- Database maintenance (updating of entries, monitoring for duplications or outdated data, and so forth)
- Agricultural work, such as caring for crops and animals, or even lawn care or park maintenance, may match the preferences of some people with autism (routine, limited social dynamics, detail oriented)

## Section 50.3

# *Possible Job Accommodations*

Excerpted from "Adult Autism and Employment: A Guide for Vocational Rehabilitation Professionals," by Scott Standifer, PhD, Office of Disability Policy and Studies, School of Health Professions, University of Missouri. © 2009 University of Missouri. Reprinted with permission.

Accommodations that are possible for employed individuals with autism spectrum disorder (ASD) may include the following:

- A co-worker as mentor to help the person understand social situations and cues and workplace culture, or help "translate" instructions or comments from others.

- Training for co-workers and supervisors about the person's characteristics, preferences, sensitivities, social skills, behavioral communication, and so forth.

- Social coaching: training in social skills.

- Gradual school-to-work transition, if possible.

- Training done on site and first day activities which match the typical routine. People with ASD often look for immediate creation of new routines. A day or two of orientation and paperwork will be very confusing. Any prompts provided during training should be the same ones used during typical work routines.

- A daily schedule prominently posted, with icons or pictures (even if reading skills are strong). The schedule should answer the questions: What am I doing? Why am I doing this? and What comes next? Even individuals who are normally well anchored in their daily routine may have occasional off days when they lose track of these details and become confused.

- A personal calendar or appointment book.

- A personal digital assistant (PDA) or smart phone with scheduling software, prompting software, and so forth.

- Advance warning of changes in routines, including a chance to practice new routines.

- Extra support in times of high staff turnover or significant changes in work tasks.

- Colored lines on the floor to identify areas of specific types of activities.

- Physical icon objects to identify tasks or areas of specific activities.

- Prominent prompts and environmental cues to signal areas of activity or transitions between activities during the day.

- Social stories for the workplace: a set of short stories or cue cards with information about what to do in different situations or explaining how people expect others to act in different situations (For example: "If I can't find a tool I need, I can ask the supervisor" [with a photo of the supervisor attached]; "If I run out of paper, I go to the copy room and ask for more;" a short paragraph on what happens when coworkers go out to lunch together, and so forth.)

- A work area with few distracting sounds, smells, or sights, possibly including the avoidance of fluorescent lights (which can hum or flicker).

- Sunglasses or tinted glasses to reduce light.

- Headphones or earplugs to reduce sound levels.

- White noise machine to mask distracting sounds.

- Dividers or partitions to reduce sound/visual clutter or help visually define discrete work areas.

- Freelance work with only brief social contact.

- Concrete, well-defined work goals.

- Concrete, well-defined feedback on quality of work.

- A limited number of job assignments at one time.

- Complex tasks broken into smaller sequences and displayed with diagrams.

- Task checklists (with symbols) derived from a careful task analysis.

- Flexibility to develop their own way of organizing a task.

- Flexibility to organize their own workspace and maintain order there.

- A safe place to retreat during times of stress.

- Routine breaks, with a chance to be alone or do something the person finds relaxing (possibly including: moving around, swinging on a swing, or jumping on a small trampoline).

- Coaching on activities to do during breaks that match their interests, the setting, and the resources available.

- A way to use writing, picture exchange, or gestures if speaking skills are weak.

- A picture exchange system, communication board or choice board if speaking skills are limited.

- A PDA or smart phone with augmentative communication or scheduling software.

- Co-worker(s) designated to help alert the person to environmental cues like telephone rings, fire alarms, honking horns, and so forth.

- Plenty of space to move between furniture, machinery.

- Work space with a limited number of things that could be knocked over by accident.

- Assistive technology for tasks involving fine motor skills.

- Extra time to think and process when receiving instructions, asking questions or answering questions.

- Self-assessment/self-rating scale (depending on functional abilities of client) to improve self-awareness and reflection of performance.

## *Portable Electronics Technology*

As of this writing (2009), the field of software designed to support people with ASD and related disabilities is just beginning to expand. A few companies have produced software for palmtop computers for a number of years, but the high cost of those devices limited the market and the number of options.

However, the recent, dramatic spread of inexpensive personal digital assistants and smart phones is changing that situation. Several augmentative and alternative communication (AAC) programs (which "speak" a person's message when the person presses icons on a screen) have been adapted to these devices. In addition, a small number of companies have begun developing scheduling, prompting, and countdown software for iPhones and other smart phones. The field is changing so rapidly that any listing of specific sources and products will be quickly outdated. But a quick internet search should provide current information.

# Part Eight

# Additional Help and Information

# Chapter 51

# *Glossary of ASD Terms and Acronyms*

## *Autism Spectrum Disorder-Related Acronyms*

**ABA:** applied behavior analysis

**ABC:** Autism Behavior Checklist—a diagnostic tool

**ADA:** Americans with Disabilities Act

**ADD:** attention deficit disorder

**ADHD:** attention deficit hyperactivity disorder

**ADI:** Autism Diagnostic Interview—a diagnostic tool developed in London by the Medical Research Council

**ADOS:** Autism Diagnostic Observation Scale

**AIT:** Auditory integration training

**AS:** Asperger syndrome

This chapter begins with autism spectrum disorders (ASD)-related acronyms from "Glossary," © 2009 Center for Autism and Related Disorders, Inc., (www.cen terforautism.com). Reprinted with permission. Terms defined under the heading "ASD Terms," include excerpts from "Glossary," National Institute on Deafness and Other Communication Disorders (NIDCD), June 7, 2010. Other terms are those marked with a [1] from *Stedman's Medical Dictionary*, 27th Edition, Copyright © 2000 Lippincott Williams & Wilkins. All rights reserved. Also, terms marked with a [2] are excerpted from "Facts about ASD," Centers for Disease Control and Prevention (CDC), May 13, 2010; and terms marked with a [3] are excerpted from "Autism Spectrum Disorders," National Institute of Mental Health (NIMH), reviewed December 8, 2010.

**ASA:** Autism Society of America

**ASD:** autism spectrum disorders

**ASL:** American sign language

**CARS:** Childhood Autism Rating Scale

**CBCL:** Achenbach Childhood Behavior Checklist—a diagnostic tool

**CHAT:** Checklist for Autism in Toddlers—a diagnostic tool

**Defeat Autism Now (DAN) doctor:** A physician who uses the DAN protocol to diagnose autism.

**DAN protocol:** An assessment protocol that examines the underlying disorders causing autism.

**DD:** Developmental disabilities

**DVD:** Developmental verbal dyspraxia

**EEG:** Electroencephalogram

**ELAP:** Early Learning Accomplishment Profile—an evaluation tool

**FC:** Facilitated communication

**FCT:** Facilitated communication training

**GARS:** Gilliam Autism Rating Scale

**HFA:** High-functioning autistic

**ICF:** Intermediate care facility

**IDEA:** Individuals with Disabilities Education Act

**IEP:** Individualized education plan

**IFSP:** Individualized family service plan

**IHP:** Individualized habilitation program

**IPP:** Individual program plan

**LCSW:** Licensed clinical social worker

**LRE:** Least restrictive environment

**MSDD:** Multi-system developmental disorder

**NT:** Neurologically typical or neurotypical

**NOS:** Not otherwise specified

**OCD:** Obsessive-compulsive disorder

**ODD:** Oppositional defiant disorder

**OT:** Occupational therapist

**PDD:** Pervasive developmental disorder

**PDDNOS:** Pervasive developmental disorder not otherwise specified

**PECS:** Picture Exchange Communication System

**PEP:** Psycho-educational profile

**PEP-R:** Psycho-educational profile revised

**PRT:** Pivotal response training

**PT:** Physical therapy

**SAS:** Specialized autism services

**SI:** Sensory integration

**SIB:** Self-injurious behavior

**SIT:** Sensory integration therapy

**TEACCH:** Treatment and Education of Autistic and Related Communication Handicapped Children

## ASD Terms

**Angelman syndrome:** Microdeletion of 15q-13, of maternal origin, resulting in mental retardation, ataxia, paroxysms of laughter, seizures, characteristic facies, and minimal speech.[1]

**Asperger disorder:** A pervasive developmental disorder characterized by severe and enduring impairment in social skills and restrictive and repetitive behaviors and interests, leading to impaired social and occupational functioning but without significant delays in language development.[1]

**assistive devices:** Technical tools and devices such as alphabet boards, text telephones, or text-to-speech conversion software used to aid individuals who have communication disorders perform actions, tasks, and activities.

**audiologist:** Health care professional who is trained to evaluate hearing loss and related disorders, including balance (vestibular) disorders and tinnitus, and to rehabilitate individuals with hearing loss and related disorders. An audiologist uses a variety of tests and procedures to assess hearing and balance function and to fit and dispense hearing aids and other assistive devices for hearing.

**augmentative devices:** Tools that help individuals with limited or absent speech to communicate, such as communication boards, pictographs (symbols that look like the things they represent), or ideographs (symbols representing ideas).

**autistic disorder (also called classic autism):** This is what most people think of when hearing the word autism. People with autistic disorder usually have significant language delays, social and communication challenges, and unusual behaviors and interests. Many people with autistic disorder also have intellectual disability.[2]

**autism spectrum disorders (ASD):** ASD demonstrate deficits in 1) social interaction, 2) verbal and nonverbal communication, and 3) repetitive behaviors or interests. In addition, they will often have unusual responses to sensory experiences, such as certain sounds or the way objects look. Each of these symptoms runs the gamut from mild to severe. There are five pervasive developmental disorders referred to as ASD.[3]

**central auditory processing disorder:** Inability to differentiate, recognize, or understand sounds; hearing and intelligence are normal.

**childhood disintegrative disorder (CDD):** Loss of such skills as vocabulary are more dramatic in CDD than they are in classical autism. The diagnosis requires extensive and pronounced losses involving motor language, and social skills. CDD is also accompanied by loss of bowel and bladder control and oftentimes seizures and a very low intelligence quotient (IQ).[3]

**cognition:** Thinking skills that include perception, memory, awareness, reasoning, judgment, intellect, and imagination.

**compulsion:** Uncontrollable thoughts or impulses to perform an act, often repetitively, as an unconscious mechanism to avoid unacceptable ideas and desires which, by themselves, arouse anxiety; the anxiety becomes fully manifest if performance of the compulsive act is prevented; may be associated with obsessive thoughts.[1]

**developmental disability:** Loss of function brought on by prenatal and postnatal events in which the predominant disturbance is in the acquisition of cognitive, language, motor, or social skills; for example, mental retardation, autistic disorder, learning disorder, and attention deficit hyperactivity disorder.[1]

**dysfluency:** Disruption in the smooth flow or expression of speech.

**dysphonia:** Any impairment of the voice or speaking ability.

**dyspraxia of speech:** In individuals with normal muscle tone and speech muscle coordination, partial loss of the ability to consistently pronounce words.

**echolalia:** Involuntary parrot-like repetition of a word or sentence just spoken by another person.[1]

**fragile X syndrome:** This disorder is the most common inherited form of mental retardation. It was so named because one part of the X chromosome has a defective piece that appears pinched and fragile when under a microscope.[3]

**genetic counselor:** A health professional who provides information and support to individuals and families who have a genetic disease or who are at risk for such a disease.

**hyperlexia:** In mentally retarded children, the presence of relatively advanced reading ability.[1]

**Landau-Kleffner syndrome:** Childhood disorder of unknown origin which often extends into adulthood and can be identified by gradual or sudden loss of the ability to understand and use spoken language.

**language:** System for communicating ideas and feelings using sounds, gestures, signs, or marks.

**language disorders:** Any of a number of problems with verbal communication and the ability to use or understand a symbol system for communication.

**learning disabilities:** Childhood disorders characterized by difficulty with certain skills such as reading or writing in individuals with normal intelligence.

**nonverbal:** Denoting communication without words, for example, by signs, symbols, facial expressions, gestures, posture.[1]

**obsession:** A recurrent and persistent idea, thought, or impulse to carry out an act that is ego-dystonic, that is experienced as senseless or repugnant, and that the individual cannot voluntarily suppress.[1]

**pervasive developmental disorder (PDD):** A group of mental disorders of infancy, childhood, or adolescence characterized by distortions in the acquisition of the multiple basic psychologic functions necessary for the elaboration of social skills, language skills, and imagination; also characterized by restricted or stereotypical activities and interests.[1]

**pervasive developmental disorder not otherwise specified (PDDNOS):** People who meet some of the criteria for autistic disorder or Asperger syndrome, but not all, may be diagnosed with PDDNOS. People with PDDNOS usually have fewer and milder symptoms than those with autistic disorder. The symptoms might cause only social and communication challenges.[2]

**Rett syndrome:** A pervasive developmental disorder characterized by the development of several specific deficits after an apparently normal prenatal and perinatal period, including deceleration in head growth, loss of purposeful hand skills with deterioration into stereotypical hand movements, impairment in expressive and receptive language, and significant psychomotor retardation.[1]

**screening:** Examination of a group of usually asymptomatic individuals to detect those with a high probability of having a given disease, typically by means of an inexpensive diagnostic test. Also, in the mental health professions, initial patient evaluation that includes medical and psychiatric history, mental status evaluation, and diagnostic formulation to determine the patient's suitability for a particular treatment modality.[1]

**sign language:** Method of communication for people who are deaf or hard of hearing in which hand movements, gestures, and facial expressions convey grammatical structure and meaning.

**specific language impairment (SLI):** Difficulty with language or the organized-symbol system used for communication in the absence of problems such as mental retardation, hearing loss, or emotional disorders.

**speech disorder:** Any defect or abnormality that prevents an individual from communicating by means of spoken words. Speech disorders may develop from nerve injury to the brain, muscular paralysis, structural defects, hysteria, or mental retardation.

**speech-language pathologist:** Health professional trained to evaluate and treat people who have voice, speech, language, or swallowing disorders (including hearing impairment) that affect their ability to communicate.

**stuttering:** Frequent repetition of words or parts of words that disrupts the smooth flow of speech.

**Tourette syndrome:** Neurological disorder characterized by recurring movements and sounds (called tics).

**tuberous sclerosis:** Tuberous sclerosis is a rare genetic disorder that causes benign tumors to grow in the brain as well as in other vital organs. It has a consistently strong association with ASD.[3]

# Chapter 52

# *Directory of Additional ASD Resources*

## Government Organizations

### *Centers for Autism and Developmental Disabilities Research and Epidemiology*
National Center on Birth Defects and Developmental Disabilities
1600 Clifton Rd.
MS E-87
Atlanta, GA 30333
Toll-Free: 800-CDC-INFO
(232-4636)
Toll-Free TTY: 888-232-6348
Website:
http://www.cdc.gov/ncbddd/
autism/caddre.html
E-mail: cdcinfo@cdc.gov

### *Centers for Disease Control and Prevention (CDC)*
1600 Clifton Rd.
Atlanta, GA 30333
Toll-Free: 800-CDC-INFO (232-4636)
Toll-Free TTY: 888-232-6348
Website: http://www.cdc.gov
E-mail: cdcinfo@cdc.gov

### *CDC Act Early*
Website:
http://www.cdc.gov/actearly

### *CDC Autism Information Center*
Toll-Free: 800-232-4636
Website: http://www.cdc.gov
/ncbddd/autism/index.html
E-mail: cdcinfo@cdc.gov

---

Resources in this chapter were compiled from several sources deemed reliable; all contact information was verified and updated in December 2010.

### Disability.gov
Office of Disability
Employment Policy (ODEP)
U.S. Department of Labor
Website:
http://www.disability.gov

### National Dissemination Center for Children with Disabilities
1825 Connecticut Ave. NW
Suite 700
Washington, DC 20009
Toll-Free: 800-695-0285
Phone: 202-884-8200
Fax: 202-884-8441
Website: http://www.nichcy.org
E-mail: nichcy@aed.org

### National Institute of Child Health and Human Development (NICHD)
Bldg. 31, Rm. 2A32
MSC 2425
31 Center Dr.
Bethesda, MD 20892
Toll-Free: 800-370-2943
Toll-Free TTY: 888-320-6942
Fax: 866-760-5947
Website:
http://www.nichd.nih.gov
E-mail:
NICHDInformationResource
Center@mail.nih.gov

### National Institute of Environmental Health Sciences (NIEHS)
111 T.W. Alexander Dr.
Research Triangle Park, NC 27709
Phone: 919-541-3345
Website:
http://www.niehs.nih.gov
E-mail: webcenter@niehs.nih.gov

### National Institute of Mental Health (NIMH)
6001 Executive Blvd.
Rm. 8184, MSC 9663
Bethesda, MD 20892
Toll-Free: 866-615-6464
Toll-Free TTY: 866-415-8051
Phone: 301-443-4513
TTY: 301-443-8431
Fax: 301-443-4279
Website:
http://www.nimh.nih.gov
E-mail: nimhinfo@nih.gov

### National Institute of Neurological Disorders and Stroke (NINDS)
P.O. Box 5801
Bethesda, MD 20824
Toll-Free: 800-352-9424
Phone: 301-496-5751
TTY: 301-468-5981
Website:
http://www.ninds.nih.gov

*National Institute on Deafness and Other Communication Disorders (NIDCD)*
Information Clearinghouse
1 Communication Ave.
Bethesda, MD 20892
Toll-Free: 800-241-1044
Toll-Free TTD/TTY:
800-241-1055
Fax: 301-770-8977
Website:
http://www.nidcd.nih.gov
E-mail:
nidcdinfo@nidcd.nih.gov

*National Dissemination Center for Children with Disabilities (NICHCY)*
1825 Connecticut Ave. NW
Suite 700
Washington, DC 20009
Toll-Free: 800-695-0285
Fax: 202-884-8441
Website: http://www.nichcy.org
E-mail: nichcy@aed.org

*NIMH National Database for Autism Research (NDAR)*
6001 Executive Blvd.
Rm. 7202, MSC 9645
Bethesda, MD 20892
Fax: 301-443-1731
(attention to NDAR)
Website: http://www.ndar.nih.gov
E-mail: ndar@mail.nih.gov

*Office for Civil Rights*
U.S. Department
of Education (DOE)
Washington, DC 20202
Toll-Free: 800-421-3481
Toll-Free TDD: 877-521-2172
Fax: 202-452-6012
Website: http://www2.ed.gov/
about/offices/list/ocr/aboutocr.html
E-mail: ocr@ed.gov

*Technical Assistance Center*
Positive Behavioral
Interventions and Supports
DOE Office of Special Education
Programs
Website: http://www.pbis.org

*U.S. Department of Education*
400 Maryland Ave., SW
Washington, DC 20202
Toll-Free: 800-872-5327
Toll-Free TTY: 800-437-0833
Website: http://www.ed.gov

## Private Organizations

*American Speech-Language-Hearing Association (ASHA)*
200 Research Blvd.
Rockville, MD 20850
Toll-Free: 800-638-8255
Phone: 301-296-5700
TTY: 301-296-5650
Fax: 301-296-8580
Website: http://www.asha.org
E-mail: actioncenter@asha.org

### Asperger Syndrome Education Network (ASPEN)
9 Aspen Circle
Edison, NJ 08820
Phone: 732-321-0880
Website:
http://www.aspennj.org/
index.asp
E-mail: info@aspennj.org

### Association for Behavioral Analysis International (ABAI)
550 W. Centre Ave.
Portage, MI 49024
Phone: 269-492-9310
Fax: 269-492-9316
Website:
http://www.abainternational.org
E-mail:
mail@abainternational.org

### Association for Science in Autism Treatment
P.O. Box 188
Crosswicks, NJ 08515
Website:
http://www.asatonline.org
E-mail: info@asatonline.org

### AutismCares
Family Financial Support
Toll-Free: 888-288-4762
Website:
http://www.autismcares.org
E-mail:
autismcares@autismspeaks.org

### Autism National Committee (AUTCOM)
Website: http://www.autcom.org

### Autism Network International
P.O. Box 35448
Syracuse, NY 13235
Website: http://www.autreat.com
E-mail: jisincla@syr.edu

### Autism Research Institute (ARI)
4182 Adams Ave.
San Diego, CA 92116
Toll-Free: 866-366-3361
Fax: 619-563-6840
Website: http://
www.autismresearchinstitute.com
E-mail: director@autism.com

### Autism Society
4340 East-West Hwy., Suite 350
Bethesda, MD 20814
Toll-Free: 800-328-8476
Phone: 301-657-0881
Website:
http://www.autism-society.org

### Autism Speaks
2 Park Ave., 11th Floor
New York, NY 10016
Phone: 212-252-8584
Fax: 212-252-8676
Website: http://www.autism
speaks.org/index2.php
ASD online video glossary:
http://www.autismspeaks.org/
video/glossary.php
E-mail:
contactus@autismspeaks.org

**Autism Support Network**
Box 1525
Fairfield, CT 06824
Phone: 203-404-4929
Fax: 203-404-4969
Website: http://www.autism
supportnetwork.com
E-mail: info@AutismSupport
Network.com

**Autism Today**
1425 Broadway #444
Seattle, WA 98122
Toll-Free: 866-9AUTISM
(928-8476)
Phone: 780-416-4448
Fax: 780-416-4330
Website:
http://www.autismtoday.com
E-mail:
support@autismtoday.com

**Autism Treatment Network**
Website: http://autismtreatment
network.org

**AWAARE Collaboration**
Working to prevent wandering
incidents and death
Website: http://www.awaare.org

**Birth Defect Research for
Children, Inc.**
800 Celebration Ave.
Suite 225
Celebration, FL 34747
Phone: 407-566-8304
Website:
http://www.birthdefects.org
E-mail: staff@birthdefects.org

**Center for Autism and
Related Disorders Inc.
(CARD)**
9019 Ventura Blvd., Suite 300
Tarzana, CA 91356
Phone: 818-345-2345
Fax: 818-758-8015
Website:
http://www.centerforautism.com
E-mail: info@centerforautism.com

**Children's Craniofacial
Association**
13140 Coit Rd., Ste. 517
Dallas, TX 75240
Toll-Free: 800-535-3643
Phone: 214-570-9099
Fax: 214-570-8811
Website: http://www.ccakids.com
E-mail: contactCCA@ccakids.com

**Disability Policy
and Studies**
University of Missouri
Website: http://www.dps
.missouri.edu

**Families and Advocates
Partnership for Education
(FAPE)**
PACER Center
8161 Normandale Blvd.
Minneapolis, MN 55437
Phone: 952-838-9000
TTY: 952-838-0190
Fax: 952-838-0199
Website: http://www.fape.org
E-mail: fape@fape.org

### Family Center on Technology and Disability (FCTD)

Academy for Educational Development (AED)
1825 Connecticut Ave.
NW 7th Fl.
Washington, DC 20009
Phone: 202-884-8068
Fax: 202-884-8441
Website: http://www.fctd.info
E-mail: fctd@aed.org

### First Signs, Inc.

P.O. Box 358
Merrimac, MA 01860
Phone: 978-346-4380
Fax: 978-346-4638
Website:
http://www.firstsigns.org
E-mail: info@firstsigns.org

### Heeling Autism

Guiding Eyes for the Blind
611 Granite Springs Rd.
Yorktown Heights, NY 10598
Toll-Free: 800-942-0149
Phone: 914-243-2228
Website:
https://www.guidingeyes.org/
prospective-students/
children-with-autism
E-mail:
heelingautism@guidingeyes.org

### Indiana Resource Center for Autism (IRCA)

Indiana Institute on Disability and Community
2853 E. Tenth St.
Bloomington, IN 47408
Phone: 812-855-6508
Website:
http://www.iidc.indiana.edu/
index.php?pageId=32
E-mail: iidc@indiana.edu

### Interactive Autism Network

Website:
http://www.ianproject.org

### International Rett Syndrome Foundation

4600 Devitt Drive
Cincinnati, OH 45246
Phone: 513-874-3020
Website:
http://www.rettsyndrome.org
E-mail:
admin@rettsyndrome.org

### Kennedy Krieger Institute

Toll-Free
Referral Line: 888-554-2080
Local Referral Line:
443-923-9400
Phone: 443-923-9200
TTY: 443-923-2645
Website:
http://www.kenneykrieger.org

*MAAP Services for Autism, Asperger Syndrome, and PDD*
P.O. Box 524
Crown Point, IN 46307
Phone: 219-662-1311
Fax: 219-662-0638
Website:
http://www.maapservices.org
E-mail: info@maapservices.org

*March of Dimes*
1275 Mamaroneck Ave.
White Plains, NY 10605
Toll-Free: 888-MODIMES
(663-4637)
Phone: 914-997-4488
Fax: 914-428-8203
Website:
http://www.marchofdimes.com
E-mail: askus@marchofdimes.com

*Moebius Syndrome Foundation*
P.O. Box 147
Pilot Grove, MO 65276
Phone: 660-834-3406
Fax: 660-882-3018
Website: http://www
.moebiussyndrome.com

*National Center for Medical Home Implementation*
c/o American Academy
of Pediatrics
141 Northwest Pt. Blvd.
Elk Grove Village, IL 60007
Toll-Free:
800-433-9016 ext. 7605
Phone: 847-434-4000
Fax: 847-228-5034
Website: http://www
.medicalhomeinfo.org
E-mail: medical_home@aap.org

*National Center on Accessible Instructional Materials at Cast, Inc.*
40 Harvard Mills Sq.
Suite 3
Wakefield, MA 01880
Phone: 781-245-2212
Website: http://aim.cast.org
E-mail: aim@cast.org

*National Organization for Rare Disorders (NORD)*
P.O. Box 1968
55 Kenosia Avenue
Danbury, CT 06813
Voice Mail:
800-999-NORD (6673)
Phone: 203-744-0100
Fax: 203-798-2291
Website: http://
www.rarediseases.org
E-mail:
orphan@rarediseases.org

*Online Asperger Syndrome Information and Support (OASIS)*
@ MAAP Services for Autism, Asperger Syndrome, and PDD
Website: http://www.aspergersyndrome.org

*Operation Autism*
Resource Guide for Military Families
Toll-Free: 866-366-9710
Website: http://www.operationautismonline.org

*Organization for Autism Research (OAR)*
2000 N. 14th St., Ste. 710
Arlington, VA 22201
Toll-Free: 866-366-9710
Phone: 703-243-9710
Website: http://www.researchautism.org/resources/reading/index.asp
E-mail: info@researchautism.org

*PEDSTest.com, LLC*
Tools for Developmental-Behavioral Screening
1013 Austin Ct.
Nolensville, TN 37135
Toll-Free: 877-296-9972
Phone: 615-776-4121
Fax: 615-776-4119
Website: http://www.pedstest.com
E-mail: evpress@pedstest.com

*Rehabilitation Engineering and Assistive Technology Society of North America (RESNA)*
Phone: 703-524-6686
Fax: 703-524-6630
Website: http://resna.org

*Rett Syndrome Research Trust*
67 Under Cliff Rd.
Trumbull, CT 06611
Phone: 203-445-0041
Website: http://www.rsrt.org
E-mail: monica@rsrt.org

*Tourette Syndrome Association*
42–40 Bell Blvd.
Suite 205
Bayside, NY 11361
Toll-Free: 888-4-TOURET (486-8738)
Phone: 718-224-2999
Fax: 718-279-9596
Website: http://tsa-usa.org
E-mail: ts@tsa-usa.org

*University of South Florida*
CARD-USF MHC2113A
13301 Bruce B. Downs Blvd.
Tampa, FL 33612
Toll-Free: 800-333-4530
Phone: 813-974-2532
Fax: 813-974-6115
Website: http://card-usf.fmhi.usf.edu

# *Index*

# Index

# Health Reference Series
## Complete Catalog
List price $93 per volume. School and library price $84 per volume.

## Adolescent Health Sourcebook, 3rd Edition

*Basic Consumer Health Information about Adolescent Growth and Development, Puberty, Sexuality, Reproductive Health, and Physical, Emotional, Social, and Mental Health Concerns of Teens and Their Parents, Including Facts about Nutrition, Physical Activity, Weight Management, Acne, Allergies, Cancer, Diabetes, Growth Disorders, Juvenile Arthritis, Infections, Substance Abuse, and More*

*Along with Information about Adolescent Safety Concerns, Youth Violence, a Glossary of Related Terms, and a Directory of Resources*

Edited by Amy L. Sutton. 600 pages. 2010. 978-0-7808-1140-9.

## Adult Health Concerns Sourcebook

*Basic Consumer Health Information about Medical and Mental Concerns of Adults, Including Facts about Choosing Healthcare Providers, Navigating Insurance Options, Maintaining Wellness, Preventing Cancer, Heart Disease, Stroke, Diabetes, and Osteoporosis, and Understanding Aging-Related Health Concerns, Including Menopause, Cognitive Changes, and Changes in the Coronary and Vascular Systems*

*Along with Tips on Caring for Aging Parents and Dealing with Health-Related Work and Travel Issues, a Glossary, and a Directory of Resources for Additional Help and Information*

Edited by Sandra J. Judd. 648 pages. 2008. 978-0-7808-0999-4.

"Provides a thorough list of topics that are important to adult health and for caregivers."
—*CHOICE, Nov '08*

"Written in easy-to-understand language... the content is well-organized and is intended to aid adults in making health care-related decisions."
—*AORN Journal, Dec '08*

## AIDS Sourcebook, 4th Edition

*Basic Consumer Health Information about Human Immunodeficiency Virus (HIV) and Acquired Immunodeficiency Syndrome (AIDS), Featuring Updated Statistics and Facts about Risks, Prevention, Screening, Diagnosis, Treatments, Side Effects, and Complications, and Including a Section about the Impact of HIV/AIDS on the Health of Women, Children, and Adolescents*

*Along with Tips on Managing Life with AIDS, Reports on Current Research Initiatives and Clinical Trials, a Glossary of Related Terms, and Resource Directories for Further Help and Information*

Edited by Ivy L. Alexander. 680 pages. 2008. 978-0-7808-0997-0.

***SEE ALSO*** *Contagious Diseases Sourcebook, 2nd Edition*

## Alcoholism Sourcebook, 3rd Edition

*Basic Consumer Health Information about Alcohol Use, Abuse, and Dependence, Featuring Facts about the Physical, Mental, and Social Health Effects of Alcohol Addiction, Including Alcoholic Liver Disease, Pancreatic Disease, Cardiovascular Disease, Neurological Disorders, and the Effects of Drinking during Pregnancy*

*Along with Information about Alcohol Treatment, Medications, and Recovery Programs, in Addition to Tips for Reducing the Prevalence of Underage Drinking, Statistics about Alcohol Use, a Glossary of Related Terms, and Directories of Resources for More Help and Information*

Edited by Joyce Brennfleck Shannon. 600 pages. 2010. 978-0-7808-1141-6.

***SEE ALSO*** *Drug Abuse Sourcebook, 3rd Edition*

## Allergies Sourcebook, 3rd Edition

*Basic Consumer Health Information about Allergic Disorders, Such as Anaphylaxis, Hives,*

Eczema, Rhinitis, Sinusitis, and Conjunctivitis, and Their Triggers, Including Pollen, Mold, Dust Mites, Animal Dander, Insects, Chemicals, Food, Food Additives, and Medications

Along with Advice about the Diagnosis and Treatment of Allergy Symptoms, a Glossary of Related Terms, a Directory of Resources for Help and Information, and Suggestions for Additional Reading

Edited by Amy L. Sutton. 588 pages. 2007. 978-0-7808-0950-5.

*SEE ALSO* Asthma Sourcebook, 2nd Edition

## Alzheimer Disease Sourcebook, 4th Edition

Basic Consumer Health Information about Alzheimer Disease, Other Dementias, and Related Disorders, Including Multi-Infarct Dementia, Dementia with Lewy Bodies, Frontotemporal Dementia (Pick Disease), Wernicke-Korsakoff Syndrome (Alcohol-Related Dementia), AIDS Dementia Complex, Huntington Disease, Creutzfeldt-Jacob Disease, and Delirium

Along with Information about Coping with Memory Loss and Forgetfulness, Maintaining Skills, and Long-Term Planning for People with Dementia, and Suggestions Addressing Common Caregiver Concerns, Updated Information about Current Research Efforts, a Glossary of Related Terms, and Directories of Sources for Additional Help and Information

Edited by Karen Bellenir. 603 pages. 2008. 978-0-7808-1001-3.

"An invaluable resource for persons who have received a diagnosis, for caregivers, and for family members dealing with this insidious disease. It is recommended for public, community college, and ready-reference sections in academic libraries."
—American Reference Books Annual, 2009

*SEE ALSO* Brain Disorders Sourcebook, 3rd Edition

## Arthritis Sourcebook, 3rd Edition

Basic Consumer Health Information about the Risk Factors, Symptoms, Diagnosis, and Treatment of Osteoarthritis, Rheumatoid Arthritis, Juvenile Arthritis, Gout, Infectious Arthritis, and Autoimmune Disorders Associated with Arthritis

Along with Facts about Medications, Surgeries, and Self-Care Techniques to Manage Pain and Disability, Tips on Living with Arthritis, a Glossary of Related Terms, and Resources for Additional Help and Information

Edited by Amy L. Sutton. 600 pages. 2010. 978-0-7808-1077-8.

## Asthma Sourcebook, 2nd Edition

Basic Consumer Health Information about the Causes, Symptoms, Diagnosis, and Treatment of Asthma in Infants, Children, Teenagers, and Adults, Including Facts about Different Types of Asthma, Common Co-Occurring Conditions, Asthma Management Plans, Triggers, Medications, and Medication Delivery Devices

Along with Asthma Statistics, Research Updates, a Glossary, a Directory of Asthma-Related Resources, and More

Edited by Karen Bellenir. 581 pages. 2006. 978-0-7808-0866-9.

*SEE ALSO* Lung Disorders Sourcebook; Respiratory Disorders Sourcebook, 2nd Edition

## Attention Deficit Disorder Sourcebook

Basic Consumer Health Information about Attention Deficit/Hyperactivity Disorder in Children and Adults, Including Facts about Causes, Symptoms, Diagnostic Criteria, and Treatment Options Such as Medications, Behavior Therapy, Coaching, and Homeopathy

Along with Reports on Current Research Initiatives, Legal Issues, and Government Regulations, and Featuring a Glossary of Related Terms, Internet Resources, and a List of Additional Reading Material

Edited by Dawn D. Matthews. 447 pages. 2002. 978-0-7808-0624-5.

"Recommended reference source."
—Booklist, Jan '03

*SEE ALSO* Learning Disabilities Sourcebook, 3rd Edition

# Autism and Pervasive Developmental Disorders Sourcebook

*Basic Consumer Health Information about Autism Spectrum and Pervasive Developmental Disorders, Such as Classical Autism, Asperger Syndrome, Rett Syndrome, and Childhood Disintegrative Disorder, Including Information about Related Genetic Disorders and Medical Problems and Facts about Causes, Screening Methods, Diagnostic Criteria, Treatments and Interventions, and Family and Education Issues*

*Along with a Glossary of Related Terms, Tips for Evaluating the Validity of Health Claims, and a Directory of Resources for Additional Help and Information*

Edited by Sandra J. Judd. 603 pages. 2007. 978-0-7808-0953-6.

"This book provides a current overview of disorders on the autism spectrum and information about various therapies, educational resources, and help for families with practical issues such as workplace adjustments, living arrangements, and estate planning. It is a useful resource for public and consumer health libraries."
—*American Reference Books Annual, 2009*

**SEE ALSO** *Learning Disabilities Sourcebook, 3rd Edition*

---

# Back and Neck Disorders Sourcebook, 2nd Edition

*Basic Consumer Health Information about Spinal Pain, Spinal Cord Injuries, and Related Disorders, Such as Degenerative Disk Disease, Osteoarthritis, Scoliosis, Sciatica, Spina Bifida, and Spinal Stenosis, and Featuring Facts about Maintaining Spinal Health, Self-Care, Pain Management, Rehabilitative Care, Chiropractic Care, Spinal Surgeries, and Complementary Therapies*

*Along with Suggestions for Preventing Back and Neck Pain, a Glossary of Related Terms, and a Directory of Resources*

Edited by Amy L. Sutton. 607 pages. 2004. 978-0-7808-0738-9.

"Recommended... An easy to use, comprehensive medical reference book."
—*E-Streams, Sep '05*

"For anyone who has back or neck problems, this book is ideal. Its easy-to-understand language and variety of topics makes this sourcebook a worthwhile read. The price... is reasonable for the amount of information contained in the book"
—*Occupational Therapy in Health Care, 2007*

---

# Blood & Circulatory Disorders Sourcebook, 3rd Edition

*Basic Consumer Health Information about Blood and Circulatory System Disorders, Such as Anemia, Leukemia, Lymphoma, Rh Disease, Hemophilia, Thrombophilia, Other Bleeding and Clotting Deficiencies, and Artery, Vascular, and Venous Diseases, Including Facts about Blood Types, Blood Donation, Bone Marrow and Stem Cell Transplants, Tests and Medications, and Tips for Maintaining Circulatory Health*

*Along with a Glossary of Related Terms and a List of Resources for Additional Help and Information*

Edited by Sandra J. Judd. 600 pages. 2010. 978-0-7808-1081-5.

**SEE ALSO** *Leukemia Sourcebook*

---

# Brain Disorders Sourcebook, 3rd Edition

*Basic Consumer Health Information about Acquired and Traumatic Brain Injuries, Brain Tumors, Cerebral Palsy and Other Genetic and Congenital Brain Disorders, Infections of the Brain, Epilepsy, and Degenerative Neurological Disorders Such as Dementia, Huntington Disease, and Amyotrophic Lateral Sclerosis (ALS)*

*Along with Information on Brain Structure and Function, Treatment and Rehabilitation Options, a Glossary of Terms Related to Brain Disorders, and a Directory of Resources for More Information*

Edited by Joyce Brennfleck Shannon. 600 pages. 2010. 978-0-7808-1083-9.

**SEE ALSO** *Alzheimer Disease Sourcebook, 4th Edition*

## Breast Cancer Sourcebook, 3rd Edition

*Basic Consumer Health Information about Breast Health and Breast Cancer, Including Facts about Environmental, Genetic, and Other Risk Factors, Prevention Efforts, Screening and Diagnostic Methods, Surgical Treatment Options and Other Care Choices, Complementary and Alternative Therapies, and Post-Treatment Concerns*

*Along with Statistical Data, News about Research Advances, a Glossary of Related Terms, and Directories of Resources for Additional Information and Support*

Edited by Karen Bellenir. 606 pages. 2009. 978-0-7808-1030-3.

**"A very useful reference for people wanting to learn more about breast cancer and how to negotiate their care or the care of a loved one. The third edition is necessary as information/ treatment options continue to evolve."**
—*Doody's Review Service, 2009*

**SEE ALSO** *Cancer Sourcebook for Women, 3rd Edition, Women's Health Concerns Sourcebook, 3rd Edition*

## Breastfeeding Sourcebook

*Basic Consumer Health Information about the Benefits of Breastmilk, Preparing to Breastfeed, Breastfeeding as a Baby Grows, Nutrition, and More, Including Information on Special Situations and Concerns Such as Mastitis, Illness, Medications, Allergies, Multiple Births, Prematurity, Special Needs, and Adoption*

*Along with a Glossary and Resources for Additional Help and Information*

Edited by Jenni Lynn Colson. 367 pages. 2002. 978-0-7808-0332-9.

**SEE ALSO** *Pregnancy and Birth Sourcebook, 3rd Edition*

## Burns Sourcebook

*Basic Consumer Health Information about Various Types of Burns and Scalds, Including Flame, Heat, Cold, Electrical, Chemical, and Sun Burns*

*Along with Information on Short-Term and Long-Term Treatments, Tissue Reconstruction, Plastic Surgery, Prevention Suggestions, and First Aid*

Edited by Allan R. Cook. 604 pages. 1999. 978-0-7808-0204-9.

**"This is an exceptional addition to the series and is highly recommended for all consumer health collections, hospital libraries, and academic medical centers."**
—*E-Streams, Mar '00*

**"This key reference guide is an invaluable addition to all health care and public libraries in confronting this ongoing health issue."**
—*American Reference Books Annual, 2000*

**SEE ALSO** *Dermatological Disorders Sourcebook, 2nd Edition*

## Cancer Sourcebook, 5th Edition

*Basic Consumer Health Information about Major Forms and Stages of Cancer, Featuring Facts about Head and Neck Cancers, Lung Cancers, Gastrointestinal Cancers, Genitourinary Cancers, Lymphomas, Blood Cell Cancers, Endocrine Cancers, Skin Cancers, Bone Cancers, Metastatic Cancers, and More*

*Along with Facts about Cancer Treatments, Cancer Risks and Prevention, a Glossary of Related Terms, Statistical Data, and a Directory of Resources for Additional Information*

Edited by Karen Bellenir. 1105 pages. 2007. 978-0-7808-0947-5.

**"The 5th, updated edition of Cancer Sourcebook should be in every public and health lending library collection... An unparalleled discussion essential for any health collections considering an all-in-one basic general reference."**
—*California Bookwatch, Aug '07*

**SEE ALSO** *Breast Cancer Sourcebook, 3rd Edition, Cancer Survivorship Sourcebook, Leukemia Sourcebook*

## Cancer Sourcebook for Women, 4th Edition

*Basic Consumer Health Information about Gynecologic Cancers and Other Cancers of Special Concern to Women, Including Cancers of the Breast, Cervix, Colon, Lung, Ovaries, Thyroid, and Uterus*

*Along with Facts about Benign Conditions of the Female Reproductive System, Cancer Risk*

Factors, Diagnostic and Treatment Procedures, Side Effects of Cancer and Cancer Treatments, Women's Issues in Cancer Survivorship, a Glossary of Related Terms, and a Directory of Resources for Additional Help and Information

Edited by Karen Bellenir. 600 pages. 2010. 978-0-7808-1139-3.

**SEE ALSO** Breast Cancer Sourcebook, 3rd Edition, Women's Health Concerns Sourcebook, 3rd Edition

# Cancer Survivorship Sourcebook

*Basic Consumer Health Information about the Physical, Educational, Emotional, Social, and Financial Needs of Cancer Patients from Diagnosis, through Cancer Treatment, and Beyond, Including Facts about Researching Specific Types of Cancer and Learning about Clinical Trials and Treatment Options, and Featuring Tips for Coping with the Side Effects of Cancer Treatments and Adjusting to Life after Cancer Treatment Concludes*

*Along with Suggestions for Caregivers, Friends, and Family Members of Cancer Patients, a Glossary of Cancer Care Terms, and Directories of Related Resources*

Edited by Karen Bellenir. 633 pages. 2007. 978-0-7808-0985-7.

**"Well organized and comprehensive in coverage, the book speaks to issues encountered both during and after cancer treatment. Recommended for consumer health and public libraries."**
*—Library Journal, Aug 1 '07*

**"Cancer Survivorship Sourcebook will be useful to anyone who has a friend or loved one with a cancer diagnosis."**
*—American Reference Books Annual, 2008*

**SEE ALSO** *Cancer Sourcebook, 5th Edition, Disease Management Sourcebook*

# Cardiovascular Disorders Sourcebook, 4th Edition

*Basic Consumer Health Information about Heart and Blood Vessel Diseases and Disorders, Such as Angina, Heart Attack, Heart Failure, Cardiomyopathy, Arrhythmias, Valve Disease, Atherosclerosis, Aneurysms, and*

Congenital Heart Defects, Including Information about Cardiovascular Disease in Women, Men, Children, Adolescents, and Minorities

Along with Facts about Diagnosing, Managing, and Preventing Cardiovascular Disease, a Glossary of Related Medical Terms, and a Directory of Resources for Additional Information

Edited by Amy L. Sutton. 600 pages. 2010. 978-0-7808-1080-8.

# Caregiving Sourcebook

*Basic Consumer Health Information for Caregivers, Including a Profile of Caregivers, Caregiving Responsibilities and Concerns, Tips for Specific Conditions, Care Environments, and the Effects of Caregiving*

*Along with Facts about Legal Issues, Financial Information, and Future Planning, a Glossary, and a Listing of Additional Resources*

Edited by Joyce Brennfleck Shannon. 583 pages. 2001. 978-0-7808-0331-2.

**"Essential for most collections."**
*—Library Journal, Apr 1 '02*

**"An ideal addition to the reference collection of any public library. Health sciences information professionals may also want to acquire the Caregiving Sourcebook for their hospital or academic library for use as a ready reference tool by health care workers interested in aging and caregiving."**
*—E-Streams, Jan '02*

# Child Abuse Sourcebook, 2nd Edition

*Basic Consumer Health Information about the Physical, Sexual, and Emotional Abuse of Children, Neglect, Münchhausen Syndrome by Proxy (MSBP), and Shaken Baby Syndrome, and Featuring Facts about Withholding Medical Care, Corporal Punishment, Child Maltreatment in Youth Sports, and Parental Substance Abuse*

*Along with Information about Child Protective Services, Foster Care, Adoption, Parenting Challenges, Abuse Prevention Programs, and Intervention, Treatment, and Recovery Guidelines, a Glossary of Related Terms, and Resources for Additional Help and Information*

Edited by Joyce Brennfleck Shannon. 600 pages. 2009. 978-0-7808-1037-2.

*SEE ALSO Domestic Violence Sourcebook, 3rd Edition*

# Childhood Diseases and Disorders Sourcebook, 2nd Edition

*Basic Consumer Health Information about the Physical, Mental, and Developmental Health of Pre-Adolescent Children, Including Facts about Infectious Diseases, Asthma, Allergies, Diabetes, and Other Acute and Chronic Conditions Affecting the Gastrointestinal Tract, Ears, Nose, Throat, Liver, Kidneys, Heart, Blood, Brain, Muscles, Bones, and Skin*

*Along with Reports on Recommended Childhood Vaccinations, Wellness Guidelines, a Glossary of Related Medical Terms, and a List of Resources for Parents*

Edited by Sandra J. Judd. 694 pages. 2009. 978-0-7808-1031-0.

**"The strength of this source is the wide range of information given about childhood health issues... It is most appropriate for public libraries and academic libraries that field medical questions."**
—*American Reference Books Annual, 2009*

*SEE ALSO Healthy Children Sourcebook*

# Colds, Flu and Other Common Ailments Sourcebook

*Basic Consumer Health Information about Common Ailments and Injuries, Including Colds, Coughs, the Flu, Sinus Problems, Headaches, Fever, Nausea and Vomiting, Menstrual Cramps, Diarrhea, Constipation, Hemorrhoids, Back Pain, Dandruff, Dry and Itchy Skin, Cuts, Scrapes, Sprains, Bruises, and More*

*Along with Information about Prevention, Self-Care, Choosing a Doctor, Over-the-Counter Medications, Folk Remedies, and Alternative Therapies, and Including a Glossary of Important Terms and a Directory of Resources for Further Help and Information*

Edited by Chad T. Kimball. 622 pages. 2001. 978-0-7808-0435-7.

**"A good starting point for research on common illnesses. It will be a useful addition to public and consumer health library collections."**
—*American Reference Books Annual, 2002*

**"Will prove valuable to any library seeking to maintain a current, comprehensive reference collection of health resources... Excellent reference."**
—*The Bookwatch, Aug '01*

*SEE ALSO Contagious Diseases Sourcebook, 2nd Edition*

# Communication Disorders Sourcebook

*Basic Information about Deafness and Hearing Loss, Speech and Language Disorders, Voice Disorders, Balance and Vestibular Disorders, and Disorders of Smell, Taste, and Touch*

Edited by Linda M. Ross. 533 pages. 1996. 978-0-7808-0077-9.

**"This is skillfully edited and is a welcome resource for the layperson. It should be found in every public and medical library."**
—*Booklist Health Sciences Supplement, Oct '97*

# Complementary & Alternative Medicine Sourcebook, 4th Edition

*Basic Consumer Health Information about Ayurveda, Acupuncture, Aromatherapy, Chiropractic Care, Diet-Based Therapies, Guided Imagery, Herbal and Vitamin Supplements, Homeopathy, Hypnosis, Massage, Meditation, Naturopathy, Pilates, Reflexology, Reiki, Shiatsu, Tai Chi, Traditional Chinese Medicine, Yoga, and Other Complementary and Alternative Medical Therapies*

*Along with Statistics, Tips for Selecting a Practitioner, Treatments for Specific Health Conditions, a Glossary of Related Terms, and a Directory of Resources for Additional Help and Information*

Edited by Amy L. Sutton. 600 pages. 2010. 978-0-7808-1082-2.

# Congenital Disorders Sourcebook, 2nd Edition

*Basic Consumer Health Information about Nonhereditary Birth Defects and Disorders*

Related to Prematurity, Gestational Injuries, Congenital Infections, and Birth Complications, Including Heart Defects, Hydrocephalus, Spina Bifida, Cleft Lip and Palate, Cerebral Palsy, and More

Along with Facts about the Prevention of Birth Defects, Fetal Surgery and Other Treatment Options, Research Initiatives, a Glossary of Related Terms, and Resources for Additional Information and Support

Edited by Sandra J. Judd. 619 pages. 2007. 978-0-7808-0945-1.

"Congenital Disorders Sourcebook provides an excellent, non-technical overview of many aspects of pregnancy with the focus on congenital disorders."
— American Reference Books Annual, 2008

"An excellent readable reference aimed at the lay public for difficult to understand medical problems. An excellent starting point for the interested parent or family member who may then be motivated to seek more information."
— Doody's Review Service, 2007

SEE ALSO Pregnancy and Birth Sourcebook, 3rd Edition

# Contagious Diseases Sourcebook, 2nd Edition

Basic Consumer Health Information about Diseases Spread from Person to Person through Direct Physical Contact, Airborne Transmissions, Sexual Contact, or Contact with Blood or Other Body Fluids, Including Pneumococcal, Staphylococcal, and Streptococcal Diseases, Colds, Influenza, Lice, Measles, Mumps, Tuberculosis, and Others

Along with Facts about Self-Care and Over-the-Counter Medications, Antibiotics and Drug Resistance, Disease Prevention, Vaccines, and Bioterrorism, a Glossary, and a Directory of Resources for More Information

Edited by Joyce Brennfleck Shannon. 600 pages. 2010. 978-0-7808-1075-4.

SEE ALSO AIDS Sourcebook, 4th Edition, Hepatitis Sourcebook

# Cosmetic and Reconstructive Surgery Sourcebook, 2nd Edition

Basic Consumer Information about Plastic Surgery and Non-Surgical Appearance-Enhancing Procedures, Including Facts about Botulinum Toxin, Collagen Replacement, Dermabrasion, Chemical Peels, Eyelid Surgery, Nose Reshaping, Lip Augmentation, Liposuction, Breast Enlargement and Reduction, Tummy Tucking, and Other Skin, Hair, Facial, and Body Shaping Procedures

Along with Information about Reconstructive Procedures for Congenital Disorders, Disfiguring Diseases, Burns, and Traumatic Injuries, a Glossary of Related Terms, and a Directory of Additional Resources

Edited by Karen Bellenir. 483 pages. 2007. 978-0-7808-0951-2.

"A comprehensive source for people considering cosmetic surgery... also recommended for medical students who will perform these procedures later in their careers; and public librarians and academic medical librarians who may assist patrons interested in this information."
— Medical Reference Services Quarterly, Fall '08

"A practical guide for health care consumers and health care workers... This easy-to-read reference guide would be useful for novice and veteran health care consumers, surgical technology students, nursing students, and perioperative nurses new to plastic and reconstructive surgery. It also may be helpful for medical-surgical nurses as a guide for patient teaching in their practices."
— AORN Journal, Aug '08

SEE ALSO Surgery Sourcebook, 2nd Edition

# Death and Dying Sourcebook, 2nd Edition

Basic Consumer Health Information about End-of-Life Care and Related Perspectives and Ethical Issues, Including End-of-Life Symptoms and Treatments, Pain Management, Quality-of-Life Concerns, the Use of Life Support, Patients' Rights and Privacy Issues, Advance Directives, Physician-Assisted Suicide, Caregiving, Organ and Tissue Donation, Autopsies, Funeral Arrangements, and Grief

Along with Statistical Data, Information about the Leading Causes of Death, a Glossary, and Directories of Support Groups and Other Resources

Edited by Joyce Brennfleck Shannon. 626 pages. 2006. 978-0-7808-0871-3.

---

# Dental Care and Oral Health Sourcebook, 3rd Edition

Basic Consumer Health Information about Dental Care and Oral Health Throughout the Lifespan, Including Facts about Cavities, Bad Breath, Cold and Canker Sores, Dry Mouth, Toothaches, Gum Disease, Malocclusion, Temporomandibular Joint and Muscle Disorders, Oral Cancers, and Dental Emergencies

Along with Information about Mouth Hygiene, Crowns, Bridges, Implants, and Fillings, Surgical, Orthodontic, and Cosmetic Dental Procedures, Pain Management, Health Conditions that Impact Oral Care, a Glossary of Related Terms, and a Directory of Additional Resources

Edited by Amy L. Sutton. 619 pages. 2008. 978-0-7808-1032-7.

"Could serve as turning point in the battle to educate consumers in issues concerning oral health. Tightly written in terms the average person can understand, yet comprehensive in scope and authoritative in tone, it is another excellent sourcebook in the Health Reference Series... Should be in the reference department of all public libraries, and in academic libraries that have a public constituency."
—American Reference Books Annual, 2009

---

# Depression Sourcebook, 2nd Edition

Basic Consumer Health Information about Unipolar Depression, Bipolar Disorder, Dysthymia, Seasonal Affective Disorder, Postpartum Depression, and Other Depressive Disorders, Including Facts about Populations at Special Risk, Coexisting Medical Conditions, Symptoms, Treatment Options, and Suicide Prevention

Along with Statistical Data, a Glossary of Related Terms, and a Directory of Resources for Additional Help and Information

Edited by Sandra J. Judd. 646 pages. 2008. 978-0-7808-1003-7.

"Recommended for public libraries."
—American Reference Books Annual, 2009

SEE ALSO Mental Health Disorders Sourcebook, 4th Edition

---

# Dermatological Disorders Sourcebook, 2nd Edition

Basic Consumer Health Information about Conditions and Disorders Affecting the Skin, Hair, and Nails, Such as Acne, Rosacea, Rashes, Dermatitis, Pigmentation Disorders, Birthmarks, Skin Cancer, Skin Injuries, Psoriasis, Scleroderma, and Hair Loss, Including Facts about Medications and Treatments for Dermatological Disorders and Tips for Maintaining Healthy Skin, Hair, and Nails

Along with Information about How Aging Affects the Skin, a Glossary of Related Terms, and a Directory of Resources for Additional Help and Information

Edited by Amy L. Sutton. 617 pages. 2006. 978-0-7808-0795-2.

"Well organized... presents a plethora of information in a manner that is appropriate in style and readability for the intended audience."
—Physical Therapy, Nov '06

"Helpfully brings together... sources in one convenient place, saving the user hours of research time."
—American Reference Books Annual, 2006

SEE ALSO Burns Sourcebook

---

# Diabetes Sourcebook, 4th Edition

Basic Consumer Health Information about Type 1 and Type 2 Diabetes Mellitus, Gestational Diabetes, Monogenic Forms of Diabetes, and Insulin Resistance, with Guidelines for Lifestyle Modifications and the Medical Management of Diabetes, Including Facts about Insulin, Insulin Delivery Devices, Oral Diabetes Medications, Self-Monitoring of Blood Glucose, Meal Planning, Physical Activity Recommendations, Foot Care, and Treatment Options for People with Kidney Failure

Along with a Section about Diabetes Complications and Co-Occurring Conditions, a Glossary of Related Terms, and Directories of Resources for Additional Help and Information

Edited by Karen Bellenir. 627 pages. 2008. 978-0-7808-1005-1.

"Completely and comprehensively covering almost everything a student or physician would need to know... well worth the investment."

—*Internet Bookwatch, Dec '08*

**SEE ALSO** *Endocrine and Metabolic Disorders Sourcebook, 2nd Edition*

---

# Diet and Nutrition Sourcebook, 3rd Edition

*Basic Consumer Health Information about Dietary Guidelines and the Food Guidance System, Recommended Daily Nutrient Intakes, Serving Proportions, Weight Control, Vitamins and Supplements, Nutrition Issues for Different Life Stages and Lifestyles, and the Needs of People with Specific Medical Concerns, Including Cancer, Celiac Disease, Diabetes, Eating Disorders, Food Allergies, and Cardiovascular Disease*

*Along with Facts about Federal Nutrition Support Programs, a Glossary of Nutrition and Dietary Terms, and Directories of Additional Resources for More Information about Nutrition*

Edited by Joyce Brennfleck Shannon. 605 pages. 2006. 978-0-7808-0800-3.

"A valuable resource tool for any individual."

—*Journal of Dental Hygiene, Apr '07*

"From different recommended eating habits to reduce disease and common ailments to nutrition advice for those with specific conditions, Diet and Nutrition Sourcebook is especially important because so much is changing in this area, and so rapidly."

—*California Bookwatch, Jun '06*

**SEE ALSO** *Eating Disorders Sourcebook, 2nd Edition, Vegetarian Sourcebook*

---

# Digestive Diseases and Disorders Sourcebook

*Basic Consumer Health Information about Diseases and Disorders that Impact the Upper and Lower Digestive System, Including Celiac Disease, Constipation, Crohn's Disease, Cyclic Vomiting Syndrome, Diarrhea, Diverticulosis and Diverticulitis, Gallstones, Heartburn, Hemorrhoids, Hernias, Indigestion (Dyspepsia), Irritable Bowel Syndrome, Lactose Intolerance, Ulcers, and More*

*Along with Information about Medications and Other Treatments, Tips for Maintaining a Healthy Digestive Tract, a Glossary, and Directory of Digestive Diseases Organizations*

Edited by Karen Bellenir. 323 pages. 2000. 978-0-7808-0327-5.

"An excellent addition to all public or patient-research libraries."

—*American Reference Books Annual,*
*2001*

"Recommended reference source."

—*Booklist, May '00*

**SEE ALSO** *Gastrointestinal Diseases and Disorders Sourcebook, 2nd Edition*

---

# Disabilities Sourcebook

*Basic Consumer Health Information about Physical and Psychiatric Disabilities, Including Descriptions of Major Causes of Disability, Assistive and Adaptive Aids, Workplace Issues, and Accessibility Concerns*

*Along with Information about the Americans with Disabilities Act, a Glossary, and Resources for Additional Help and Information*

Edited by Dawn D. Matthews. 602 pages. 2000. 978-0-7808-0389-3.

"A must for libraries with a consumer health section."

—*American Reference Books Annual, 2002*

"A much needed addition to the Omnigraphics Health Reference Series. A current reference work to provide people with disabilities, their families, caregivers or those who work with them, a broad range of information in one volume, has not been available until now... It is recommended for all public and academic library reference collections."

—*E-Streams, May '01*

"An excellent source book in easy-to-read format covering many current topics; highly recommended for all libraries."

—*CHOICE, Jan '01*

# Disease Management Sourcebook

*Basic Consumer Health Information about Coping with Chronic and Serious Illnesses, Navigating the Health Care System, Communicating with Health Care Providers, Assessing Health Care Quality, and Making Informed Health Care Decisions, Including Facts about Second Opinions, Hospitalization, Surgery, and Medications*

*Along with a Section about Children with Chronic Conditions, Information about Legal, Financial, and Insurance Issues, a Glossary of Related Terms, and Directories of Additional Resources*

Edited by Joyce Brennfleck Shannon. 621 pages. 2008. 978-0-7808-1002-0.

"Consumers need to know how to manage their health care the same way they manage anything else in their lives. The text is very readable and is written for the layperson and consumer. The cost is not prohibitive. This book should be in all collections of health care libraries and public libraries."
— *American Reference Books Annual, 2009*

"The information is very current, and the selection of font and layout make the book easy to read. A hardback that will stand up to much usage, this is an excellent resource for consumers... Recommended. General readers."
*—CHOICE, Nov '08*

"Intended for lay readers, this resource clarifies the many confusing and overwhelming details associated with chronic disease care. Meticulous and clearly explained, the book even includes diagrams intended to ease comprehension of over-the-counter medication labels. An essential guide to navigating the health-care rapids."
*—Library Journal, Aug '08*

# Domestic Violence Sourcebook, 3rd Edition

*Basic Consumer Health Information about Warning Signs, Risk Factors, and Health Consequences of Intimate Partner Violence, Sexual Violence and Rape, Stalking, Human Trafficking, Child Maltreatment, Teen Dating Violence, and Elder Abuse*

*Along with Facts about Victims and Perpetrators, Strategies for Violence Prevention, and Emergency Interventions, Safety Plans, and Financial and Legal Tips for Victims, a Glossary of Related Terms, and Directories of Resources for Additional Information and Support*

Edited by Joyce Brennfleck Shannon. 634 pages. 2009. 978-0-7808-1038-9.

"A recommended pick for any library interested in consumer health and social issues... A 'must' for any serious health collection."
*—California Bookwatch, Jul '09*

*SEE ALSO Child Abuse Sourcebook, 2nd Edition*

# Drug Abuse Sourcebook, 3rd Edition

*Basic Consumer Health Information about the Abuse of Cocaine, Club Drugs, Hallucinogens, Heroin, Inhalants, Marijuana, and Other Illicit Substances, Prescription Medications, and Over-the-Counter Medicines*

*Along with Facts about Addiction and Related Health Effects, Drug Abuse Treatment and Recovery, Drug Testing, Prevention Programs, Glossaries of Drug-Related Terms, and Directories of Resources for More Information*

Edited by Joyce Brennfleck Shannon. 600 pages. 2010. 978-0-7808-1079-2.

*SEE ALSO Alcoholism Sourcebook, 3rd Edition*

# Ear, Nose, and Throat Disorders Sourcebook, 2nd Edition

*Basic Consumer Health Information about Disorders of the Ears, Hearing Loss, Vestibular Disorders, Nasal and Sinus Problems, Throat and Vocal Cord Disorders, and Otolaryngologic Cancers, Including Facts about Ear Infections and Injuries, Genetic and Congenital Deafness, Sensorineural Hearing Disorders, Tinnitus, Vertigo, Ménière Disease, Rhinitis, Sinusitis, Snoring, Sore Throats, Hoarseness, and More*

*Along with Reports on Current Research Initiatives, a Glossary of Related Medical Terms, and a Directory of Sources for Further Help and Information*

Edited by Sandra J. Judd. 631 pages. 2007. 978-0-7808-0872-0.

614

"A resource book for the general public that provides comprehensive coverage of basic up-to-date medical information about the causes, symptoms, diagnosis, and treatment of diseases and disorders that affect the ears, nose, sinuses, throat, and voice... The majority of information is presented in question and answer format, much like questions a patient might ask of a health care provider. An extensive index facilitates the reader's ability to easily access information on any specific topic."
—*Journal of Dental Hygiene, Oct '07*

"A handy compilation of information on common and some not so common ailments of the ears, nose, and throat."
—*Doody's Review Service, 2007*

# Eating Disorders Sourcebook, 2nd Edition

*Basic Consumer Health Information about Anorexia Nervosa, Bulimia, Binge Eating, Compulsive Exercise, Female Athlete Triad, and Other Eating Disorders, Including Facts about Body Image and Other Cultural and Age-Related Risk Factors, Prevention Efforts, Adverse Health Effects, Treatment Options, and the Recovery Process*

*Along with Guidelines for Healthy Weight Control, a Glossary, and Directories of Additional Resources*

Edited by Joyce Brennfleck Shannon. 557 pages. 2007. 978-0-7808-0948-2.

"Recommended for the reference collection of large public libraries."
—*American Reference Books Annual, 2008*

"A basic health reference any health or general library needs."
—*Internet Bookwatch, Jun '07*

**SEE ALSO** *Diet and Nutrition Sourcebook, 3rd Edition, Mental Health Disorders Sourcebook, 4th Edition*

# Emergency Medical Services Sourcebook

*Basic Consumer Health Information about Preventing, Preparing for, and Managing Emergency Situations, When and Who to Call for Help, What to Expect in the Emergency Room, the Emergency Medical Team,*

*Patient Issues, and Current Topics in Emergency Medicine*

*Along with Statistical Data, a Glossary, and Sources of Additional Help and Information*

Edited by Jenni Lynn Colson. 472 pages. 2002. 978-0-7808-0420-3.

"Handy and convenient for home, public, school, and college libraries. Recommended."
—*CHOICE, Apr '03*

"This reference can provide the consumer with answers to most questions about emergency care in the United States, or it will direct them to a resource where the answer can be found."
—*American Reference Books Annual, 2003*

**SEE ALSO** *Injury and Trauma Sourcebook*

# Endocrine and Metabolic Disorders Sourcebook, 2nd Edition

*Basic Consumer Health Information about Hormonal and Metabolic Disorders that Affect the Body's Growth, Development, and Functioning, Including Disorders of the Pancreas, Ovaries and Testes, and Pituitary, Thyroid, Parathyroid, and Adrenal Glands, with Facts about Growth Disorders, Addison Disease, Cushing Syndrome, Conn Syndrome, Diabetic Disorders, Multiple Endocrine Neoplasia, Inborn Errors of Metabolism, and More*

*Along with Information about Endocrine Functioning, Diagnostic and Screening Tests, a Glossary of Related Terms, and Directories of Additional Resources*

Edited by Joyce Brennfleck Shannon. 597 pages. 2007. 978-0-7808-0952-9.

**SEE ALSO** *Diabetes Sourcebook, 4th Edition*

# Environmental Health Sourcebook, 3rd Edition

*Basic Consumer Health Information about the Environment and Its Effects on Human Health, Including Facts about Air, Water, and Soil Contamination, Hazardous Chemicals, Foodborne Hazards and Illnesses, Household Hazards Such as Radon, Mold, and Carbon Monoxide, Consumer Hazards from Toxic Products and Imported Goods, and Disorders*

Linked to Environmental Causes, Including Chemical Sensitivity, Cancer, Allergies, and Asthma

Along with Information about the Impact of Environmental Hazards on Specific Populations, a Glossary of Related Terms, and Resources for Additional Help and Information.

Edited by Laura Larsen. 600 pages. 2010. 978-0-7808-1078-5

# Ethnic Diseases Sourcebook

Basic Consumer Health Information for Ethnic and Racial Minority Groups in the United States, Including General Health Indicators and Behaviors, Ethnic Diseases, Genetic Testing, the Impact of Chronic Diseases, Women's Health, Mental Health Issues, and Preventive Health Care Services

Along with a Glossary and a Listing of Additional Resources

Edited by Joyce Brennfleck Shannon. 648 pages. 2001. 978-0-7808-0336-7.

"Not many books have been written on this topic to date, and the Ethnic Diseases Sourcebook is a strong addition to the list. It will be an important introductory resource for health consumers, students, health care personnel, and social scientists. It is recommended for public, academic, and large hospital libraries."
— American Reference Books Annual, 2002

"Will prove valuable to any library seeking to maintain a current, comprehensive reference collection of health resources... An excellent source of health information about genetic disorders which affect particular ethnic and racial minorities in the U.S."
—The Bookwatch, Aug '01

# Eye Care Sourcebook, 3rd Edition

Basic Consumer Health Information about Eye Care and Eye Disorders, Including Facts about the Diagnosis, Prevention, and Treatment of Refractive Disorders, Cataracts, Glaucoma, Macular Degeneration, and Problems Affecting the Cornea, Retina, and Lacrimal Glands

Along with Advice about Preventing Eye Injuries and Tips for Living with Low Vision or Blindness, a Glossary of Related Terms, and Directories of Resources for More Help and Information

Edited by Amy L. Sutton. 646 pages. 2008. 978-0-7808-1000-6.

"A solid reference tool for eye care and a valuable addition to a collection."
—American Reference Books Annual, 2009

# Family Planning Sourcebook

Basic Consumer Health Information about Planning for Pregnancy and Contraception, Including Traditional Methods, Barrier Methods, Hormonal Methods, Permanent Methods, Future Methods, Emergency Contraception, and Birth Control Choices for Women at Each Stage of Life

Along with Statistics, a Glossary, and Sources of Additional Information

Edited by Amy Marcaccio Keyzer. 503 pages. 2001. 978-0-7808-0379-4.

"Recommended for public, health, and undergraduate libraries as part of the circulating collection."
—E-Streams, Mar '02

"Will prove valuable to any library seeking to maintain a current, comprehensive reference collection of health resources... Excellent reference."
—The Bookwatch, Aug '01

SEE ALSO Pregnancy and Birth Sourcebook, 3rd Edition

# Fitness and Exercise Sourcebook, 3rd Edition

Basic Consumer Health Information about the Physical and Mental Benefits of Fitness, Including Cardiorespiratory Endurance, Muscular Strength, Muscular Endurance, and Flexibility, with Facts about Sports Nutrition and Exercise-Related Injuries and Tips about Physical Activity and Exercises for People of All Ages and for People with Health Concerns

Along with Advice on Selecting and Using Exercise Equipment, Maintaining Exercise Motivation, a Glossary of Related Terms, and a Directory of Resources for More Help and Information

Edited by Amy L. Sutton. 635 pages. 2007. 978-0-7808-0946-8.

"Updates the consumer information on the physical and mental benefits of physical activity throughout the lifespan offered in earlier editions... Recommended. All readers; all levels."
—*CHOICE, Oct '07*

"An exceptionally well-rounded coverage perfect for any concerned about developing and understanding a fitness program."
—*California Bookwatch, Jun '07*

SEE ALSO *Sports Injuries Sourcebook, 3rd Edition*

## Food Safety Sourcebook

*Basic Consumer Health Information about the Safe Handling of Meat, Poultry, Seafood, Eggs, Fruit Juices, and Other Food Items, and Facts about Pesticides, Drinking Water, Food Safety Overseas, and the Onset, Duration, and Symptoms of Foodborne Illnesses, Including Types of Pathogenic Bacteria, Parasitic Protozoa, Worms, Viruses, and Natural Toxins*

*Along with the Role of the Consumer, the Food Handler, and the Government in Food Safety, a Glossary, and Resources for Additional Help and Information*

Edited by Dawn D. Matthews. 327 pages. 1999. 978-0-7808-0326-8.

"Recommended reference source."
—*Booklist, May '00*

"This book takes the complex issues of food safety and foodborne pathogens and presents them in an easily understood manner. [It does] an excellent job of covering a large and often confusing topic."
— *American Reference Books Annual, 2000*

## Forensic Medicine Sourcebook

*Basic Consumer Information for the Layperson about Forensic Medicine, Including Crime Scene Investigation, Evidence Collection and Analysis, Expert Testimony, Computer-Aided Criminal Identification, Digital Imaging in the Courtroom, DNA Profiling, Accident Reconstruction, Autopsies, Ballistics, Drugs and Explosives Detection, Latent Fingerprints,*

*Product Tampering, and Questioned Document Examination*

*Along with Statistical Data, a Glossary of Forensics Terminology, and Listings of Sources for Further Help and Information*

Edited by Annemarie S. Muth. 574 pages. 1999. 978-0-7808-0232-2.

"Given the expected widespread interest in its content and its easy to read style, this book is recommended for most public and all college and university libraries."
—*E-Streams, Feb '01*

"A wealth of information, useful statistics, references are up-to-date and extremely complete. This wonderful collection of data will help students who are interested in a career in any type of forensic field. It is a great resource for attorneys who need information about types of expert witnesses needed in a particular case. It also offers useful information for fiction and nonfiction writers whose work involves a crime. A fascinating compilation. All levels."
—*CHOICE, Jan '00*

"There are several items that make this book attractive to consumers who are seeking certain forensic data... This is a useful current source for those seeking general forensic medical answers."
—*American Reference Books Annual, 2000*

## Gastrointestinal Diseases and Disorders Sourcebook, 2nd Edition

*Basic Consumer Health Information about the Upper and Lower Gastrointestinal (GI) Tract, Including the Esophagus, Stomach, Intestines, Rectum, Liver, and Pancreas, with Facts about Gastroesophageal Reflux Disease, Gastritis, Hernias, Ulcers, Celiac Disease, Diverticulitis, Irritable Bowel Syndrome, Hemorrhoids, Gastrointestinal Cancers, and Other Diseases and Disorders Related to the Digestive Process*

*Along with Information about Commonly Used Diagnostic and Surgical Procedures, Statistics, Reports on Current Research Initiatives and Clinical Trials, a Glossary, and Resources for Additional Help and Information*

Edited by Sandra J. Judd. 654 pages. 2006. 978-0-7808-0798-3.

"The text is designed for the general reader seeking information on prevention, disease warning signs, diagnostic and therapeutic questions... It is an excellent resource for the general reader to conveniently locate credible, coordinated and indexed information... The sourcebook will prove very helpful for patients, caregivers and should be available in every physician waiting room."

—*Doody's Review Service, 2006*

**SEE ALSO** *Diet and Nutrition Sourcebook, 3rd Edition, Digestive Diseases and Disorders Sourcebook*

# Genetic Disorders Sourcebook, 4th Edition

*Basic Consumer Health Information about Hereditary Diseases and Disorders, Including Facts about the Human Genome, Genetic Inheritance Patterns, Disorders Associated with Specific Genes, Such as Sickle Cell Disease, Hemophilia, and Cystic Fibrosis, Chromosome Disorders, Such as Down Syndrome, Fragile X Syndrome, and Turner Syndrome, and Complex Diseases and Disorders Resulting from the Interaction of Environmental and Genetic Factors, Such as Allergies, Cancer, and Obesity*

*Along with Facts about Genetic Testing, Suggestions for Parents of Children with Special Needs, Reports on Current Research Initiatives, a Glossary of Genetic Terminology, and Resources for Additional Help and Information*

Edited by Sandra J. Judd. 600 pages. 2010. 978-0-7808-1076-1.

# Head Trauma Sourcebook

*Basic Information for the Layperson about Open-Head and Closed-Head Injuries, Treatment Advances, Recovery, and Rehabilitation*

*Along with Reports on Current Research Initiatives*

Edited by Karen Bellenir. 414 pages. 1997. 978-0-7808-0208-7.

# Headache Sourcebook

*Basic Consumer Health Information about Migraine, Tension, Cluster, Rebound and Other Types of Headaches, with Facts about the Cause and Prevention of Headaches, the Effects of Stress and the Environment, Headaches during Pregnancy and Menopause, and Childhood Headaches*

*Along with a Glossary and Other Resources for Additional Help and Information*

Edited by Dawn D. Matthews. 342 pages. 2002. 978-0-7808-0337-4.

**"Highly recommended for academic and medical reference collections."**

—*Library Bookwatch, Sep '02*

**SEE ALSO** *Pain Sourcebook, 3rd Edition*

# Healthy Aging Sourcebook

*Basic Consumer Health Information about Maintaining Health through the Aging Process, Including Advice on Nutrition, Exercise, and Sleep, Help in Making Decisions about Midlife Issues and Retirement, and Guidance Concerning Practical and Informed Choices in Health Consumerism*

*Along with Data Concerning the Theories of Aging, Different Experiences in Aging by Minority Groups, and Facts about Aging Now and Aging in the Future; and Featuring a Glossary, a Guide to Consumer Help, Additional Suggested Reading, and Practical Resource Directory*

Edited by Jenifer Swanson. 537 pages. 1999. 978-0-7808-0390-9.

**"Recommended reference source."**

—*Booklist, Feb '00*

**SEE ALSO** *Adult Health Sourcebook, Physical and Mental Issues in Aging Sourcebook*

# Healthy Children Sourcebook

*Basic Consumer Health Information about the Physical and Mental Development of Children between the Ages of 3 and 12, Including Routine Health Care, Preventative Health Services, Safety and First Aid, Healthy Sleep, Dental Care, Nutrition, and Fitness, and Featuring Parenting Tips on Such Topics as Bedwetting, Choosing Day Care, Monitoring TV and Other Media, and Establishing a Foundation for Substance Abuse Prevention*

*Along with a Glossary of Commonly Used Pediatric Terms and Resources for Additional Help and Information.*

Edited by Chad T. Kimball. 624 pages. 2003. 978-0-7808-0247-6.

"Should be required reading for parents and teachers."
—E-Streams, Jun '04

"It is hard to imagine that any other single resource exists that would provide such a comprehensive guide of timely information on health promotion and disease prevention for children aged 3 to 12."
—American Reference Books Annual, 2004

"This easy-to-read volume is a tremendous resource."
—AORN Journal, May '05

SEE ALSO Childhood Diseases and Disorders Sourcebook, 2nd Edition

# Healthy Heart Sourcebook for Women
Basic Consumer Health Information about Cardiac Issues Specific to Women, Including Facts about Major Risk Factors and Prevention, Treatment and Control Strategies, and Important Dietary Issues

Along with a Special Section Regarding the Pros and Cons of Hormone Replacement Therapy and Its Impact on Heart Health, and Additional Help, Including Recipes, a Glossary, and a Directory of Resources

Edited by Dawn D. Matthews. 321 pages. 2000. 978-0-7808-0329-9.

"A good reference source and recommended for all public, academic, medical, and hospital libraries."
—Medical Reference Services Quarterly, Summer '01

"Contains very important information about coronary artery disease that all women should know. The information is current and presented in an easy-to-read format. The book will make a good addition to any library."
—American Medical Writers Association Journal, Summer '00

SEE ALSO Cardiovascular Diseases and Disorders Sourcebook, 4th Edition, Women's Health Concerns Sourcebook, 3rd Edition

# Hepatitis Sourcebook
Basic Consumer Health Information about Hepatitis A, Hepatitis B, Hepatitis C, and Other Forms of Hepatitis, Including Autoimmune Hepatitis, Alcoholic Hepatitis, Nonalcoholic Steatohepatitis, and Toxic Hepatitis, with Facts about Risk Factors, Screening Methods, Diagnostic Tests, and Treatment Options

Along with Information on Liver Health, Tips for People Living with Chronic Hepatitis, Reports on Current Research Initiatives, a Glossary of Terms Related to Hepatitis, and a Directory of Sources for Further Help and Information

Edited by Sandra J. Judd. 570 pages. 2006. 978-0-7808-0749-5.

"The breadth of information found in this one book would not be readily found in another source. Highly recommended."
—American Reference Books Annual, 2006

SEE ALSO Contagious Diseases Sourcebook, 2nd Edition

# Household Safety Sourcebook
Basic Consumer Health Information about Household Safety, Including Information about Poisons, Chemicals, Fire, and Water Hazards in the Home

Along with Advice about the Safe Use of Home Maintenance Equipment, Choosing Toys and Nursery Furniture, Holiday and Recreation Safety, a Glossary, and Resources for Further Help and Information

Edited by Dawn D. Matthews. 587 pages. 2002. 978-0-7808-0338-1.

"As a sourcebook on household safety this book meets its mark. It is encyclopedic in scope and covers a wide range of safety issues that are commonly seen in the home."
—E-Streams, Jul '02

# Hypertension Sourcebook
Basic Consumer Health Information about the Causes, Diagnosis, and Treatment of High Blood Pressure, with Facts about Consequences, Complications, and Co-Occurring Disorders, Such as Coronary Heart Disease, Diabetes, Stroke, Kidney Disease, and Hypertensive Retinopathy, and Issues in Blood Pressure

Control, Including Dietary Choices, Stress Management, and Medications

Along with Reports on Current Research Initiatives and Clinical Trials, a Glossary, and Resources for Additional Help and Information

Edited by Dawn D. Matthews and Karen Bellenir. 588 pages. 2004. 978-0-7808-0674-0.

**"Academic, public, and medical libraries will want to add the Hypertension Sourcebook to their collections."**
— *E-Streams, Aug '05*

**"The strength of this source is the wide range of information given about hypertension."**
— *American Reference Books Annual, 2005*

**SEE ALSO** *Stroke Sourcebook, 2nd Edition*

# Immune System Disorders Sourcebook, 2nd Edition
*Basic Consumer Health Information about Disorders of the Immune System, Including Immune System Function and Response, Diagnosis of Immune Disorders, Information about Inherited Immune Disease, Acquired Immune Disease, and Autoimmune Diseases, Including Primary Immune Deficiency, Acquired Immunodeficiency Syndrome (AIDS), Lupus, Multiple Sclerosis, Type 1 Diabetes, Rheumatoid Arthritis, and Graves' Disease*

*Along with Treatments, Tips for Coping with Immune Disorders, a Glossary, and a Directory of Additional Resources*

Edited by Joyce Brennfleck Shannon. 643 pages. 2005. 978-0-7808-0748-8.

**"Highly recommended for academic and public libraries."**
— *American Reference Books Annual, 2006*

**"The updated second edition is a 'must' for any consumer health library seeking a solid resource covering the treatments, symptoms, and options for immune disorder sufferers... An excellent guide."**
— *MBR Bookwatch, Jan '06*

**SEE ALSO** *AIDS Sourcebook, 4th Edition, Arthritis Sourcebook, 3rd Edition*

# Infant and Toddler Health Sourcebook
*Basic Consumer Health Information about the Physical and Mental Development of Newborns, Infants, and Toddlers, Including Neonatal Concerns, Nutrition Recommendations, Immunization Schedules, Common Pediatric Disorders, Assessments and Milestones, Safety Tips, and Advice for Parents and Other Caregivers*

*Along with a Glossary of Terms and Resource Listings for Additional Help*

Edited by Jenifer Swanson. 570 pages. 2000. 978-0-7808-0246-9.

**"As a reference for the general public, this would be useful in any library."**
— *E-Streams, May '01*

**"Recommended reference source."**
— *Booklist, Feb '01*

# Infectious Diseases Sourcebook
*Basic Consumer Health Information about Non-Contagious Bacterial, Viral, Prion, Fungal, and Parasitic Diseases Spread by Food and Water, Insects and Animals, or Environmental Contact, Including Botulism, E. Coli, Encephalitis, Legionnaires' Disease, Lyme Disease, Malaria, Plague, Rabies, Salmonella, Tetanus, and Others, and Facts about Newly Emerging Diseases, Such as Hantavirus, Mad Cow Disease, Monkeypox, and West Nile Virus*

*Along with Information about Preventing Disease Transmission, the Threat of Bioterrorism, and Current Research Initiatives, with a Glossary and Directory of Resources for More Information*

Edited by Karen Bellenir. 610 pages. 2004. 978-0-7808-0675-7.

**"This reference continues the excellent tradition of the Health Reference Series in consolidating a wealth of information on a selected topic into a format that is easy to use and accessible to the general public."**
— *American Reference Books Annual, 2005*

**"Recommended for public and academic libraries."**
— *E-Streams, Jan '05*

SEE ALSO *Environmental Health Sourcebook, 3rd Edition*

# Injury and Trauma Sourcebook

*Basic Consumer Health Information about the Impact of Injury, the Diagnosis and Treatment of Common and Traumatic Injuries, Emergency Care, and Specific Injuries Related to Home, Community, Workplace, Transportation, and Recreation*

*Along with Guidelines for Injury Prevention, a Glossary, and a Directory of Additional Resources*

Edited by Joyce Brennfleck Shannon. 675 pages. 2002. 978-0-7808-0421-0.

"Practitioners should be aware of guides such as this in order to facilitate their use by patients and their families."
*—Doody's Health Sciences Book Review Journal, Sep-Oct '02*

"Recommended reference source."
*—Booklist, Sep '02*

"Highly recommended for academic and medical reference collections."
*—Library Bookwatch, Sep '02*

**SEE ALSO** *Emergency Medical Services Sourcebook, Sports Injuries Sourcebook, 3rd Edition*

# Learning Disabilities Sourcebook, 3rd Edition

*Basic Consumer Health Information about Dyslexia, Auditory and Visual Processing Disorders, Communication Disorders, Dyscalculia, Dysgraphia, and Other Conditions That Impede Learning, Including Attention Deficit/Hyperactivity Disorder, Autism Spectrum Disorders, Hearing and Visual Impairments, Chromosome-Based Disorders, and Brain Injury*

*Along with Facts about Brain Function, Assessment, Therapy and Remediation, Accommodations, Assistive Technology, Legal Protections, and Tips about Family Life, School Transitions, and Employment Strategies, a Glossary of Related Terms, and Directories of Additional Resources*

Edited by Joyce Brennfleck Shannon. 613 pages. 2009. 978-0-7808-1039-6.

"Intended to be a starting point for people who need to know about learning disabilities. Each chapter on a specific disability includes readable, well-organized descriptions... The book is well indexed and a glossary is included. Chapters on organizations and helpful websites will aid the reader who needs more information."
*—American Reference Books Annual, 2009*

"This book provides the necessary information to better understand learning disabilities and work with children who have them... It would be difficult to find another book that so comprehensively explains learning disabilities without becoming incomprehensible to the average parent who needs this information."
*—Doody's Review Service, 2009*

**SEE ALSO** *Attention Deficit Disorder Sourcebook, Autism and Pervasive Developmental Disorders Sourcebook*

# Leukemia Sourcebook

*Basic Consumer Health Information about Adult and Childhood Leukemias, Including Acute Lymphocytic Leukemia (ALL), Chronic Lymphocytic Leukemia (CLL), Acute Myelogenous Leukemia (AML), Chronic Myelogenous Leukemia (CML), and Hairy Cell Leukemia, and Treatments Such as Chemotherapy, Radiation Therapy, Peripheral Blood Stem Cell and Marrow Transplantation, and Immunotherapy*

*Along with Tips for Life During and After Treatment, a Glossary, and Directories of Additional Resources*

Edited by Joyce Brennfleck Shannon. 564 pages. 2003. 978-0-7808-0627-6.

"Unlike other medical books for the layperson... the language does not talk down to the reader... This volume is highly recommended for all libraries."
*—American Reference Books Annual, 2004*

"A fine title which ranges from diagnosis to alternative treatments, staging, and tips for life during and after diagnosis."
*—The Bookwatch, Dec '03*

**SEE ALSO** *Blood & Circulatory Disorders Sourcebook, 3rd Edition, Cancer Sourcebook, 5th Edition*

# Liver Disorders Sourcebook

*Basic Consumer Health Information about the Liver and How It Works; Liver Diseases, Including Cancer, Cirrhosis, Hepatitis, and*

*Toxic and Drug Related Diseases; Tips for Maintaining a Healthy Liver; Laboratory Tests, Radiology Tests, and Facts about Liver Transplantation*

*Along with a Section on Support Groups, a Glossary, and Resource Listings*

Edited by Joyce Brennfleck Shannon. 580 pages. 2000. 978-0-7808-0383-1.

**"This title is recommended for health sciences and public libraries with consumer health collections."**
—*E-Streams, Oct '00*

**"Recommended reference source."**
—*Booklist, Jun '00*

**SEE ALSO** *Gastrointestinal Diseases and Disorders Sourcebook, 2nd Edition, Hepatitis Sourcebook*

## Lung Disorders Sourcebook

*Basic Consumer Health Information about Emphysema, Pneumonia, Tuberculosis, Asthma, Cystic Fibrosis, and Other Lung Disorders, Including Facts about Diagnostic Procedures, Treatment Strategies, Disease Prevention Efforts, and Such Risk Factors as Smoking, Air Pollution, and Exposure to Asbestos, Radon, and Other Agents*

*Along with a Glossary and Resources for Additional Help and Information*

Edited by Dawn D. Matthews. 657 pages. 2002. 978-0-7808-0339-8.

**"Highly recommended for academic and medical reference collections."**
—*Library Bookwatch, Sep '02*

**SEE ALSO** *Asthma Sourcebook, 2nd Edition, Respiratory Disorders Sourcebook, 2nd Edition*

## Medical Tests Sourcebook, 3rd Edition

*Basic Consumer Health Information about X-Rays, Blood Tests, Stool and Urine Tests, Biopsies, Mammography, Endoscopic Procedures, Ultrasound Exams, Computed Tomography, Magnetic Resonance Imaging (MRI), Nuclear Medicine, Genetic Testing, Home-Use Tests, and More*

*Along with Facts about Preventive Care and Screening Test Guidelines, Screening and*

*Assessment Tests Associated with Such Specific Concerns as Cancer, Heart Disease, Allergies, Diabetes, Thyroid Disfunction, and Infertility, a Glossary of Related Terms, and a Directory of Resources for Additional Help and Information*

Edited by Karen Bellenir. 627 pages. 2008. 978-0-7808-1040-2

**"This volume has a wide scope that makes it useful... Can be a valuable reference guide."**
—*American Reference Books Annual, 2009*

**"Would be a valuable contribution to any consumer health or public library."**
—*Doody's Book Review Service, 2009*

## Men's Health Concerns Sourcebook, 3rd Edition

*Basic Consumer Health Information about Wellness in Men and Gender-Related Differences in Health, With Facts about Heart Disease, Cancer, Traumatic Injury, and Other Leading Causes of Death in Men, Reproductive Concerns, Sexual Dysfunction, Disorders of the Prostate, Penis, and Testes, Sex-Linked Genetic Disorders, and Other Medical and Mental Concerns of Men*

*Along with Statistical Data, a Glossary of Related Terms, and a Directory of Resources for Additional Information*

Edited by Sandra J. Judd. 632 pages. 2009. 978-0-7808-1033-4.

**"A good addition to any reference shelf in academic, consumer health, or hospital libraries."**
—*ARBAOnline, Oct '09*

**SEE ALSO** *Prostate and Urological Disorders Sourcebook*

## Mental Health Disorders Sourcebook, 4th Edition

*Basic Consumer Health Information about the Causes and Symptoms of Mental Health Problems, Including Depression, Bipolar Disorder, Anxiety Disorders, Posttraumatic Stress Disorder, Obsessive-Compulsive Disorder, Eating Disorders, Addictions, and Personality and Psychotic Disorders*

*Along with Information about Medications and Treatments, Mental Health Concerns in*

*Children, Adolescents, and Adults, Tips on Living with Mental Health Disorders, a Glossary of Related Terms, and a Directory of Resources for Additional Help and Information*

Edited by Amy L. Sutton. 680 pages. 2009. 978-0-7808-1041-9.

"Mental health concerns are presented in everyday language and intended for patients and their families as well as the general public... This resource is comprehensive and up to date... The easy-to-understand writing style helps to facilitate assimilation of needed facts and specifics on often challenging topics."
—*ARBAOnline, Oct '09*

"No health collection should be without this resource, which will reach into many a general lending library as well."
—*Internet Bookwatch, Oct '09*

*SEE ALSO Depression Sourcebook, 2nd Edition, Stress-Related Disorders Sourcebook, 2nd Edition*

# Mental Retardation Sourcebook

*Basic Consumer Health Information about Mental Retardation and Its Causes, Including Down Syndrome, Fetal Alcohol Syndrome, Fragile X Syndrome, Genetic Conditions, Injury, and Environmental Sources*

*Along with Preventive Strategies, Parenting Issues, Educational Implications, Health Care Needs, Employment and Economic Matters, Legal Issues, a Glossary, and a Resource Listing for Additional Help and Information*

Edited by Joyce Brennfleck Shannon. 627 pages. 2000. 978-0-7808-0377-0.

"Public libraries will find the book useful for reference and as a beginning research point for students, parents, and caregivers."
—*American Reference Books Annual, 2001*

"The strength of this work is that it compiles many basic fact sheets and addresses for further information in one volume. It is intended and suitable for the general public."
—*E-Streams, Nov '00*

"An invaluable overview."
—*Reviewer's Bookwatch, Jul '00*

# Movement Disorders Sourcebook, 2nd Edition

*Basic Consumer Health Information about the Symptoms and Causes of Movement Disorders, Including Parkinson Disease, Amyotrophic Lateral Sclerosis, Cerebral Palsy, Muscular Dystrophy, Multiple Sclerosis, Myasthenia, Myoclonus, Spina Bifida, Dystonia, Essential Tremor, Choreatic Disorders, Huntington Disease, Tourette Syndrome, and Other Disorders That Cause Slowed, Absent, or Excessive Movements*

*Along with Information about Surgical and Nonsurgical Interventions, Physical Therapies, Strategies for Independent Living, a Glossary of Related Terms, and a Directory of Resources for Additional Help and Information*

Edited by Amy L. Sutton. 618 pages. 2009. 978-0-7808-1034-1.

"The second updated edition of Movement Disorders Sourcebook is a winner, providing the latest research and health findings on all kinds of movement disorders in children and adults... a top pick for any health or general lending library's health reference collection."
—*California Bookwatch, Aug '09*

*SEE ALSO Muscular Dystrophy Sourcebook*

# Multiple Sclerosis Sourcebook

*Basic Consumer Health Information about Multiple Sclerosis (MS) and Its Effects on Mobility, Vision, Bladder Function, Speech, Swallowing, and Cognition, Including Facts about Risk Factors, Causes, Diagnostic Procedures, Pain Management, Drug Treatments, and Physical and Occupational Therapies*

*Along with Guidelines for Nutrition and Exercise, Tips on Choosing Assistive Equipment, Information about Disability, Work, Financial, and Legal Issues, a Glossary of Related Terms, and a Directory of Additional Resources*

Edited by Joyce Brennfleck Shannon. 553 pages. 2007. 978-0-7808-0998-7.

# Muscular Dystrophy Sourcebook

*Basic Consumer Health Information about Congenital, Childhood-Onset, and Adult-Onset*

Forms of Muscular Dystrophy, Such as Duchenne, Becker, Emery-Dreifuss, Distal, Limb-Girdle, Facioscapulohumeral (FSHD), Myotonic, and Ophthalmoplegic Muscular Dystrophies, Including Facts about Diagnostic Tests, Medical and Physical Therapies, Management of Co-Occurring Conditions, and Parenting Guidelines

Along with Practical Tips for Home Care, a Glossary, and Directories of Additional Resources

Edited by Joyce Brennfleck Shannon. 552 pages. 2004. 978-0-7808-0676-4.

**"This book is highly recommended for public and academic libraries as well as health care offices that support the information needs of patients and their families."**
—E-Streams, Apr '05

**"Excellent reference."**
—The Bookwatch, Jan '05

**SEE ALSO** Movement Disorders Sourcebook, 2nd Edition

# Obesity Sourcebook

Basic Consumer Health Information about Diseases and Other Problems Associated with Obesity, and Including Facts about Risk Factors, Prevention Issues, and Management Approaches

Along with Statistical and Demographic Data, Information about Special Populations, Research Updates, a Glossary, and Source Listings for Further Help and Information

Edited by Wilma Caldwell and Chad T. Kimball. 360 pages. 2001. 978-0-7808-0333-6.

**"The book synthesizes the reliable medical literature on obesity into one easy-to-read and useful resource for the general public."**
—American Reference Books Annual, 2002

**"Well suited for the health reference collection of a public library or an academic health science library that serves the general population."**
—E-Streams, Sep '01

# Osteoporosis Sourcebook

Basic Consumer Health Information about Primary and Secondary Osteoporosis and Juvenile Osteoporosis and Related Conditions, Including Fibrous Dysplasia, Gaucher Disease, Hyperthyroidism, Hypophosphatasia,

Myeloma, Osteopetrosis, Osteogenesis Imperfecta, and Paget's Disease

Along with Information about Risk Factors, Treatments, Traditional and Non-Traditional Pain Management, a Glossary of Related Terms, and a Directory of Resources

Edited by Allan R. Cook. 568 pages. 2001. 978-0-7808-0239-1.

**"This resource is recommended as a great reference source for public, health, and academic libraries, and is another triumph for the editors of Omnigraphics."**
—American Reference Books Annual, 2002

**"Will prove valuable to any library seeking to maintain a current, comprehensive reference collection of health resources... From prevention to treatment and associated conditions, this provides an excellent survey."**
—The Bookwatch, Aug '01

**SEE ALSO** Healthy Aging Sourcebook, Women's Health Concerns Sourcebook, 3rd Edition

# Pain Sourcebook, 3rd Edition

Basic Consumer Health Information about Acute and Chronic Pain, Including Nerve Pain, Bone Pain, Muscle Pain, Cancer Pain, and Disorders Characterized by Pain, Such as Arthritis, Temporomandibular Muscle and Joint (TMJ) Disorder, Carpal Tunnel Syndrome, Headaches, Heartburn, Sciatica, and Shingles, and Facts about Diagnostic Tests and Treatment Options for Pain, Including Over-the-Counter and Prescription Drugs, Physical Rehabilitation, Injection and Infusion Therapies, Implantable Technologies, and Complementary Medicine

Along with Tips for Living with Pain, a Glossary of Related Terms, and a Directory of Additional Resources

Edited by Joyce Brennfleck Shannon. 644 pages. 2008. 978-0-7808-1006-8.

**"Excellent for ready-reference users and can be used for beginning students in health fields... appropriate for the consumer health collection in both public and academic libraries."**
—American Reference Books Annual, 2009

SEE ALSO Arthritis Sourcebook, 3rd Edition; Back and Neck Sourcebook, 2nd Edition;

*Headache Sourcebook; Sports Injuries Sourcebook, 3rd Edition*

# Pediatric Cancer Sourcebook

*Basic Consumer Health Information about Leukemias, Brain Tumors, Sarcomas, Lymphomas, and Other Cancers in Infants, Children, and Adolescents, Including Descriptions of Cancers, Treatments, and Coping Strategies*

*Along with Suggestions for Parents, Caregivers, and Concerned Relatives, a Glossary of Cancer Terms, and Resource Listings*

Edited by Edward J. Prucha. 575 pages. 1999. 978-0-7808-0245-2.

**"An excellent source of information. Recommended for public, hospital, and health science libraries with consumer health collections."**
—*E-Streams, Jun '00*

**"A valuable addition to all libraries specializing in health services and many public libraries."**
—*American Reference Books Annual, 2000*

**SEE ALSO** *Childhood Diseases and Disorders Sourcebook, 2nd Edition, Healthy Children Sourcebook*

# Physical and Mental Issues in Aging Sourcebook

*Basic Consumer Health Information on Physical and Mental Disorders Associated with the Aging Process, Including Concerns about Cardiovascular Disease, Pulmonary Disease, Oral Health, Digestive Disorders, Musculoskeletal and Skin Disorders, Metabolic Changes, Sexual and Reproductive Issues, and Changes in Vision, Hearing, and Other Senses*

*Along with Data about Longevity and Causes of Death, Information on Acute and Chronic Pain, Descriptions of Mental Concerns, a Glossary of Terms, and Resource Listings for Additional Help*

Edited by Jenifer Swanson. 660 pages. 1999. 978-0-7808-0233-9.

**"This is a treasure of health information for the layperson."**
—*CHOICE Health Sciences Supplement, May '00*

**"Recommended for public libraries."**
—*American Reference Books Annual, 2000*

**SEE ALSO** *Healthy Aging Sourcebook*

# Podiatry Sourcebook, 2nd Edition

*Basic Consumer Health Information about Disorders, Diseases, and Deformities that Affect the Foot and Ankle, Including Sprains, Corns, Calluses, Bunions, Plantar Warts, Plantar Fasciitis, Neuromas, Clubfoot, Flat Feet, Achilles Tendonitis, and Much More*

*Along with Information about Selecting a Foot Care Specialist, Foot Fitness, Shoes and Socks, Diagnostic Tests and Corrective Procedures, Financial Assistance for Corrective Devices, a Glossary of Related Terms, and a Directory of Resources for Additional Help and Information*

Edited by Ivy L. Alexander. 516 pages. 2007. 978-0-7808-0944-4.

**"An excellent resource... Although there have been various types of 'foot books' published in the past, none are as comprehensive as this one. 5 Stars (out of 5)!"**
—*Doody's Review Service, 2007*

**"Perfect for both health libraries and general-interest lending collections."**
—*Internet Bookwatch, Jul '07*

# Pregnancy and Birth Sourcebook, 3rd Edition

*Basic Consumer Health Information about Pregnancy and Fetal Development, Including Facts about Fertility and Conception, Physical and Emotional Changes during Pregnancy, Prenatal Care and Diagnostic Tests, High-Risk Pregnancies and Complications, Labor, Delivery, and the Postpartum Period*

*Along with Tips on Maintaining Health and Wellness during Pregnancy and Caring for Newborn Infants, a Glossary of Related Terms, and Directories of Resources for Additional Help and Information*

Edited by Amy L. Sutton. 645 pages. 2009. 978-0-7808-1074-7.

**SEE ALSO** *Breastfeeding Sourcebook, Congenital Disorders Sourcebook, 2nd Edition, Family Planning Sourcebook, Women's Health Concerns Sourcebook, 3rd Edition*

## Prostate and Urological Disorders Sourcebook

*Basic Consumer Health Information about Urogenital and Sexual Disorders in Men, Including Prostate and Other Andrological Cancers, Prostatitis, Benign Prostatic Hyperplasia, Testicular and Penile Trauma, Cryptorchidism, Peyronie Disease, Erectile Dysfunction, and Male Factor Infertility, and Facts about Commonly Used Tests and Procedures, Such as Prostatectomy, Vasectomy, Vasectomy Reversal, Penile Implants, and Semen Analysis*

*Along with a Glossary of Andrological Terms and a Directory of Resources for Additional Information*

Edited by Karen Bellenir. 604 pages. 2006. 978-0-7808-0797-6.

**"Certain to be a popular pick among library reference holdings... No prior knowledge is assumed for any of the conditions or terms herein, making it a most accessible general-interest reference."**
—*California Bookwatch, Apr '06*

**SEE ALSO** *Men's Health Concerns Sourcebook, 3rd Edition, Urinary Tract and Kidney Diseases and Disorders Sourcebook, 2nd Edition*

## Prostate Cancer Sourcebook

*Basic Consumer Health Information about Prostate Cancer, Including Information about the Associated Risk Factors, Detection, Diagnosis, and Treatment of Prostate Cancer*

*Along with Information on Non-Malignant Prostate Conditions, and Featuring a Section Listing Support and Treatment Centers and a Glossary of Related Terms*

Edited by Dawn D. Matthews. 340 pages. 2001. 978-0-7808-0324-4.

**"Recommended reference source."**
—*Booklist, Jan '02*

**"A valuable resource for health care consumers seeking information on the subject... All text is written in a clear, easy-to-understand language that avoids technical jargon. Any library that collects consumer health resources would strengthen their collection with the addition of the Prostate Cancer Sourcebook."**
—*American Reference Books Annual, 2002*

**SEE ALSO** *Cancer Sourcebook, 5th Edition, Men's Health Concerns Sourcebook, 3rd Edition*

## Rehabilitation Sourcebook

*Basic Consumer Health Information about Rehabilitation for People Recovering from Heart Surgery, Spinal Cord Injury, Stroke, Orthopedic Impairments, Amputation, Pulmonary Impairments, Traumatic Injury, and More, Including Physical Therapy, Occupational Therapy, Speech/Language Therapy, Massage Therapy, Dance Therapy, Art Therapy, and Recreational Therapy*

*Along with Information on Assistive and Adaptive Devices, a Glossary, and Resources for Additional Help and Information*

Edited by Dawn D. Matthews. 519 pages. 2000. 978-0-7808-0236-0.

**"This is an excellent resource for public library reference and health collections."**
—*American Reference Books Annual, 2001*

**"Recommended reference source."**
—*Booklist, May '00*

## Respiratory Disorders Sourcebook, 2nd Edition

*Basic Consumer Health Information about Infectious, Inflammatory, and Chronic Conditions Affecting the Lungs and Respiratory System, Including Pneumonia, Bronchitis, Influenza, Tuberculosis, Sarcoidosis, Asthma, Cystic Fibrosis, Chronic Obstructive Pulmonary Disease, Lung Abscesses, Pulmonary Embolism, Occupational Lung Diseases, and Other Bacterial, Viral, and Fungal Infections*

*Along with Facts about the Structure and Function of the Lungs and Airways, Methods of Diagnosing Respiratory Disorders, and Treatment and Rehabilitation Options, a Glossary of Related Terms, and a Directory of Resources for Additional Help and Information*

Edited by Sandra L. Judd. 638 pages. 2008. 978-0-7808-1007-5.

**"An excellent book for patients, their families, or for those who are just curious about respiratory disease. Public libraries and physician offices would find this a valuable resource as well. 4 Stars! (out of 5)"**
—*Doody's Review Service, 2009*

**"A great addition for public and school libraries because it provides concise health information... readers can start with this reference source and get satisfactory answers before proceeding to other medical reference tools for**

more in depth information... A good guide for health education on lung disorders."
—*American Reference Books Annual, 2009*

**SEE ALSO** *Asthma Sourcebook, 2nd Edition, Lung Disorders Sourcebook*

## Sexually Transmitted Diseases Sourcebook, 4th Edition

*Basic Consumer Health Information about Chlamydial Infections, Gonorrhea, Hepatitis, Herpes, HIV/AIDS, Human Papillomavirus, Pubic Lice, Scabies, Syphilis, Trichomoniasis, Vaginal Infections, and Other Sexually Transmitted Diseases, Including Facts about Risk Factors, Symptoms, Diagnosis, Treatment, and the Prevention of Sexually Transmitted Infections*

*Along with Updates on Current Research Initiatives, a Glossary of Related Terms, and Resources for Additional Help and Information*

Edited by Laura Larsen. 623 pages. 2009. 978-0-7808-1073-0.

"**Extremely beneficial... The question-and-answer format along with the index and table of contents make this well-organized resource extremely easy to reference, read, and comprehend... an invaluable medical reference source for lay readers, and a highly appropriate addition for public library collections, health clinics, and any library with a consumer health collection"**
—*ARBAOnline, Oct '09*

**SEE ALSO** *AIDS Sourcebook, 4th Edition, Contagious Diseases Sourcebook, 2nd Edition, Men's Health Concerns Sourcebook, 3rd Edition, Women's Health Concerns Sourcebook, 3rd Edition*

## Sleep Disorders Sourcebook, 3rd Edition

*Basic Consumer Health Information about Sleep Disorders, Including Insomnia, Sleep Apnea and Snoring, Jet Lag and Other Circadian Rhythm Disorders, Narcolepsy, and Parasomnias, Such as Sleep Walking and Sleep Talking, and Featuring Facts about Other Health Problems that Affect Sleep, Why Sleep Is Necessary, How Much Sleep Is Needed, the Physical and Mental Effects of Sleep Deprivation, and Pediatric Sleep Issues*

*Along with Tips for Diagnosing and Treating Sleep Disorders, a Glossary of Related Terms, and a List of Resources for Additional Help and Information*

Edited by Sandra J. Judd. 600 pages. 2010. 978-0-7808-1084-6.

## Smoking Concerns Sourcebook

*Basic Consumer Health Information about Nicotine Addiction and Smoking Cessation, Featuring Facts about the Health Effects of Tobacco Use, Including Lung and Other Cancers, Heart Disease, Stroke, and Respiratory Disorders, Such as Emphysema and Chronic Bronchitis*

*Along with Information about Smoking Prevention Programs, Suggestions for Achieving and Maintaining a Smoke-Free Lifestyle, Statistics about Tobacco Use, Reports on Current Research Initiatives, a Glossary of Related Terms, and Directories of Resources for Additional Help and Information*

Edited by Karen Bellenir. 595 pages. 2004. 978-0-7808-0323-7.

"**Provides everything needed for the student or general reader seeking practical details on the effects of tobacco use."**
—*The Bookwatch, Mar '05*

"**Public libraries and consumer health care libraries will find this work useful."**
—*American Reference Books Annual, 2005*

**SEE ALSO** *Respiratory Disorders Sourcebook, 2nd Edition*

## Sports Injuries Sourcebook, 3rd Edition

*Basic Consumer Health Information about Sprains and Strains, Fractures, Growth Plate Injuries, Overtraining Injuries, and Injuries to the Head, Face, Shoulders, Elbows, Hands, Spinal Column, Knees, Ankles, and Feet, and with Facts about Heat-Related Illness, Steroids and Sport Supplements, Protective Equipment, Diagnostic Procedures, Treatment Options, and Rehabilitation*

*Along with a Glossary of Related Terms and a Directory of Resources for Additional Help and Information*

Edited by Sandra J. Judd. 623 pages. 2007. 978-0-7808-0949-9.

SEE ALSO *Fitness and Exercise Sourcebook, 3rd Edition, Podiatry Sourcebook, 2nd Edition*

## Stress-Related Disorders Sourcebook, 2nd Edition

*Basic Consumer Health Information about Stress and Stress-Related Disorders, Including Types of Stress, Sources of Acute and Chronic Stress, the Impact of Stress on the Body's Systems, and Mental and Emotional Health Problems Associated with Stress, Such as Depression, Anxiety Disorders, Substance Abuse, Posttraumatic Stress Disorder, and Suicide*

*Along with Advice about Getting Help for Stress-Related Disorders, Information about Stress Management Techniques, a Glossary of Stress-Related Terms, and a Directory of Resources for Additional Help and Information*

Edited by Amy L. Sutton. 608 pages. 2007. 978-0-7808-0996-3.

"Accessible to the lay reader. Highly recommended for medical and psychiatric collections."
—*Library Journal, Mar '08*

"Well-written for a general readership, the 2nd Edition of Stress-Related Disorders Sourcebook is a useful addition to the health reference literature."
—*American Reference Books Annual, 2008*

SEE ALSO *Mental Health Disorders Sourcebook, 4th Edition*

## Stroke Sourcebook, 2nd Edition

*Basic Consumer Health Information about Stroke, Including Ischemic, Hemorrhagic, and Mini Strokes, as Well as Risk Factors, Prevention Guidelines, Diagnostic Tests, Medications and Surgical Treatments, and Complications of Stroke*

*Along with Rehabilitation Techniques and Innovations, Tips on Staying Healthy and Maintaining Independence after Stroke, a Glossary of Related Terms, and a Directory of Resources for Stroke Survivors and Their Families*

Edited by Amy L. Sutton. 626 pages. 2008. 978-0-7808-1035-8.

"An encyclopedic handbook on stroke that is written in a language the layperson can understand... This is one of the most helpful, readable books on stroke. This volume is highly recommended and should be in every medical, hospital and public library; in addition, every family practitioner should have a copy in his or her office."
—*American Reference Books Annual, 2009*

SEE ALSO *Brain Disorders Sourcebook, 3rd Edition, Hypertension Sourcebook*

## Surgery Sourcebook, 2nd Edition

*Basic Consumer Health Information about Common Inpatient and Outpatient Surgeries, Including Critical Care and Trauma, Gastrointestinal, Gynecologic and Obstetric, Cardiac and Vascular, Neurologic, Ophthalmologic, Orthopedic, Reconstructive and Cosmetic, and Other Major and Minor Surgeries*

*Along with Information about Anesthesia and Pain Relief Options, Risks and Complications, Postoperative Recovery Concerns, and Innovative Surgical Techniques and Tools, a Glossary of Related Terms, and a Directory of Additional Resources*

Edited by Amy L. Sutton. 645 pages. 2008. 978-0-7808-1004-4.

"Large public libraries and medical libraries would benefit from this material in their reference collections."
—*American Reference Books Annual, 2009*

SEE ALSO *Cosmetic and Reconstructive Surgery Sourcebook, 2nd Edition*

## Thyroid Disorders Sourcebook

*Basic Consumer Health Information about Disorders of the Thyroid and Parathyroid Glands, Including Hypothyroidism, Hyperthyroidism, Graves Disease, Hashimoto Thyroiditis, Thyroid Cancer, and Parathyroid Disorders, Featuring Facts about Symptoms, Risk Factors, Tests, and Treatments*

*Along with Information about the Effects of Thyroid Imbalance on Other Body Systems, Environmental Factors That Affect the Thyroid Gland, a Glossary, and a Directory of Additional Resources*

Edited by Joyce Brennfleck Shannon. 573 pages. 2005. 978-0-7808-0745-7.

**"Recommended for consumer health collections."**
*—American Reference Books Annual, 2006*

**"Highly recommended pick for Basic Consumer health reference holdings at all levels."**
*—The Bookwatch, Aug '05*

***SEE ALSO*** *Endocrine and Metabolic Disorders Sourcebook, 2nd Edition*

---

# Transplantation Sourcebook
*Basic Consumer Health Information about Organ and Tissue Transplantation, Including Physical and Financial Preparations, Procedures and Issues Relating to Specific Solid Organ and Tissue Transplants, Rehabilitation, Pediatric Transplant Information, the Future of Transplantation, and Organ and Tissue Donation*

*Along with a Glossary and Listings of Additional Resources*

Edited by Joyce Brennfleck Shannon. 610 pages. 2002. 978-0-7808-0322-0.

**"Recommended for libraries with an interest in offering consumer health information."**
*—E-Streams, Jul '02*

**"This is a unique and valuable resource for patients facing transplantation and their families."**
*—Doody's Review Service, Jun '02*

---

# Traveler's Health Sourcebook
*Basic Consumer Health Information for Travelers, Including Physical and Medical Preparations, Transportation Health and Safety, Essential Information about Food and Water, Sun Exposure, Insect and Snake Bites, Camping and Wilderness Medicine, and Travel with Physical or Medical Disabilities*

*Along with International Travel Tips, Vaccination Recommendations, Geographical Health Issues, Disease Risks, a Glossary, and a Listing of Additional Resources*

Edited by Joyce Brennfleck Shannon. 619 pages. 2000. 978-0-7808-0384-8.

**"Recommended reference source."**
*—Booklist, Feb '01*

**"This book is recommended for any public library, any travel collection, and especially any collection for the physically disabled."**
*—American Reference Books Annual, 2001*

***SEE ALSO*** *Worldwide Health Sourcebook*

---

# Urinary Tract and Kidney Diseases and Disorders Sourcebook, 2nd Edition
*Basic Consumer Health Information about the Urinary System, Including the Bladder, Urethra, Ureters, and Kidneys, with Facts about Urinary Tract Infections, Incontinence, Congenital Disorders, Kidney Stones, Cancers of the Urinary Tract and Kidneys, Kidney Failure, Dialysis, and Kidney Transplantation*

*Along with Statistical and Demographic Information, Reports on Current Research in Kidney and Urologic Health, a Summary of Commonly Used Diagnostic Tests, a Glossary of Related Terms, and a Directory of Resources for Additional Help and Information*

Edited by Ivy L. Alexander. 621 pages. 2005. 978-0-7808-0750-1.

**"A good choice for a consumer health information library or for a medical library needing information to refer to their patients."**
*—American Reference Books Annual, 2006*

***SEE ALSO*** *Prostate and Urological Disorders Sourcebook*

---

# Vegetarian Sourcebook
*Basic Consumer Health Information about Vegetarian Diets, Lifestyle, and Philosophy, Including Definitions of Vegetarianism and Veganism, Tips about Adopting Vegetarianism, Creating a Vegetarian Pantry, and Meeting Nutritional Needs of Vegetarians, with Facts Regarding Vegetarianism's Effect on Pregnant and Lactating Women, Children, Athletes, and Senior Citizens*

*Along with a Glossary of Commonly Used Vegetarian Terms and Resources for Additional Help and Information*

Edited by Chad T. Kimball. 337 pages. 2002. 978-0-7808-0439-5.

"Organizes into one concise volume the answers to the most common questions concerning vegetarian diets and lifestyles. This title is recommended for public and secondary school libraries."

—E-Streams, Apr '03

**"Invaluable reference for public and school library collections alike."**
—Library Bookwatch, Apr '03

**"The articles in this volume are easy to read and come from authoritative sources. The book does not necessarily support the vegetarian diet but instead provides the pros and cons of this important decision... Recommended for public libraries and consumer health libraries."**
—American Reference Books Annual, 2003

**SEE ALSO** Diet and Nutrition Sourcebook, 3rd Edition

■

# Women's Health Concerns Sourcebook, 3rd Edition

Basic Consumer Health Information about Issues and Trends in Women's Health and Health Conditions of Special Concern to Women, Including Endometriosis, Uterine Fibroids, Menstrual Irregularities, Menopause, Sexual Dysfunction, Infertility, Cancer in Women, and Other Such Chronic Disorders as Lupus, Fibromyalgia, and Thyroid Disease

Along with Statistical Data, Tips for Maintaining Wellness, a Glossary, and a Directory of Resources for Further Help and Information

Edited by Sandra J. Judd. 679 pages. 2009. 978-0-7808-1036-5.

**"This useful resource provides information about a wide range of topics that will help women understand their bodies, prevent or treat disease, and maintain health... A detailed index helps readers locate information. This is a useful addition to public and consumer health library collections"**
—ARBAOnline, Jun '09

**SEE ALSO** Breast Cancer Sourcebook, 3rd Edition, Cancer Sourcebook for Women, 4th Edition, Healthy Heart Sourcebook for Women

■

# Workplace Health and Safety Sourcebook

Basic Consumer Health Information about Workplace Health and Safety, Including the Effect of Workplace Hazards on the Lungs,

Skin, Heart, Ears, Eyes, Brain, Reproductive Organs, Musculoskeletal System, and Other Organs and Body Parts

Along with Information about Occupational Cancer, Personal Protective Equipment, Toxic and Hazardous Chemicals, Child Labor, Stress, and Workplace Violence

Edited by Chad T. Kimball. 610 pages. 2000. 978-0-7808-0231-5.

**"As a reference for the general public, this would be useful in any library."**
—E-Streams, Jun '01

**"Provides helpful information for primary care physicians and other caregivers interested in occupational medicine... General readers; professionals."**
—CHOICE, May '01

■

# Worldwide Health Sourcebook

Basic Information about Global Health Issues, Including Malnutrition, Reproductive Health, Disease Dispersion and Prevention, Emerging Diseases, Risky Health Behaviors, and the Leading Causes of Death

Along with Global Health Concerns for Children, Women, and the Elderly, Mental Health Issues, Research and Technology Advancements, and Economic, Environmental, and Political Health Implications, a Glossary, and a Resource Listing for Additional Help and Information

Edited by Joyce Brennfleck Shannon. 597 pages. 2001. 978-0-7808-0330-5.

**"Named an Outstanding Academic Title."**
—CHOICE, Jan '02

**"Yet another handy but also unique compilation in the extensive Health Reference Series, this is a useful work because many of the international publications reprinted or excerpted are not readily available. Highly recommended."**
—CHOICE, Nov '01

**SEE ALSO** Traveler's Health Sourcebook

# Teen Health Series
## Complete Catalog
List price $69 per volume. School and library price $62 per volume.

## Abuse and Violence Information for Teens

*Health Tips about the Causes and Consequences of Abusive and Violent Behavior*

Including Facts about the Types of Abuse and Violence, the Warning Signs of Abusive and Violent Behavior, Health Concerns of Victims, and Getting Help and Staying Safe

Edited by Sandra Augustyn Lawton. 411 pages. 2008. 978-0-7808-1008-2.

"A useful resource for schools and organizations providing services to teens and may also be a starting point in research projects."
— *Reference and Research Book News, Aug '08*

"Violence is a serious problem for teens... This resource gives teens the information they need to face potential threats and get help—either for themselves or for their friends."
— *American Reference Books Annual, 2009*

## Accident and Safety Information for Teens

*Health Tips about Medical Emergencies, Traumatic Injuries, and Disaster Preparedness*

Including Facts about Motor Vehicle Accidents, Burns, Poisoning, Firearms, Natural Disasters, National Security Threats, and More

Edited by Karen Bellenir. 420 pages. 2008. 978-0-7808-1046-4.

"Aimed at teenage audiences, this guide provides practical information for handling a comprehensive list of emergencies, from sport injuries and auto accidents to alcohol poisoning and natural disasters."
— *Library Journal, Apr 1, '09*

"Useful in the young adult collections of public libraries as well as high school libraries."
— *American Reference Books Annual, 2009*

**SEE ALSO** Sports Injuries Information for Teens, 2nd Edition

## Alcohol Information for Teens, 2nd Edition

*Health Tips about Alcohol and Alcoholism*

Including Facts about Alcohol's Effects on the Body, Brain, and Behavior, the Consequences of Underage Drinking, Alcohol Abuse Prevention and Treatment, and Coping with Alcoholic Parents

Edited by Lisa Bakewell. 410 pages. 2009. 978-0-7808-1043-3.

"This handbook, written for a teenage audience, provides information on the causes, effects, and preventive measures related to alcohol abuse among teens... The chapters are quick to make a connection to their teenage reading audience. The prose is straightforward and the book lends itself to spot reading. It should be useful both for practical information and for research, and it is suitable for public and school libraries."
— *ARBAOnline, Jun '09*

**SEE ALSO** Drug Information for Teens, 2nd Edition

## Allergy Information for Teens

*Health Tips about Allergic Reactions Such as Anaphylaxis, Respiratory Problems, and Rashes*

Including Facts about Identifying and Managing Allergies to Food, Pollen, Mold, Animals, Chemicals, Drugs, and Other Substances

Edited by Karen Bellenir. 410 pages. 2006. 978-0-7808-0799-0.

"This is a comprehensive, readable text on the subject of allergic diseases in teenagers. 5 Stars (out of 5)!"
— *Doody's Review Service, Jun '06*

"This authoritative and useful self-help title is a solid addition to YA collections, whether for personal interest or reports."
— *School Library Journal, Jul '06*

## Asthma Information for Teens, 2nd Ed.

*Health Tips about Managing Asthma and Related Concerns*

*Including Facts about Asthma Causes, Triggers and Symptoms, Diagnosis, and Treatment*

Edited by Kim Wohlenhaus. 400 pages. 2010. 978-0-7808-1086-0.

# Body Information for Teens
**Health Tips about Maintaining Well-Being for a Lifetime**
*Including Facts about the Development and Functioning of the Body's Systems, Organs, and Structures and the Health Impact of Lifestyle Choices*

Edited by Sandra Augustyn Lawton. 458 pages. 2007. 978-0-7808-0443-2.

# Cancer Information for Teens, 2nd Edition
**Health Tips about Cancer Awareness, Symptoms, Prevention, Diagnosis, and Treatment**
*Including Facts about Common Cancers Affecting Teens, Causes, Detection, Coping Strategies, Clinical Trials, Nutrition and Exercise, Cancer in Friends or Family, and More*

Edited by Karen Bellenir and Lisa Bakewell. 445 pages. 2010. 978-0-7808-1085-3.

# Complementary and Alternative Medicine Information for Teens
**Health Tips about Non-Traditional and Non-Western Medical Practices**
*Including Information about Acupuncture, Chiropractic Medicine, Dietary and Herbal Supplements, Hypnosis, Massage Therapy, Prayer and Spirituality, Reflexology, Yoga, and More*

Edited by Sandra Augustyn Lawton. 407 pages. 2007. 978-0-7808-0966-6.

"This volume covers CAM specifically for teenagers but of general use also. It should be a welcome addition to both public and academic libraries."
—*American Reference Books Annual, 2008*

"This volume provides a solid foundation for further investigation of the subject, making it useful for both public and high school libraries."
—*VOYA: Voice of Youth Advocates, Jun '07*

# Diabetes Information for Teens
**Health Tips about Managing Diabetes and Preventing Related Complications**
*Including Information about Insulin, Glucose Control, Healthy Eating, Physical Activity, and Learning to Live with Diabetes*

Edited by Sandra Augustyn Lawton. 410 pages. 2006. 978-0-7808-0811-9.

"A comprehensive instructional guide for teens... some of the material may also be directed towards parents or teachers. 5 stars (out of 5)!"
—*Doody's Review Service, 2006*

"Students dealing with their own diabetes or that of a friend or family member or those writing reports on the topic will find this a valuable resource."
—*School Library Journal, Aug '06*

"This text is directed to the teen population and would be an excellent library resource for a health class or for the teacher as a reference for class preparation. It can, however, serve a much wider audience. The clinical educator on diabetes may find it valuable to educate the newly diagnosed client regardless of age. It also would be an excellent reference and education tool for a preventive medicine seminar on diabetes."
—*Physical Therapy, Mar '07*

# Diet Information for Teens, 2nd Edition
**Health Tips about Diet and Nutrition**
*Including Facts about Dietary Guidelines, Food Groups, Nutrients, Healthy Meals, Snacks, Weight Control, Medical Concerns Related to Diet, and More*

Edited by Karen Bellenir. 432 pages. 2006. 978-0-7808-0820-1.

"A very quick and pleasant read in spite of the fact that it is very detailed in the information it gives... A book for anyone concerned about diet and nutrition."
—*American Reference Books Annual, 2007*

**SEE ALSO** *Eating Disorders Information for Teens, 2nd Edition*

# Drug Information for Teens, 2nd Edition
### Health Tips about the Physical and Mental Effects of Substance Abuse
*Including Information about Marijuana, Inhalants, Club Drugs, Stimulants, Hallucinogens, Opiates, Prescription and Over-the-Counter Drugs, Herbal Products, Tobacco, Alcohol, and More*

Edited by Sandra Augustyn Lawton. 468 pages. 2006. 978-0-7808-0862-1.

"As with earlier installments in Omnigraphics' Teen Health Series, Drug Information for Teens is designed specifically to meet the needs and interests of middle and high school students... Strongly recommended for both academic and public libraries."
—*American Reference Books Annual, 2007*

"Solid thoughtful advice is given about how to handle peer pressure, drug-related health concerns, and treatment strategies."
—*School Library Journal, Dec '06*

**SEE ALSO** *Alcohol Information for Teens, 2nd Edition, Tobacco Information for Teens, 2nd Edition*

# Eating Disorders Information for Teens, 2nd Edition
### Health Tips about Anorexia, Bulimia, Binge Eating, And Other Eating Disorders
*Including Information about Risk Factors, Diagnosis and Treatment, Prevention, Related Health Concerns, and Other Issues*

Edited by Sandra Augustyn Lawton. 377 pages. 2009. 978-0-7808-1044-0.

"This handy reference offers basic information and addresses specific disorders, consequences, prevention, diagnosis and treatment, healthy eating, and more. It is written in a conversational style that is easy to understand... Will provide plenty of facts for reports as well as browsing potential for students with an interest in the topic.
—*School Library Journal, Jun '09*

"Written in a straightforward style that will appeal to its teenage audience. The author does not play down the danger of living with an eating disorder and urges those struggling with this problem to seek professional help.

This work, as well as others in this series, will be a welcome addition to high school and undergraduate libraries."
—*American Reference Books Annual, 2009*

**SEE ALSO** *Diet Information for Teens, 2nd Edition*

# Fitness Information for Teens, 2nd Edition
### Health Tips about Exercise, Physical Well-Being, and Health Maintenance
*Including Facts about Conditioning, Stretching, Strength Training, Body Shape and Body Image, Sports Nutrition, and Specific Activities for Athletes and Non-Athletes*

Edited by Lisa Bakewell. 432 pages. 2009. 978-0-7808-1045-7.

"This no-nonsense guide packs a great deal into its pages... This is a helpful reference for basic diet and exercise information for health reports or personal use."
—*School Library Journal, April 2009*

"An excellent source for general information on why teens should be active, making time to exercise, the equipment people might need, various types of activities to try, how to maintain health and wellness, and how to avoid barriers to becoming healthier... This would still be an excellent addition to a public library ready-reference collection or a high school health library collection."
—*American Reference Books Annual, 2009*

"This easy to read, well-written, up-to-date overview of fitness for teenagers provides excellent wellness and exercise tips, information, and directions... It is a useful tool for them to obtain a base knowledge in fitness topics and different sports."
—*Doody's Review Service, 2009*

**SEE ALSO** *Diet Information for Teens, 2nd Edition, Sports Injuries Information for Teens, 2nd Edition*

# Learning Disabilities Information for Teens
### Health Tips about Academic Skills Disorders and Other Disabilities That Affect Learning

Including Information about Common Signs of Learning Disabilities, School Issues, Learning to Live with a Learning Disability, and Other Related Issues

Edited by Sandra Augustyn Lawton. 400 pages. 2006. 978-0-7808-0796-9.

"This book provides a wealth of information for any reader interested in the signs, causes, and consequences of learning disabilities, as well as related legal rights and educational interventions... Public and academic libraries should want this title for both students and general readers."
—*American Reference Books Annual, 2006*

## Mental Health Information for Teens, 3rd Edition
*Health Tips about Mental Wellness and Mental Illness*
Including Facts about Mental and Emotional Health, Depression and Other Mood Disorders, Anxiety Disorders, Behavior Disorders, Self-Injury, Psychosis, Schizophrenia, and More

Edited by Karen Bellenir. 400 pages. 2010. 978-0-7808-1087-7.

*SEE ALSO* Stress Information for Teens, Suicide Information for Teens, 2nd Edition

## Pregnancy Information for Teens
*Health Tips about Teen Pregnancy and Teen Parenting*
Including Facts about Prenatal Care, Pregnancy Complications, Labor and Delivery, Postpartum Care, Pregnancy-Related Lifestyle Concerns, and More

Edited by Sandra Augustyn Lawton. 434 pages. 2007. 978-0-7808-0984-0.

## Sexual Health Information for Teens, 2nd Edition
*Health Tips about Sexual Development, Reproduction, Contraception, and Sexually Transmitted Infections*
Including Facts about Puberty, Sexuality, Birth Control, Chlamydia, Gonorrhea, Herpes, Human Papillomavirus, Syphilis, and More

Edited by Sandra Augustyn Lawton. 430 pages. 2008. 978-0-7808-1010-5.

"This offering represents the most up-to-date information available on an array of topics including abstinence-only sexual education and pregnancy-prevention methods... The range of coverage—from puberty and anatomy to sexually transmitted diseases—is thorough and extensive. Each chapter includes a bibliographic citation, and the three back sections containing additional resources, further reading, and the index are all first-rate... This volume will be well used by students in need of the facts, whether for educational or personal reasons."
—*School Library Journal, Nov '08*

"Presents information related to the emotional, physical, and biological development of both males and females that occurs during puberty. It also strives to address some of the issues and questions that may arise... The text is easy to read and understand for young readers, with satisfactory definitions within the text to explain new terms."
—*American Reference Books Annual, 2009*

## Skin Health Information for Teens, 2nd Edition
*Health Tips about Dermatological Concerns and Skin Cancer Risks*
Including Facts about Acne, Warts, Hives, and Other Conditions and Lifestyle Choices, Such as Tanning, Tattooing, and Piercing, That Affect the Skin, Nails, Scalp, and Hair

Edited by Edited by Kim Wohlenhaus. 418 pages. 2009. 978-0-7808-1042-6.

"The material in this work will be easily understood by teenagers and young adults. The publisher has liberally used bulleted lists and sidebars to keep the reader's attention... A useful addition to school and public library collections."
—*ARBAOnline, Oct '09*

## Sleep Information for Teens
*Health Tips about Adolescent Sleep Requirements, Sleep Disorders, and the Effects of Sleep Deprivation*
Including Facts about Why People Need Sleep, Sleep Patterns, Circadian Rhythms, Dreaming, Insomnia, Sleep Apnea, Narcolepsy, and More

Edited by Karen Bellenir. 355 pages. 2008. 978-0-7808-1009-9.

"Clear, concise, and very readable and would be a good source of sleep information for anyone—not just teenagers. This work is highly recommended for medical libraries, public school libraries, and public libraries."
—*American Reference Books Annual, 2009*

**SEE ALSO** *Body Information for Teens*

---

# Sports Injuries Information for Teens, 2nd Edition
*Health Tips about Acute, Traumatic, and Chronic Injuries in Adolescent Athletes*
*Including Facts about Sprains, Fractures, and Overuse Injuries, Treatment, Rehabilitation, Sport-Specific Safety Guidelines, Fitness Suggestions, and More*

Edited by Karen Bellenir. 429 pages. 2008. 978-0-7808-1011-2.

"An engaging selection of informative articles about the prevention and treatment of sports injuries... The value of this book is that the articles have been vetted and are often augmented with inserts of useful facts, definitions of technical terms, and quick tips. Sensitive topics like injuries to genitalia are discussed openly and responsibly. This revised edition contains updated articles and defines sport more broadly than the first edition."
—*School Library Journal, Nov '08*

"This work will be useful in the young adult collections of public libraries as well as high school libraries... A useful resource for student research."
—*American Reference Books Annual, 2009*

**SEE ALSO** *Accident and Safety Information for Teens*

---

# Stress Information for Teens
*Health Tips about the Mental and Physical Consequences of Stress*
*Including Information about the Different Kinds of Stress, Symptoms of Stress, Frequent Causes of Stress, Stress Management Techniques, and More*

Edited by Sandra Augustyn Lawton. 392 pages. 2008. 978-0-7808-1012-9.

"Understanding what stress is, what causes it, how the body and the mind are impacted by it, and what teens can do are the general categories addressed here... The chapters are brief but informative, and the list of community-help organizations is exhaustive. Report writers will find information quickly and easily, as will those who have personal concerns. The print is clear and the format is readable, making this an accessible resource for struggling readers and researchers."
—*School Library Journal, Dec '08*

"The articles selected will specifically appeal to young adults and are designed to answer their most common questions."
— *American Reference Books Annual, 2009*

**SEE ALSO** *Mental Health Information for Teens, 3rd Edition*

---

# Suicide Information for Teens, 2nd Edition
*Health Tips about Suicide Causes and Prevention*
*Including Facts about Depression, Risk Factors, Getting Help, Survivor Support, and More*

Edited by Kim Wohlenhaus. 400 pages. 2010. 978-0-7808-1088-4.

**SEE ALSO** *Mental Health Information for Teens, 3rd Edition*

---

# Tobacco Information for Teens, 2nd Edition
*Health Tips about the Hazards of Using Cigarettes, Smokeless Tobacco, and Other Nicotine Products*
*Including Facts about Nicotine Addiction, Nicotine Delivery Systems, Secondhand Smoke, Health Consequences of Tobacco Use, Related Cancers, Smoking Cessation, and Tobacco Use Statistics*

Edited by Karen Bellenir. 400 pages. 2010. 978-0-7808-1153-9.

**SEE ALSO Drug Information for Teens, 2nd Edition**

# Health Reference Series

# FOOTLIGHTS AND SPOTLIGHTS

*Cambridge*
*1858*